Treatment of Fracture-Related Infection

Nieves Vanaclocha
Editor

Treatment of Fracture-Related Infection

An Orthoplastic Approach

Foreword by Volker Alt

Springer

Editor
Nieves Vanaclocha
Orthoplastics Unit and Department of Plastic
and Reconstructive Surgery
University and Polytechnic Hospital La Fe
Valencia, Spain

ISBN 978-3-031-92451-4 ISBN 978-3-031-92452-1 (eBook)
https://doi.org/10.1007/978-3-031-92452-1

This Springer imprint is published by the registered company Springer Nature Switzerland AG
The registered company address is: Gewerbestrasse 11, 6330 Cham, Switzerland

Foreword

I am honored to have been asked to write the foreword to the textbook *Surgical Management of Fracture Related Infection: An Orthoplastic Approach.*

Infection complication after fracture has accompanied mankind from its very beginning and the different terminology for this complication has been used in the past, such as osteomyelitis, osteitis, etc. Only in the last decade, the definition of the specific term "fracture-related infection" (FRI) has put a more specific focus on this entity both on clinical and scientific aspects. This led to a clearer approach in diagnostics and decision-making and dedicated treatment algorithms. Recently, the development and introduction of the FRI-classification has achieved a better categorization of FRI patients, which is of importance due to the high variability in the clinical presentation from uncomplicated infections with healed fractures to complex situations with severe soft tissue defects or major bone defects.

I believe that FRI is one of the most, if not the most complex and most demanding situation for a patient and the treating surgeon after fracture fixation. The treatment and the course of FRI has been described in the literature to be complex and to be related with surgical re-interventions and high costs for the healthcare system. The most important thing for me is the fact that FRI is not just a somatic complication but that it often has a severe negative impact on the psychological situation of the patient with a high risk of depression and other disorders associated with significant reduction of quality of life. Furthermore, prolonged treatment or recurrence of infection can have far-reaching effects beyond just physical health. The emotional, financial, and social toll can be significant, leading to a loss of livelihood, strained relationships, and feelings of isolation. Therefore, all efforts should be undertaken to achieve successful outcome in FRI patients with a targeted and evidence-based treatment approach. I am very delighted to see that the current textbook entitled *Surgical Treatment of Fracture Related Infection: An Orthoplastic Approach* is dedicated to that topic and relies on the most recent and significant literature on FRI.

The high variability of clinical appearances of FRI cases requires individual treatment decisions. However, these individual decisions should be based on general principles with good underlying clinical evidence. A major achievement in the last years was the introduction of a multidisciplinary team approach in FRI treatment, which has been clearly shown in the literature to be beneficial for FRI patients with significant reduction in amputation rates and the reduction of revision procedures. Besides the important medical input of non-surgical expertise, e.g., from microbiology, infectious disease etc., the collaboration between orthopedic and orthopedic trauma surgeons on one side and plastic surgeons on the other side is of utmost importance for FRI patients as a high percentage of patients face both bone infection and soft tissue defects. Only the dedicated and targeted approach of both problems can lead to clinical success, for which the term "orthoplastic approach" was established in clinical practice and also in the scientific literature. This crucial improvement in the management of FRI patient is acknowledged by the current textbook as it does not only focus on the infected bone and implant but also on the soft tissue management and reliable wound coverage.

The textbook's structure is excellent. The reader is introduced into epidemiology, pathogenesis, and classification of FRI followed by a chapter on diagnostics. The core of the book is the surgical management of FRI, which is based on the recently published FRI-classification. To my best knowledge, this is the first textbook that uses this FRI-classification to present treatment options based on the different categories of the FRI-classification. It gives specific insights into the management of critical bone loss situations and addresses the important aspect of limb salvage options versus amputation in devastating situations. An important chapter is dedicated to the soft tissue management in the context of the above-mentioned orthoplastic approach. Furthermore, systemic and local antibiotic therapy and the aspects of postoperative care for FRI patients are given.

I congratulate the editor and all authors for this important book to advance treatment of FRI. I am deeply convinced that the readers will benefit from the evidence and expert opinions that have been pulled together in this outstanding textbook.

Regensburg, Germany Volker Alt

Preface

Fracture-related infection (FRI) has been a long-standing problem, there having been found archeological evidence of its presence millions of years ago. Technological advancements and policy changes over the years have not managed to reduce its burden, which remains high, both in monetary terms and in terms of disability and lost quality of life. Teams all over the world struggle, surgery after surgery, to cure the patient of this devastating complication.

It is often difficult for surgeons to confidently answer questions regarding the optimal management of an individual FRI patient, even in the context of experienced multidisciplinary teams and after extensive literature searches. This is mainly because, on the one hand, the available literature is scarce, with much being yet unknown, and on the other hand, the great heterogeneity among publications considerably impairs data comparison between them. FRI itself is a very heterogeneous pathology, encompassing uncomplicated infections of healed fractures which resolve after implant removal, large infected bone defects and unsalvageable joints (which require much more complex treatments for FRI resolution), and everything in between, with variable host status and condition of the soft tissue envelope. Since no classification system has yet been validated or uniformly accepted, different studies use different classifications, making inter-study comparisons and data aggregation (something of particular importance, given the often small sample sizes) difficult. These difficulties are coupled with the high variability of outcome measure reporting and overall low quality of the evidence (most study designs are retrospective and do not report on the authors' rationale for the use of one treatment or another). The result is that the available clinical evidence to support decision-making is scarce, fragmented, and difficult to aggregate in a way that will inform clinical decision-making.

However, the situation is slowly changing, following the increased focus on classification and reporting of outcomes in order to facilitate inter-study data comparison and aggregation. It is my hope that this book will contribute toward those efforts and toward achieving the best possible treatment for every FRI patient based on the currently available evidence by clearly summarizing and organizing what is known about FRI in a way that is meaningful and useful to answer the questions that arise during clinical practice. Let us advance together.

Valencia, Spain Nieves Vanaclocha

Acknowledgments

This book would not have been possible without the inestimable help of many people.

I must start with the authors of the chapters, who are not only committed to the care of fracture-related infection patients but also have made a special effort writing this book so other surgeons can benefit from their expertise as well. I am particularly thankful to my colleague Dr. Cristina Ojeda-Thies, for whom, despite not yet having met in person, I have developed such deep respect in the course of this project. Her expertise and dedication proved immensely valuable, and working together has been a privilege. In addition to her, three authors deserve a special mention as well: Dr. Alessandro Thione, who first suggested the idea of writing this book and encouraged me to, Dr. Alberto Pérez-García, a mentor and a friend who has continuously challenged me and supported my professional development in this and other projects, and Dr. Joan Ferràs-Tarragó, who has juggled his participation in this book with a host of other professional and personal challenges.

I also wish to express my deepest gratitude to the team at Springer for the opportunity to write this book, as well as for their illustrations and meticulous reviews for enhanced clarity.

Last but not least, Dr. Pablo Jordà Gómez has read draft after draft with patience, focusing on practicality and clinical applicability for maximum added value and counterbalancing my view, inevitably influenced by my Plastic Surgery training, with his Traumatology and Orthopedics perspective, bettering subsequent versions. This book would not be what it is today if not for him.

Thank you all for your support and commitment to making this book the best it could be.

Contents

Part II Management of Fracture-Related Infections (FRI)

Part I

General Knowledge of Fracture-Related Infections (FRI)

1 Introduction: Epidemiology, Pathogenesis, and Classification of Fracture-Related Infection

Pablo Jordà Gómez and Nieves Vanaclocha

Introduction

Fracture-related infection (FRI) is a bone disease caused by pathogenic organisms after trauma to that bone [1, 2]. Unspecific terms that have been traditionally used to refer to it in the literature include "deep infection," "osteitis" (bone infection that begins in the cortex), and "osteomyelitis" (bone infection that begins in the marrow) [3]. However, these terms are not accurate to describe the entire pathological process, both due to the presence of microbes in the bone and due to the presence of implants, which interact with the pathogenic microorganisms and with the fracture area. Thus, they are being displaced by the term FRI, which describes and encompasses the pathological process more accurately and facilitates literature research on the topic [4]. FRI is one of the most challenging complications of fractures and their treatment, requiring a complex multidisciplinary approach that usually combines one or more surgical procedures and pathogen-directed antibiotic therapy. It is associated to disability, and its treatment usually extends over months, with long recovery periods and significant morbidity associated to its treatments [1, 5]. As a consequence, the impact on the patient's quality of life cannot be understated [6, 7].

The lack of a clear definition of FRI until 2018, when it was given its own diagnostic criteria and a therapeutic approach [6], has impeded correct diagnosis, quantification of its impact, and the building of good-quality evidence to support decision-making [5, 6, 8]. Another problem is the great heterogeneity among treatment protocols and reported outcome variables, impairing comparison and data pooling. Additionally, it is difficult to understand the rationale behind the use of any particular technique based on the data that are published. This situation mimics that with prosthetic joint infections (PJI) some years ago, the addressing of which has led to an improvement in the homogenization of studies on PJI, and a consequent advance in its diagnostic and therapeutic approach [9]. In FRI, in large part thanks to the efforts of the Fracture-Related Infection Consensus Group, greater homogenization among studies is expected in the coming years, with consequent advances in the therapeutic approach and improvement in clinical results.

Epidemiology

Understanding epidemiological characteristics allows identification of incidence patterns, which can be used to design stratified prevention strate-

P. Jordà Gómez
Department of Orthopedic Surgery and Traumatology, Hospital General Universitari de Castelló, Castelló, Spain

N. Vanaclocha (✉)
Orthoplastics Unit and Department of Plastic and Reconstructive Surgery, University and Polytechnic Hospital La Fe, Valencia, Spain

N. Vanaclocha (ed.), *Treatment of Fracture-Related Infection*,
https://doi.org/10.1007/978-3-031-92452-1_1

gies, and of risk factors, some of which are amenable to optimization to improve clinical outcomes. Unfortunately, the incidence of FRI has not been precisely determined, partly owing to the absence of a consensus on diagnostic criteria until recently and partly due to the many factors that influence its occurrence.

For instance, high-energy trauma and more severe soft tissue injury have been found to increase the risk of FRI [2, 10, 11]. The reported risk of FRI ranges from 1% to 2% for closed fractures to over 30% for Gustilo–Anderson type III open tibia fractures [12].

Another factor influencing FRI incidence is the location of the fracture. It has been reported that over 70% of FRIs occur in the lower limb [13]. This could be related to the poorer soft tissue envelope in that anatomical location (especially, in the leg), because soft tissues have a higher irrigation density than bone, so a poorer soft tissue envelope means less blood flow to support both fracture healing and the eradication of microbes [14]. Within the lower limb, there are also different FRI rates for fractures in different locations in accordance with their soft tissue envelopes, ranging from 1.5% for distal femur fractures to 6% for ankle fractures and 7% for tibial plateau fractures [2].

Patient status is another important factor affecting the risk of FRI development, with the typical patient being a middle-aged male (male: female ratio is about 2:1, in line with the higher incidence of open fractures in men) [13, 15]. A literature review estimated that fracture-fixation device infections comprise just under 5% of all implant-associated infections [16], but the data varies greatly (3–18% [17]) depending on the patient's characteristics. For instance, the presence of concomitant injuries, especially in the context of polytrauma, has been found to be associated with a higher risk of FRI [18]. This is, on one hand, because the musculoskeletal injuries in these patients tend to be complex, and on the other, because the associated systemic inflammatory response syndrome compromises the immune response. Moreover, patient-related factors that are known to negatively impact wound healing, such as smoking or diabetes mellitus, also confer a higher risk of FRI [2]. The higher prevalence of obesity and an aging population have been identified as the main contributors to the 28% increase in FRI prevalence in the European region over the past decade [19]. Now that uniform diagnostic criteria are available, research is expected to shed more light on this and other epidemiological phenomena in the coming years.

FRI Epidemiology

Fractures with the highest risk of FRI:

- High degree of bone and soft-tissue injury (high-energy trauma), polytrauma
- Osteosynthesis present
- Comorbid host (smoker, diabetic)

Pathogenesis

FRIs are most often caused by bacterial contamination in the fracture area. In open fractures, this situation is the result of the production mechanism, while in closed fractures, the most frequent origin is the inoculation of pathogens into the surgical wound at the time of surgery [20]. Other, less common infection routes are contiguous spread from adjacent skin (wound healing problems, late soft tissue coverage) and hematogenous spread [14, 18].

In most cases, FRI is caused by pyogenic bacteria, especially *Staphylococcus aureus* (*S. aureus*), the most common etiologic germ. *S. aureus* accounts for about a third of FRIs (32–37%), regardless of time to onset, location of the injury, severity of the fracture, or host characteristics (age, comorbidities, body mass index) [5, 13, 21, 22]. The next most frequent causative microorganisms are coagulase-negative staphylococci (20–39%), followed by enterobacteria (14–27%), anaerobes (16%), and streptococci (11%) [23, 24].

Some series have found the prevalence of coagulase-negative staphylococci to be higher in late-onset FRIs than in early FRIs, and a higher proportion of more virulent bacteria (*S. aureus*, Gram-negative bacilli) and of antibiotic-resistant bacteria in early FRIs [13, 25]. However, other research groups have not found any differences in the microbial species found in early and late-onset FRIs [26, 27]. As a result of this, and given the high incidence of antibiotic-resistant microorganisms in FRIs, which are related to poor outcomes, intravenous empirical therapy is currently only recommended immediately after surgery while waiting for a microbiological diagnosis, but for exceptional cases (e.g., sepsis) [1, 24].

Polymicrobial infections account for 25–38% of all FRIs and are typical of open fractures [13, 26, 28]. The main microorganisms present in them are Gram-negative bacilli, and they are related to worse outcomes compared to monomicrobial FRIs [28].

Timeline

Healthy intact bone can generally resist infection well, but trauma exposes molecules which are inaccessible under normal circumstances and to which microorganisms can bind to infect the bone. This is especially true of *S. aureus*, as it is able to bind to collagen and cartilage through its adhesins, adhere to bone matrix and osteosynthesis material through the fibronectin and laminin it expresses, and survive inside osteoblasts [21, 29]. Once bacteria colonize susceptible bone or implants at the fracture site, the colonies become surrounded by an area of reactive hyperemia. Both pathogens and leukocytes produce pro-inflammatory factors, which cause local bone destruction [30]. The resulting avascular area is scarcely accessible by immune cells and systemic antimicrobials, which reach at subinhibitory concentrations, so the microbes proliferate and develop antimicrobial tolerance [21]. This situation is further worsened by the formation of biofilm and other immune-privileged sites.

Over time, prolonged inflammation results in osteoclast activation and osteoblast inhibition and apoptosis at the fracture site, producing more osteolysis and bone marrow fibrosis. At the periosteum, osteoblasts deposit new bone (involucrum) in an effort to heal the fracture, but at the fracture site remodeling is not induced, and nonunion ensues. Thus, a deleterious spiral of increasing bone involvement and biofilm over time is produced [18].

Biofilm Formation and Other Immune-Privileged Sites

Biofilm is a colony-like aggregation of microorganic cells embedded in an exopolysaccharide matrix mixed with extracellular products, firmly attached to non-vital surfaces such as implants or necrotic tissue [18, 31]. It plays a central role in FRI pathogenesis, because it allows the bacteria in it to reduce their metabolic and generational rate, which, together with the avascular location, results in systemic antibiotics not reaching therapeutic values in the biofilm [24]. Over time (2–6 weeks in the case of *S. aureus*) biofilm matures and its antibiotic resistance increases [18, 32]. The consequence is, on one hand, that infectious outbreaks can occur after long periods of apparent inactivity, and on the other, that *both* medical (antimicrobials) and surgical therapies are needed for infection eradication [24, 29, 33].

Other immune-privileged bacterial reservoirs include the osteocyte lacuno-canalicular network (OLCN), intracellular reservoirs (osteoblasts, macrophages), and staphylococcal abscess communities. These reservoirs have been found to play a significant role in microorganisms' ability for antimicrobial evasion and persistence, with systemic antibiotics reaching the OLCN at subinhibitory concentrations [34]. As with biofilm, animal studies suggest that bacterial colonization of the OLCN can happen within 2 weeks, so *the window of opportunity to prevent biofilm formation and bacterial infiltration of OLCN is narrow*. This situation is further worsened by delayed neutrophil recruitment after a fracture, giving bacteria a head start in creating and colonizing immune-privileged sites, and by the fact that even small amounts (3 mm) of inflammation severely reduce the penetration of systemic antibiotics in animal models. Preventative strategies are still under study to utilize this early, narrow window to decrease the risk of FRI.

In addition, due to the existence of these reservoirs, a small degree of microscopic illness (residual bacterial colonies) beyond the surgical margins is to be expected even after the best of debridements [35]. This must be taken into account when planning treatment, and underscores the need for proper sampling to guide postoperative antibiotic therapy that will correctly target the residual microbes [14].

FRI Pathogenesis

The typical pathogenesis of FRI is the following:

1. A fracture is produced, exposing molecules that are usually inaccessible to which microbes can bind.
2. Pyogenic bacteria (*S. aureus*, coagulase-negative staphylococci, enterobacteria, anaerobes, streptococci) contaminate the fracture and any implants at the site. They immediately start building biofilm on non-vital surfaces (necrotic tissue, implants) and colonizing the OLCN and eukaryotic cells.
3. Reactive hyperemia (reduces penetration of systemic antimicrobials). Delayed neutrophil recruitment.
4. Both pathogens and leukocytes produce pro-inflammatory cytokines that cause osteolysis, providing more avascular surfaces on which biofilm can develop.
5. Biofilm matures and antibiotic tolerance increases.
6. Over time, more inflammation produces more osteolysis, creating a cycle of increasing bone involvement and biofilm formation.
7. Bacterial reservoirs in immune-privileged sites periodically cause recurrences despite antibiotic therapy.
8. Non-union ensues.

Classification

Classification is important to stratify patients in a way that guides treatment, informs on prognosis, and allows data comparison amongst different research publications [36]. Although several classifications have been proposed, so far, none has been uniformly accepted [33, 37].

The oldest classification is based on the time of onset after surgery, by Willenegger and Roth, dividing FRIs in early or acute (<2 weeks), delayed (2–10 weeks), and late-onset infections (>10 weeks) [38]. This classification aimed at reflecting the pathophysiological changes over time (increasing bone involvement and biofilm formation) and is one of the most commonly used clinically [18]. However, these time cutoffs are arbitrary, they do not reflect the continuity of the process (the pathophysiological changes over time occur gradually), and no association has been found with prognosis, so this classification does not help guide treatment [39].

The depth of bacterial colonization has also been used to classify infected fractures, but the differentiation between "superficial infections" (which only affect the overlying soft tissue without bone involvement) and "deep infections" (bone is involved) can only be made after obtaining tissue samples from the fracture site, so it does not inform initial management [40].

Most classifications are based on bone involvement and host status, plus or minus other factors. The Cierny–Mader osteomyelitis classification [41], which considers bone involvement and host status solely, is currently the most frequently used in published studies [33, 42]. However, it does not consider the status of the soft tissue envelope, which is critical in FRI, so newer classifications incorporating this item have been proposed. For example, the BACH classification (which also takes into account soft tissue coverage and antibiotic resistance—an item often known only postsurgically) [43], Romanò classification (aimed at maximal comprehensiveness, but not necessarily clinical utility, by evaluating seven items: clinical presentation, etiology, anatomical location, host type, microorganism, bone defect, and soft tissue defect, with a subclassification for fracture healing) [44], and the FRI classification [36] (so far, the most recent). Out of these, the FRI classification is the most tailored to aiding treatment decisions in FRI patients, so it will be discussed in further detail and used throughout this book.

The FRI classification was designed to include all the relevant aspects for decision-making on the therapeutic management of these injuries by the FRI Consensus Group, and named after the three elements that it assesses [36]:

- Fracture (F): state of the fracture (healed vs. not healed, and healing potential).
- Related patient factors (R): patient systemic factors and comorbidities (number, with or without organ damage) that impact both bone and soft tissue healing, as well as the available treatments.
- Impairment of soft tissues (I): condition of the soft tissues adjacent to the fracture.

Each element is subdivided into five categories, numbered 1–5 according to complexity, with "1" representing the least complex circumstance of each element and "5" describing the most complex situation (Table 1.1).

FRI Classifications

None uniformly accepted so far. The main ones are:

- Based on time of onset: Willenegger and Roth (early/acute, delayed, late).
- Based on the depth of bacterial colonization: superficial vs. deep.
- Based on bone involvement and host status: Cierny-Mader (most frequently used in publications), FRI classification (+ soft tissue impairment), BACH classification (+ soft tissue impairment + antimicrobial options), Romanò (+ clinical presentation, etiology, anatomical location, microorganism, soft tissue defect).

Conclusions

FRI is a severe complication involving bone infections, often requiring complex treatment. The lack of a clear definition until 2018 hindered proper diagnosis and research on the topic.

FRI occurs mostly in the lower limb. Its incidence varies from 1% to 2% for closed fractures to over 30% for Gustilo–Anderson type III open

Table 1.1 FRI classification

	1	2	3	4	5
F Fracture	Fracture healed	Unhealed fracture, good bone healing potential	Unhealed fracture, poor bone healing potential	Unhealed fracture, major bone defect	Unhealed fracture, bone reconstruction not possible
R Relevant patient factors	Fit for surgery	1/2 systemic comorbidities, without end-organ damage	3/+ systemic comorbidities without end-organ damage	Established end-organ damage	Unfit for surgery or declines treatment
I Impairment of soft tissues	Robust direct wound closure possible	Direct wound closure possible but fragile	Loco-regional tissue transfer needed	Free tissue transfer needed	Soft tissue reconstruction not possible

tibia fractures. Relevant patient-related factors such as smoking or *diabetes mellitus* also increase the risk of FRI after a fracture.

FRI is mainly caused by pyogenic bacteria. The most common etiologic germ is *S. aureus*, affecting about a third of cases, but Gram-negative bacteria (around a fifth of cases) and polymicrobial infections (approximately 1 in every 4 cases, typical of open fractures) are not rare.

Biofilm grows on non-vital surfaces: necrotic tissue and implants. It plays a vital role in FRI pathogenesis because systemic antibiotics can reach the microorganisms in it only at subtherapeutic levels. Over time, more inflammation produces more osteolysis, creating a cycle of increasing bone involvement, and biofilm matures, increasing the pathogens' potential for antimicrobial evasion and persistence.

Other immune-privileged bacterial reservoirs include the OLCN and intracellular reservoirs, which result in residual colonies beyond the surgical margins even after proper debridement. Proper sampling is indispensable for antibiotic therapy to accurately target these colonies.

Although several classification systems have been proposed, none have gained widespread acceptance in clinical practice. The new FRI classification system holds promise in this regard, as it includes the three critical elements that determine prognosis and guide treatment: Fracture (F), Related patient factors (R), and Impairment of soft tissues (I).

References

1. McNally M, Govaert G, Dudareva M, Morgenstern M, Metsemakers W-J. Definition and diagnosis of fracture-related infection. EFORT Open Rev. 2020;5:614–9.
2. He S-Y, Yu B, Jiang N. Current concepts of fracture-related infection. Int J Clin Pract. 2023;2023:4839701.
3. Tiemann AH, Hofmann GO. Principles of the therapy of bone infections in adult extremities. Strategies Trauma Limb Reconstr. 2009;4:57–64.
4. Walter N, Orbenes N, Rupp M, Alt V. The state of research in fracture-related infection—a bibliometric analysis. Medicina. 2022;58:1170.
5. Iliadis AD, Shivji F, Debuka E, Trompeter A, Narayan B, Heidari N. Current concepts in the prevention, diagnosis and treatment of fracture-related infection (FRI). Eur J Orthop Surg Traumatol. 2021;31:957–66.
6. Metsemakers WJ, Morgenstern M, McNally MA, et al. Fracture-related infection: a consensus on definition from an international expert group. Injury. 2018;49:505–10.
7. Hotchen AJ, Dudareva M, Corrigan RA, Ferguson JY, McNally MA. Can we predict outcome after treatment of long bone osteomyelitis? Bone Joint J. 2020;102-B:1587–96.
8. Prada C, Bengoa F, Bhandari M. The management of fracture related infections: what practices can be supported by high-level evidence? J Orthop Surg (Hong Kong). 2022;30:10225536221119580.
9. Zimmerli W, Trampuz A, Ochsner PE. Prosthetic-joint infections. N Engl J Med. 2004;351:1645–54.
10. Pollak AN, Jones AL, Castillo RC, Bosse MJ, MacKenzie EJ, LEAP Study Group. The relationship between time to surgical debridement and incidence of infection after open high-energy lower extremity trauma. J Bone Joint Surg Am. 2010;92:7–15.
11. Lu V, Zhang J, Patel R, Zhou AK, Thahir A, Krkovic M. Fracture related infections and their risk factors for treatment failure-a major trauma centre perspective. Diagnostics (Basel). 2022;12:1289.
12. Ktistakis I, Giannoudi M, Giannoudis PV. Infection rates after open tibial fractures: are they decreasing? Injury. 2014;45:1025–7.
13. Depypere M, Sliepen J, Onsea J, Debaveye Y, Govaert GAM, IJpma FFA, Zimmerli W, Metsemakers W-J. The microbiological etiology of fracture-related infection. Front Cell Infect Microbiol. 2022;12:934485.
14. Moriarty TF, Metsemakers W-J, Morgenstern M, Hofstee MI, Vallejo Diaz A, Cassat JE, Wildemann B, Depypere M, Schwarz EM, Richards RG. Fracture-related infection. Nat Rev Dis Primers. 2022;8:67.
15. Shah A, Judge A, Griffin XL. Incidence and quality of care for open fractures in England between 2008 and 2019: a cohort study using data collected by the Trauma Audit and Research Network. Bone Joint J. 2022;104-B:736–46.
16. Metsemakers WJ, Kortram K, Morgenstern M, et al. Definition of infection after fracture fixation: a systematic review of randomized controlled trials to evaluate current practice. Injury. 2018;49:497–504.
17. Fernandes MDC, Peres LR, Queiroz Neto ACD, Lima Neto JQ, Turíbio FM, Matsumoto MH. Open fractures and the incidence of infection in the surgical debridement 6 hours after trauma. Acta Ortop Bras. 2015;23:38–42.
18. Morgenstern M, Clauss M, Sendi P, Cadosch D, Osinga R, Metsemakers W-J. Treatment of fracture-related infections. In: Pape H-C, Borrelli J, Moore EE, Pfeifer R, Stahel PF, editors. Textbook of polytrauma management. Cham: Springer; 2022. p. 573–81.

19. Walter N, Rupp M, Lang S, Alt V. The epidemiology of fracture-related infections in Germany. Sci Rep. 2021;11:10443.
20. Rupp M, Walter N, Bärtl S, Heyd R, Hitzenbichler F, Alt V. Fracture-related infection—epidemiology, etiology, diagnosis, prevention, and treatment. Dtsch Arztebl Int. 2024; https://doi.org/10.3238/arztebl.m2023.0233.
21. Masters EA, Ricciardi BF, de Mesy Bentley KL, Moriarty TF, Schwarz EM, Muthukrishnan G. Skeletal infections: microbial pathogenesis, immunity and clinical management. Nat Rev Microbiol. 2022;20:385–400.
22. Zimmerly W. Bone and joint infections: from microbiology to diagnostics and treatment. 2nd ed. Hoboken: Wiley-Blackwell; 2021.
23. Rupp M, Baertl S, Walter N, Hitzenbichler F, Ehrenschwender M, Alt V. Is there a difference in microbiological epidemiology and effective empiric antimicrobial therapy comparing fracture-related infection and periprosthetic joint infection? A retrospective comparative study. Antibiotics (Basel). 2021;10:921.
24. Depypere M, Morgenstern M, Kuehl R, Senneville E, Moriarty TF, Obremskey WT, Zimmerli W, Trampuz A, Lagrou K, Metsemakers W-J. Pathogenesis and management of fracture-related infection. Clin Microbiol Infect. 2020;26:572–8.
25. Kuehl R, Tschudin-Sutter S, Morgenstern M, Dangel M, Egli A, Nowakowski A, Suhm N, Theilacker C, Widmer AF. Time-dependent differences in management and microbiology of orthopaedic internal fixation-associated infections: an observational prospective study with 229 patients. Clin Microbiol Infect. 2019;25:76–81.
26. Corrigan RA, Sliepen J, Dudareva M, IJpma FFA, Govaert G, Atkins BL, Rentenaar R, Wouthuyzen-Bakker M, McNally M. Causative pathogens do not differ between early, delayed or late fracture-related infections. Antibiotics (Basel). 2022;11:943.
27. Baertl S, Walter N, Engelstaedter U, Ehrenschwender M, Hitzenbichler F, Alt V, Rupp M. What is the most effective empirical antibiotic treatment for early, delayed, and late fracture-related infections? Antibiotics (Basel). 2022;11:287.
28. Jorge LS, Fucuta PS, Oliveira MGL, Nakazone MA, de Matos JA, Chueire AG, Salles MJC. Outcomes and risk factors for polymicrobial posttraumatic osteomyelitis. J Bone Jt Infect. 2018;3:20–6.
29. Kremers HM, Nwojo ME, Ransom JE, Wood-Wentz CM, Melton LJ, Huddleston PM. Trends in the epidemiology of osteomyelitis. J Bone Joint Surg Am. 2015;97:837–45.
30. Lew DP, Waldvogel FA. Osteomyelitis. Lancet. 2004;364:369–79.
31. Costerton JW, Lewandowski Z, Caldwell DE, Korber DR, Lappin-Scott HM. Microbial biofilms. Ann Rev Microbiol. 1995;49:711–45.
32. Stevenson MC, Slater JC, Sagi HC, Palacio Bedoya F, Powers-Fletcher MV. Diagnosing fracture-related infections: where are we now? J Clin Microbiol. 2022;60:e0280720.
33. Panteli M, Giannoudis PV. Chronic osteomyelitis: what the surgeon needs to know. EFORT Open Rev. 2016;1:128–35.
34. Masters EA, de Mesy Bentley KL, Gill AL, et al. Identification of penicillin binding protein 4 (PBP4) as a critical factor for Staphylococcus aureus bone invasion during osteomyelitis in mice. PLoS Pathog. 2020;16:e1008988.
35. de Mesy Bentley KL, Trombetta R, Nishitani K, et al. Evidence of Staphylococcus aureus deformation, proliferation and migration in canaliculi of live cortical bone in murine models of osteomyelitis. J Bone Miner Res. 2017;32:985–90.
36. Alt V, McNally M, Wouthuyzen-Bakker M, Metsemakers W-J, Marais L, Zalavras C, Morgenstern M. The FRI classification—a new classification of fracture-related infections. Injury. 2024;55:111831.
37. Hotchen AJ, McNally MA, Sendi P. The classification of long bone osteomyelitis: a systemic review of the literature. J Bone Jt Infect. 2017;2:167–74.
38. Willenegger H, Roth B. Treatment tactics and late results in early infection following osteosynthesis. Unfallchirurgie. 1986;12:241–6.
39. McNally M, Corrigan R, Sliepen J, Dudareva M, Rentenaar R, IJpma F, Atkins BL, Wouthuyzen-Bakker M, Govaert G. What factors affect outcome in the treatment of fracture-related infection? Antibiotics. 2022;11:946.
40. Metsemakers WJ, Kuehl R, Moriarty TF, Richards RG, Verhofstad MHJ, Borens O, Kates S, Morgenstern M. Infection after fracture fixation: current surgical and microbiological concepts. Injury. 2018;49:511–22.
41. Bezstarosti H, Van Lieshout EMM, Voskamp LW, Kortram K, Obremskey W, McNally MA, Metsemakers WJ, Verhofstad MHJ. Insights into treatment and outcome of fracture-related infection: a systematic literature review. Arch Orthop Trauma Surg. 2019;139:61–72.
42. Cierny G, Mader JT. Adult chronic osteomyelitis. Orthopedics. 1984;7:1557–64.
43. Hotchen AJ, Dudareva M, Ferguson JY, Sendi P, McNally MA. The BACH classification of long bone osteomyelitis. Bone Joint Res. 2019;8:459–68.
44. Romanò CL, Romanò D, Logoluso N, Drago L. Bone and joint infections in adults: a comprehensive classification proposal. Eur Orthop Traumatol. 2011;1:207.

Diagnosis of Fracture-Related Infection

2

Joan Ferràs-Tarragó and Nieves Vanaclocha

Introduction

The diagnosis of fracture-related infection (FRI) can be complex, hindering both efficient patient management and research in this field. In most cases, FRI develops in the weeks following the traumatic event, when it is challenging to determine whether the fracture's sluggish evolution is due to an infection or due to other reasons such as unstable osteosynthesis, delayed consolidation, or tissue damage resulting from the traumatic event and/or its treatment. In research, the lack of standardization in FRI (name of the pathology itself, definition, diagnostic criteria, outcome variables) has been pointed out as an impediment to the scientific advancement in FRI, and thus, to better patient outcomes [1].

Accordingly, the most important advancement in FRI in recent years was the consensus established in 2018 by members of the AO Foundation and the EBJIS, where, through an expert opinion process, a definition and diagnostic criteria of FRI were established [2]. They proposed four confirmatory criteria, two clinical and two based on microorganism identification in tissue samples, and a variety of suggestive criteria, which should prompt further investigation looking for confirmatory criteria (Table 2.1). It is on these criteria on which diagnosis of FRI is currently based.

The suggestive criteria include clinical, radiological, laboratory, microbiological, and histo-

J. Ferràs-Tarragó (✉)
Department of Orthopaedic Surgery, Hospital La Fe, Valencia, Spain

N. Vanaclocha
Orthoplastics Unit and Department of Plastic and Reconstructive Surgery, University and Polytechnic Hospital La Fe, Valencia, Spain

N. Vanaclocha (ed.), *Treatment of Fracture-Related Infection*,
https://doi.org/10.1007/978-3-031-92452-1_2

Table 2.1 Diagnostic criteria for FRI

	Confirmatory criteria	Suggestive criteria
Clinical signs	Fistula, sinus, wound breakdown Pus or purulent drainage	Local/systemic (e.g., local redness, swelling, fever) New-onset joint effusion Persistent, increasing or new-onset wound drainage
Microbiology	Phenotypically indistinguishable pathogens from at least two separate deep tissue/implant specimens	Pathogenic microorganism from one deep tissue/implant specimen
Others	Presence of microorganisms in deep tissue specimens, confirmed histopathologically by using specific stains for bacteria and fungi Presence of >5 polymorphonuclear neutrophils per high-power field (late-onset FRI)	Elevated serum inflammatory markers (ESR, WBC, CRP) Radiological and/or nuclear imaging signs

CRP C-reactive protein, *ESR* erythrocyte sedimentation rate, *WBC* white blood cell count

pathological signs. Given the variety of clinical presentations available for FRI and the normal and abnormal variability in some of these signs (e.g., serum inflammatory biomarkers), it is their combination that strengthens or weakens the suspicion of FRI. At the time of this writing, there is no combination of laboratory and/or radiographic parameters that confirms the diagnosis of FRI. However, often the patient does not present any confirmatory criteria preoperatively, so suggestive signs increase the strength of the diagnostic suspicion and support surgical action before the infection progresses and its consequences become more severe.

The precision and reliability of the AO-EBJIS consensus diagnostic scheme (Fig. 2.1) is still being validated, but results so far are promising [3].

Knowledge of all the signs and possible tests for FRI diagnosis, their value, and their significance is crucial for a precise and accurate diagnosis. In this chapter, we will discuss preoperative, intraoperative, and postoperative possibilities for FRI diagnosis.

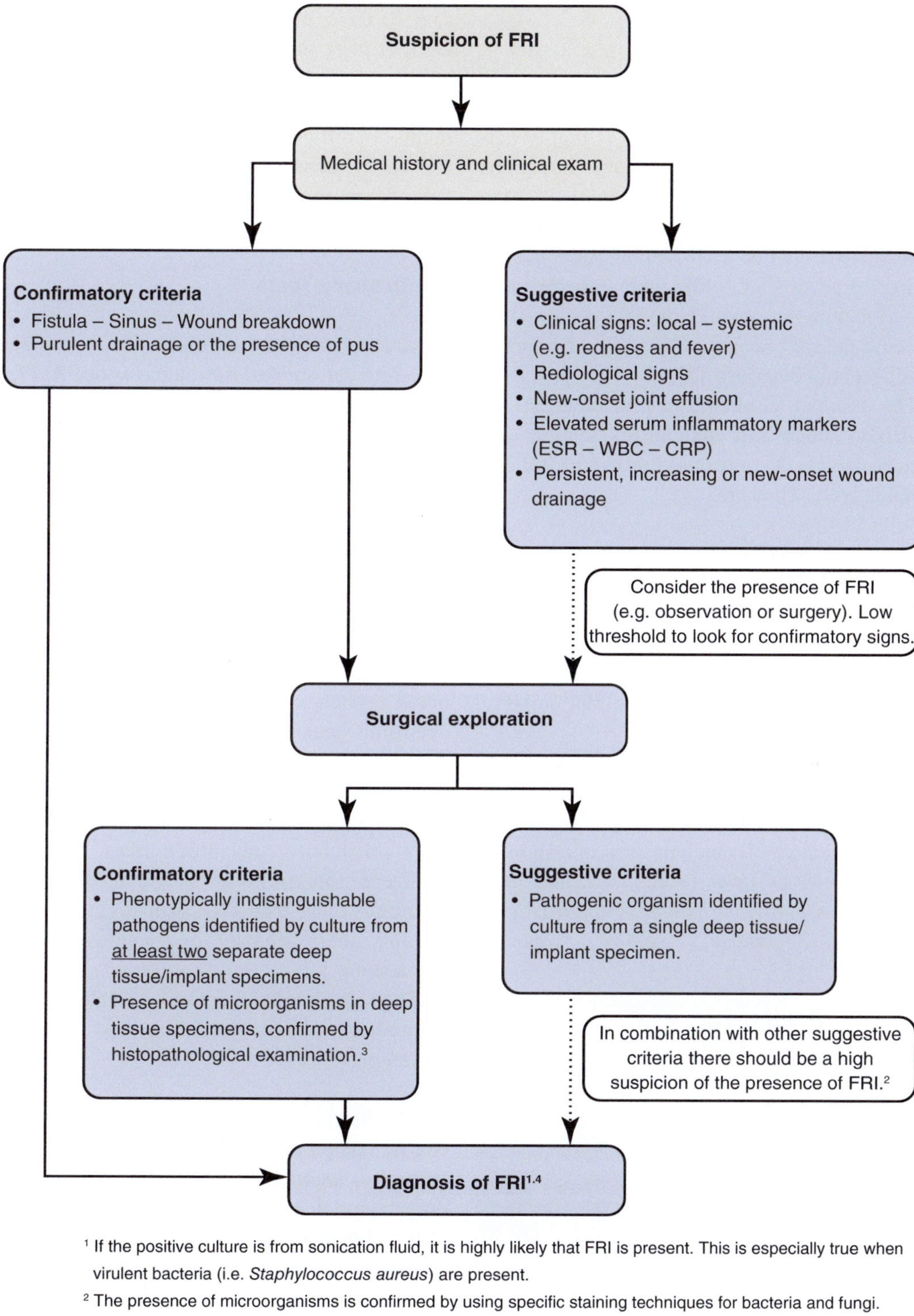

Fig. 2.1 The AO-EBJIS consensus diagnostic scheme. (Adapted from [2])

Preoperative Diagnosis

Clinical Diagnosis

The clinical presentation of FRIs is highly heterogeneous, spanning easily treatable infections in healed fractures to large segmental bone defects and other complex scenarios that pose reconstructive challenges [4]. Some patients have obvious signs of FRI, while others present only with a fracture nonunion. Note that, in any fracture with delayed healing, FRI should be part of the differential diagnosis [5].

The clinical confirmatory criteria of the AO-EBJIS consensus diagnostic scheme are (almost always) the only ones that can be fulfilled preoperatively. They are:

- The presence of a fistula (Fig. 2.2), sinus, or wound dehiscence with communication to the bone or implant (regardless of whether any drainage is associated to the wound breakdown).
- The presence of purulent drainage through the surgical wound or pus observed during surgery.

Approximately 75% of FRI patients present confirmatory criteria upon presentation [6].

The suggestive clinical signs that should elicit suspicion of FRI include systemic signs of infection, such as fever (>38.3 °C), and local signs such as erythema, edema, phlogosis, prolonged postoperative serous drainage (>7–10 days, or progressively increasing drainage), or pain outside of what would be expected in the postoperative recovery (e.g., increasing, pain without weight-bearing). Some of these elements are difficult to quantify, but they are generally easily identifiable by surgeons as deviations from the normal postoperative recovery.

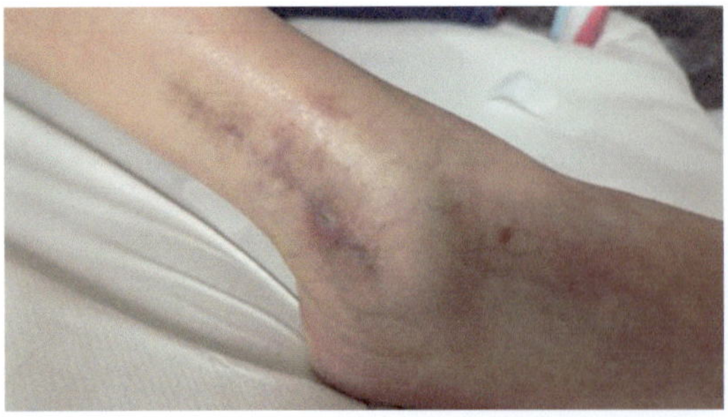

Fig. 2.2 Fistula in an FRI of an ankle fracture, 12 weeks after osteosynthesis implantation. The patient had suffered a fibula fracture after twisting his ankle. Note the poor soft tissue envelope in this patient, which must be taken into account during diagnosis and treatment planning

Laboratory Tests

Laboratory findings are unspecific, but suggestive signs can support the diagnosis of FRI [7, 8].

Serum erythrocyte sedimentation rate (ESR), C-reactive protein (CRP), and white blood cell (WBC) count are the three main laboratory parameters described for diagnosing FRI [9]. Out of the three, CRP is the most reliable molecule in a single evaluation for the early diagnosis of FRI, but its sensitivity values range from 60% to 100%, and its specificity ranges from 30% to 85%, according to various studies [7, 10]. The importance of these serum biomarkers lies not so much in their value but rather in their behavior over time, because:

- Ranges for their non-pathologic values change between laboratories, making it difficult to establish universal cutoff points.
- These biomarkers' levels rise in multiple conditions other than FRI, so it is challenging to unify their behavior in fractures across all patients.
- Their use as dichotomous variables does not predict positive culture results in surgical samples.

The behavior of these biomarkers over time can be compared with the normal postoperative pattern to identify deviations from the expected progression that support the diagnostic suspicion of FRI. For example, the normal behavior of CRP is to peak at 48 h post-trauma and return to normal values by the third postoperative week [10]. ESR has a slower curve, peaking approximately 5–7 days postoperatively and returning to preoperative values around 2 months post-trauma [10]. Depending on the type of surgical procedure, the characteristics of the trauma, and the type of patient, these values may vary, but abnormal temporal patterns can support the suspicion of FRI.

Other described biomarkers include leukocytosis, alpha-1 acid glycoprotein, or procalcitonin, but they are unreliable indicators [7, 11].

The use of immune biomarkers, including antimicrobial peptides, specific cytokines related to inflammatory profiles, and immunoglobulins (against one or multiple microbial targets), is currently under research [12]. Studies on this are promising, but their potential use and usefulness in diagnosing FRI are yet to be determined.

Imaging

Imaging tests are essential in the evaluation of FRIs, not only from a diagnostic point of view, but also because they provide crucial information for management, such as the presence and extent of osteonecrosis, the stability of the osteosynthetic construct, and the degree of fracture consolidation. So far, there is no consensus on the best imaging modality.

Upon clinical suspicion, conventional radiography is the first imaging test requested almost without exception, due to its widespread availability and low cost. It allows the surgeon to evaluate the stability of the osteosynthetic construct and the progression of bone healing. X-ray signs mimic pathogenesis: unhealed fracture, osteolysis at the fracture site or around the implant, involucrum, and implant loosening, among others [5].

Computed tomography (CT) is recommended in all patients with a suspicion of FRI as it allows evaluation of osteosynthesis instability, osteolysis, delayed consolidation, sequestra, and reactive periosteal bone formation. Additionally, it enables the assessment of the patient's anatomical particularities and estimation of the bone defect size, if any is present or expected, to plan for subsequent reconstruction options.

Magnetic resonance imaging (MRI) is another key test in FRI, complementing the information that can be obtained with CT. Specifically, it allows evaluation of the presence of soft-tissue abscesses, bone defects (including sequestra, fistulae, or cloacae), and subcortical abscesses. Both MRI and CT are best used in combination with clinical data for maximal diagnostic accuracy, so high-quality communication with the radiology team, providing plenty of clinical information, is necessary.

Nuclear medicine techniques are useful in complex diagnostic cases in which a latent or subclinical infection of an unhealed fracture is suspected, but there are minimal suggestive signs to support this suspicion. In such cases, preoperative diagnosis is key, because the presence of an underlying infection will greatly influence the surgical technique to be used, as well as the morbidity associated with the therapeutic process. Nuclear imaging techniques, though less specific, are generally more sensitive and less susceptible to metal implant-induced scattering than CT or MRI, so they are especially suitable for these diagnostically challenging cases. The best-described technique is WBC scintigraphy plus single photon emission computed tomography (SPECT), with a sensitivity of 79–100% and a specificity of 89–97% [10]. WBC scintigraphy is not affected by postoperative changes, which poses a significant advantage over other nuclear medicine techniques. Its main drawbacks are the time and resources it consumes and its lower precision in certain locations, such as the axial skeleton. Another, less precise nuclear medicine technique is fluorodeoxyglucose positron emission tomography (FDG-PET). It has better spatial resolution than WBC scintigraphy-SPECT and requires only one scan (scintigraphy requires two scans, 20 h apart), but there is increased FDG uptake during the first postoperative month, making it unsuitable for early FRI diagnosis. The combination of FDG-PET/CT, which utilizes the increased sensitivity of FDG-PET and the anatomical detail of CT, has been reported to have a sensitivity of 65–94% and a specificity of 76–100%, depending on the series. The use of nuclear imaging is limited by its availability and cost, but expected to take a stronger role in diagnosing FRI as evidence on it accumulates [5].

Microbiological Diagnosis

The microbiological confirmatory criterion of FRI is the identification of two identical pathogens (including their antimicrobial resistance profile) in at least two deep tissue samples taken with independent sterile instruments. The gold standard is for these samples to be obtained during surgical debridement and so this information—which both allows identification of the causative pathogen and guides the antibiotic therapy—is obtained *postoperatively* (see Section "How to collect tissue samples appropriately?" below).

However, in FRI cases in which the surgical treatment entails high morbidity and mortality, image-guided culture sampling by the interventional radiology team is a highly useful preoperative diagnostic element. It is important to note that both image-guided aspiration and biopsy have low diagnostic yields because they sample a limited area that may not contain the pathogen. Thus, a negative result does not rule out infection, but a positive result does confirm FRI. Additionally, if positive, the microbiological evaluation will inform the team on the pathogen's aggressiveness, an information that can then be used in the subsequent therapeutic planning. Another issue with image-guided sampling is that the risk of sample contamination during extraction is higher than if the sample is obtained from an open surgical field, and local bleeding after sample collection can contaminate the area. Given these risks, meticulous sample collection is crucial, and only appropriate in selected cases.

The use of swabs is contraindicated due to the high likelihood of contamination during the sampling process.

If the patient has a fever (>38.3 °C), it is advisable to extract blood cultures, especially in acute infections. In chronic infectious processes, bacteremia is uncommon, and its diagnostic yield is significantly lower.

Preoperative Diagnosis of FRI

Confirmed diagnosis:

- Clinical confirmatory signs: fistula, sinus, wound dehiscence exposing bone or implant, or purulent drainage.
- Microbiological confirmation: identification of identical pathogens by culture of at least 2 separate samples (obtention guided by imaging). Only in selected patients (low yield, risk of contamination).

Suspected diagnosis (suggestive signs):

- Clinical: systemic (fever) or local (erythema, swelling, abnormal wound drainage) signs of infection.
- Laboratory: abnormal temporal pattern (increasing levels after initial decrease, persistent elevation) of CRP, ESR and WBC count.
- Imaging (usually, X-rays, CT and MRI): unhealed fracture, osteolysis, implant loosening, involucrum, sequestra, fistulae. Nuclear imaging (WBC-SPECT, FDG-PET) is more sensitive but provides less anatomical detail than CT and MRI, it is useful in cases with minimal suggestive signs and symptoms.

Intraoperative Diagnosis

There are cases where it is not possible to establish a confirmed diagnosis of FRI preoperatively. When suggestive but not confirmatory criteria are present, the threshold for surgical exploration should be low [2, 12].

The first sample collection and debridement surgery is the best opportunity to achieve a diagnosis and identify the causative pathogen. All surgeries in FRI patients are accompanied by a cycle of potent antibiotics, so if the pathogen is not identified in the first surgery, it is likely that subsequent antibiotic cycles will favor the development of antimicrobial resistances in the colony. This occurs because the incorrect detection of the pathogen or its resistance profile leads to the application of empirical or nontargeted treatments, which, if the pathogen is not susceptible, result in doses below the minimal inhibitory concentration threshold, thereby generating resistance. Thus, adequate tissue sample collection is essential.

How to Collect Tissue Samples Appropriately?

The methodology for intraoperative culture sampling is the cornerstone of a rigorous microbiological diagnosis. Microbiological specimens must be collected meticulously after exposure of the FRI site [12, 13]:

Whenever possible, withdraw antibiotics preoperatively for at least 2 weeks.

- Obtain at least five tissue specimens, including liquid and solid samples, from the bone–metal interface for culture, as well as two samples for histological analysis.
- Swabs or samples from any soft tissue fistulae or sinus tracts present should be avoided.
- Reduce the risk of cross-contamination by using a different, sterile instrument for each sample, making sure neither the sample nor the instrument touches the patient's skin, and introducing the samples immediately into the culture tube ("no-touch technique").
- Minimize manipulation of the surgical field by the team until sample collection is completed.
- Transfer samples rapidly to the laboratory.
- Send any removed implants for sonication.

Some publications alert to insufficient compliance with these recommendations, with sampling not being performed properly in almost half of cases [14]. Improper sampling can lead to false-negative or false-positive results, which then result in inadequate treatment decisions, so sampling should be standardized and adequate [5].

There is controversy regarding the appropriate timing for the administration of intraoperative antibiotic prophylaxis. Some groups prefer to delay it until after sample collection to theoretically promote a higher culture yield, though the available literature reports no differences between its administration during the anesthetic induction process and after sample collection.

Reamed bone obtained through the reamer-irrigator-aspirator system has been reported to provide a high diagnostic yield for infections involving the medullary canal, with additional pathogens found in almost one in every five patients [15]. However, these results are yet to be validated for this maneuver to become standard.

Intraoperative Tissue Sample Collection
Key points:

- No antibiotics during at least the 2 weeks prior.
- At least 5 specimens for culture +2 for histopathology from the site of interest (bone-implant interface). No swabs, no samples from fistulae or sinus tracts.
- Avoid cross-contamination: different and unused instrument for each sample, "no-touch technique".
- Rapid and appropriate transfer to laboratory (do not wait until the end of the surgery for the samples to be sent).

The diagnostic value of sonication is unclear, but it is routinely performed if implants are removed.

Samples from reamed bone can be useful.

Intraoperative Histopathology

Surgical treatments of FRI are generally aggressive for the patient and demanding for the surgeon, because it is crucial to be sufficiently aggressive to achieve curation but also to not increase morbidity any more than necessary. The condition of the soft tissues and the bone stock quality are both generally suboptimal (Fig. 2.3) and may worsen as a consequence of the surgical treatment, imposing the need to define the action plan well, be meticulous in all surgical gestures and steps, and be respectful toward the soft tissues. Given this situation, the authors of this chapter believe that therapeutic surgery must always follow a *confirmed diagnosis* of FRI, especially if the osteosynthesis material is to be exchanged or treatment of a nonunion is necessary. Thus, in cases with a strong, unconfirmed preoperative suspicion of FRI, it is best to attempt histological confirmation of FRI before proceeding with any other surgical actions that add aggression.

FRI is confirmed if histopathological examination of deep tissue samples reveals the presence of pathogens or more than 5 polymorphonuclear neutrophils (PMNs) per high-power field (HPF) (×400 magnification). They have been used for a long time with a large body of literature supporting them, and recent studies have quantified the sensitivity and specificity of these criteria around 90% [16], so these criteria are highly reliable. Where available, intraoperative histopathology represents a highly effective additional step before making decisions about the course of surgery. In institutions in which it is not possible to perform histopathological analysis intraoperatively, this examination is performed postoperatively, and the surgery may have to be staged.

Postoperative Diagnosis

Cultures

Tissue cultures are the gold standard for FRI diagnosis, identification of two phenotypically indistinguishable pathogens by culture being one of the four confirmatory criteria for FRI in the AO-EBJIS consensus diagnostic scheme. Moreover, as previously pointed out, identification of the pathogen responsible for FRI is essential not only to confirm FRI, but also to guide targeted postoperative antimicrobial therapy, which is key for success.

Of note, slow-growing pathogens can take between 10 and 14 days to yield positive results, so it is prudent to maintain cultures until that time has passed.

Multidisciplinary protocols with infectious diseases and microbiology specialists should be established for proper handling and preparation of the samples, as well as employing individual cultures for each sample, enriched culture media, and systems for biofilm disruption prior to culture.

Sonication

Sonication of removed osteosynthesis material is a useful adjuvant in FRIs, offering potentially earlier identification of the causative pathogen, and is routinely performed [17, 18].

However, its diagnostic value in FRI is yet unclear [17, 19]. Moreover, implant removal is often laborious, and, during the process, contamination of the material is likely. Therefore, cautious interpretation is advised.

Molecular Diagnostics

Pathogen identification through tissue cultures and sonication can (and sometimes does) fail. This happens mainly due to antibiotic therapy prior to sample collection, other reasons for failure including sample transportation and processing problems, or the presence of fastidious microorganisms. This has prompted the search for methods of pathogen identification that are unaffected by preoperative antibiotic therapy, such as molecular diagnostic techniques.

Molecular methods include targeted polymerase chain reaction (PCR), broad-range PCR, and next-generation sequencing. These techniques, as well as being unaffected by antimicrobial administration, allow a faster diagnosis (usually, a few days) than tissue cultures, and easier identification of fastidious microbes. However, so far, they have not demonstrated clear superiority over properly conducted conventional culture techniques (most studies have been carried out in periprosthetic joint infection, PJI), are considerably more expensive (their cost-effectiveness in FRI is yet to be determined), and have higher risk of contamination and analytical complexity [7, 12]. They also do not distinguish between viable and non-viable bacteria (which may have been transferred from sterilized instruments), and do not provide information on antimicrobial sensitivity other than the presence or absence of genes that confer resistance. Thus, they complement but not substitute tissue cultures, and their use is currently reserved for specific cases in which slow-growing pathogens are suspected to accelerate the diagnostic process, when tissue cultures are negative, or in cases of antibiotic therapy prior to sample collection.

Targeted PCR detects a specific gene of a particular microorganism and/or resistance mechanism (singleplex), or multiple genes of different microorganisms and resistance mechanisms (multiplex). Though commercial kits exist, most laboratories carry out multiple custom-targeted PCRs tailored to local microbial patterns. However, this is becoming a challenge as regulations regarding in vitro medical devices are becoming stricter. Targeted PCR can provide fast results (48 h) and has been observed to be highly sensitive, but it will only detect the targets included.

Broad-range PCR allows detection of genes that are universally present in microorganisms, the most frequent target being 16S ribosomal RNA (other targets exist for fungi). It has an additional step compared to targeted PCR, as first screening and amplification are carried out, then sequencing is performed. The sequence is then compared to a database. Unlike targeted PCR, it is not limited to targets, but the risk of contamination is higher, resulting in a relatively high proportion of false positives in the available literature (mostly, studying PJI). Additionally, genes from any potential nonviable bacteria in sterilized instruments will be detected too. Other limitations include little added value in comparison with conventional cultures, its high cost and time consumption, and its requirement of highly qualified staff to perform it.

A system combining broad-range PCR with electrospray ionization mass spectrometry has been developed to address multiple microbial species simultaneously [20], but its use is experimental and the two published studies on it (different from the publication describing the instrument) investigate bacteria on inert materials, not live cells or organisms which have a much more complex environment.

Unbiased next-generation sequencing does not require a priori prediction of which pathogens will be detected (unlike conventional tissue cultures or PCR-based techniques). It has attracted attention in FRI, where the variability of germs is high. However, host DNA (as well as microbial DNA) will be detected, and to filter it out is a time-consuming process as deep sequencing is required, so the usefulness of targeted metagenomics is under research. It has a lower cost and less complex analysis. Preliminary data suggests that both approaches are useful to increase diagnostic yield of sonication fluid, but the evidence is very heterogeneous and there are many open questions, including which is the optimal specimen (e.g., tissue samples, sonication fluid), what value does it add to conventional tissue cultures and/or PCR techniques (which are cheaper), and which patients benefit from next-generation sequencing techniques.

Current research investigating the use of molecular techniques for pathogen identification is likely to shed light on these and the many other unanswered questions regarding these techniques in the coming years.

Postoperative Diagnosis of FRI

- Cultures: identification of phenotypically indistinguishable pathogens by culture (gold standard) of at least 2 separate deep tissue or implant (sonication fluid) samples.
- Histopathological confirmation: identification of pathogens in a deep tissue sample, > 5 PMNs/HPF.

Molecular diagnostics can be used if antimicrobials prior to sample collection, negative cultures, or fastidious microbes suspected: PCR (broad-range, targeted), next generation sequencing (unbiased, targeted).

Conclusions

The AO-EBJIS consensus described four confirmatory criteria for FRI diagnosis: two clinical (presence of a fistula/sinus/wound breakdown, or presence of pus) and two based on microorganism identification in deep tissue samples (identification of two phenotypically identical pathogens from two separate cultures, or identification of microorganisms or > 5 PMNs/HPF by histopathology).

Suggestive criteria include clinical, radiological, laboratory, microbiological, and histopathological signs. They strengthen or weaken the suspicion of FRI. The threshold for surgical exploration should be low.

Suggestive clinical signs include local or systemic signs of infection (e.g., local redness, swelling, fever), a new-onset joint effusion, or persistent, increasing or new-onset wound drainage.

Suggestive laboratory signs include abnormal behavior of inflammatory biomarkers *over time* (e.g., levels increase after an initial decrease, persistent elevation): CRP, ESR, and WBC count.

Suggestive radiological signs include osteolysis, implant loosening, sequestration, nonunion, involucrum. There is no consensus on the best imaging modality, but usually X-rays, CT, and MRI are obtained. Nuclear imaging techniques are useful in cases of an oligosymptomatic FRI with few signs of infection, because they are more sensitive than other imaging techniques. The best-studied technique is WBC-SPECT.

Tissue cultures are the gold standard for FRI diagnosis. They are essential to guide targeted postoperative antimicrobial therapy, which is key for success. The first sample collection and debridement surgery is the best opportunity to identify and characterize the causative pathogen, so adequate sample collection is essential.

Sonication is routinely performed, but its diagnostic value is yet uncertain.

Molecular diagnostic technologies are promising, but further research is needed to understand how to best utilize them and which patients benefit best. Currently, they are reserved for patients in whom fastidious microbes are suspected, those with negative cultures or those in whom antimicrobials have been administered preoperatively, and always in combination with conventional tissue cultures.

References

1. McNally M, Corrigan R, Sliepen J, Dudareva M, Rentenaar R, Ijpma F, Atkins BL, Wouthuyzen-Bakker M, Govaert G. What factors affect outcome in the treatment of fracture-related infection? Antibiotics (Basel). 2022;11:946.
2. Metsemakers WJ, Morgenstern M, McNally MA, et al. Fracture-related infection: a consensus on definition from an international expert group. Injury. 2018;49:505–10.
3. Walter N, Orbenes N, Rupp M, Alt V. The state of research in fracture-related infection-a bibliometric analysis. Medicina (Kaunas). 2022;58:1170.
4. Alt V, McNally M, Wouthuyzen-Bakker M, Metsemakers W-J, Marais L, Zalavras C, Morgenstern M. The FRI classification – a new classification of fracture-related infections. Injury. 2024;55:111831.
5. Govaert GAM, Kuehl R, Atkins BL, Trampuz A, Morgenstern M, Obremskey WT, Verhofstad MHJ, McNally MA, Metsemakers W-J. Diagnosing fracture-related infection: current concepts and recommendations. J Orthop Trauma. 2020;34:8–17.
6. Natoli RM, Malek S. Fracture-related infection blood-based biomarkers: diagnostic strategies. Injury. 2024;55(Suppl 6):111823.
7. Stevenson MC, Slater JC, Sagi HC, Palacio Bedoya F, Powers-Fletcher MV. Diagnosing fracture-related infections: where are we now? J Clin Microbiol. 2022;60:e0280720.
8. van den Kieboom J, Bosch P, Plate JDJ, IJpma FFA, Kuehl R, McNally MA, Metsemakers W-J, Govaert GAM. Diagnostic accuracy of serum inflammatory markers in late fracture-related infection: a systematic review and meta-analysis. Bone Joint J. 2018;100-B:1542–50.
9. McNally M, Govaert G, Dudareva M, Morgenstern M, Metsemakers W-J. Definition and diagnosis of fracture-related infection. EFORT Open Rev. 2020;5:614–9.
10. Vicenti G, Buono C, Albano F, Ladogana T, Pesare E, Colasuonno G, Passarelli AC, Solarino G. Early management for fracture-related infection: a literature review. Healthcare (Basel). 2024;12:1306.
11. Mouzopoulos G, Kanakaris NK, Kontakis G, Obakponovwe O, Townsend R, Giannoudis PV. Management of bone infections in adults: the surgeon's and microbiologist's perspectives. Injury. 2011;42(Suppl 5):S18–23.
12. Morgenstern M, Kühl R, Eckardt H, Acklin Y, Stanic B, Garcia M, Baumhoer D, Metsemakers W-J. Diagnostic challenges and future perspectives

in fracture-related infection. Injury. 2018;49(Suppl 1):S83–90.
13. Govaert GA, Ijpma FF, McNally M, McNally E, Reininga IH, Glaudemans AW. Accuracy of diagnostic imaging modalities for peripheral post-traumatic osteomyelitis – a systematic review of the recent literature. Eur J Nucl Med Mol Imaging. 2017;44:1393–407.
14. Scotcher M, Uren N, Qureshi A, Hancock N, Round J. Fracture-related infection in revision proximal femoral intramedullary nails. Injury. 2024;55:111338.
15. Onsea J, Pallay J, Depypere M, et al. Intramedullary tissue cultures from the reamer-irrigator-aspirator system for diagnosing fracture-related infection. J Orthop Res. 2021;39:281–90.
16. Sigmund IK, McNally MA, Luger M, Böhler C, Windhager R, Sulzbacher I. Diagnostic accuracy of neutrophil counts in histopathological tissue analysis in periprosthetic joint infection using the ICM, IDSA, and EBJIS criteria. Bone Joint Res. 2021;10:536–47.
17. Moriarty TF, Metsemakers W-J, Morgenstern M, Hofstee MI, Vallejo Diaz A, Cassat JE, Wildemann B, Depypere M, Schwarz EM, Richards RG. Fracture-related infection. Nat Rev Dis Primers. 2022;8:67.
18. Morgenstern M, Clauss M, Sendi P, Cadosch D, Osinga R, Metsemakers W-J. Treatment of fracture-related infections. In: Textbook of polytrauma management: a multidisciplinary approach. 3rd ed. Berlin: Springer; 2022. p. 573–81.
19. Wildemann B, Ignatius A, Leung F, Taitsman LA, Smith RM, Pesántez R, Stoddart MJ, Richards RG, Jupiter JB. Non-union bone fractures. Nat Rev Dis Primers. 2021;7:57.
20. Ecker DJ, Sampath R, Massire C, Blyn LB, Hall TA, Eshoo MW, Hofstadler SA. Ibis T5000: a universal biosensor approach for microbiology. Nat Rev Microbiol. 2008;6:553–8.

Part II

Management of Fracture-Related Infections (FRI)

General Aspects of Treatment of Fracture-Related Infection

3

Cristina Ojeda-Thies, Pilar Hernández-Jiménez, Mikel Mancheño-Losa, and Nieves Vanaclocha

Introduction

The treatment of fracture-related infection (FRI) remains one of the greatest challenges in orthopedic surgery. Due to the presence of biofilm on implants and necrotic tissue, antibiotic treatment alone is insufficient for complete resolution of the infection. Surgery is also required for infection eradication [1]. Whether surgery is the best option for a particular patient, its optimal timing and what type of surgical strategy is best will vary greatly from one patient to another.

The goals of treatment are fracture union, infection eradication, healing of the soft tissue envelope and restoration of limb function [2]. While the 2018 consensus [3] improved the diagnosis of FRI through the definition of confirmatory and suggestive diagnostic criteria, the optimal treatment of this condition remains to be established. As a biofilm-associated infection, most principles have been derived from periprosthetic infections (PJI), where the body of literature is much more established. However, there are significant differences between PJI and FRI that are relevant for treatment, such as the presence of a (usually nonunited) fracture, or the possibility of implant removal without functional loss once the fracture is healed in FRI.

Surgical strategies for FRI can prioritize fracture union (debridement and suppression until union and eventual implant removal), eradication of the infection (resection of the fractured segment and management of the bony defect), simultaneous approach to both (fracture debridement and revision of fracture stabilization if needed), or none (antibiotic suppression). This chapter will focus on the commonalities among the different strategies of FRI treatment.

Regardless of the chosen strategy, several principles remain as cornerstones of treatment: (1) surgical debridement and irrigation, (2) tissue sampling, (3) fracture stabilization, (4) dead space management, (5) soft tissue coverage, and (6) appropriate antimicrobial therapy [2]. Clinical equipoise remains regarding several of these principles, particularly regarding the techniques required to address bone loss, the choice of fixation and the duration and delivery of antimicrobial therapy, and randomized trials regarding surgical management are lacking. Treatment

C. Ojeda-Thies (✉)
Bone Infection Unit, Department of Traumatology and Orthopedic Surgery, 12 de Octubre University Hospital, Madrid, Spain

Department of Surgery, School of Medicine, Complutense University, Madrid, Spain
e-mail: cristina.ojeda@salud.madrid.org

P. Hernández-Jiménez · M. Mancheño-Losa
Musculoskeletal Infection Consultation Unit, Department of Internal Medicine, Hospital Universitario 12 de Octubre, Madrid, Spain

N. Vanaclocha
Orthoplastics Unit and Department of Plastic and Reconstructive Surgery, University and Polytechnic Hospital La Fe, Valencia, Spain

N. Vanaclocha (ed.), *Treatment of Fracture-Related Infection*,
https://doi.org/10.1007/978-3-031-92452-1_3

should be tailored to the individual characteristics of the fracture, pathogens involved, and host, making comparisons of published research difficult. In all cases, preoperative planning and multidisciplinary management including orthopedic surgeons, infectious disease specialists, microbiologists, radiologists, and plastic surgeons has been proven to improve results after FRI [4].

Based on the heterogeneous collection of published studies, in this chapter we will address:

- Preoperative considerations: who (which patients), when (surgical timing), by whom (when should the patient be evaluated by a multidisciplinary team), how (when is a single-stage advisable).
- Intraoperative considerations: how to properly debride, how to manage dead space, and other technical details.

For information on postoperative care, refer to Chap. 11.

Principles of FRI Treatment

- Eradication requires a combination of surgery and pathogen-directed antimicrobial therapy.
- As well as infection eradication, treatment goals include fracture union, healing of the soft tissue envelope and restoration of limb function.

Preoperative Considerations

Surgical Indication

A combination of surgery and pathogen-directed antimicrobial therapy is needed to achieve infection eradication, so it is recommended in patients in whom FRI has been diagnosed (confirmatory criteria including wound breakdown exposing bone or implants) or is suspected (suggestive clinical, laboratory, or radiological findings) [3].

However, many surgical strategies for FRI entail significant morbidity, so it is important to consider the risk–benefit relationship between the morbidity of treatment versus the morbidity of the infection, and the long-term risks of each. Patients unfit for surgery or with a reduced life expectancy (R4 and R5 in the FRI classification [5], or Cierny–Mader type C hosts) usually benefit more from conservative treatments such as antibiotic suppression [6, 7]. Suppressive treatment also has drawbacks, including a high rate of complications such as adverse drug reactions and antimicrobial resistance. For more information on these issues, the reader is referred to Chap. 10.

Surgical Timing

As the duration of FRI increases, so does the biofilm maturation and bone involvement [8]. Thus, surgery should be performed as soon as possible on an optimized patient (*early elective surgery*) [9]. If implants are retained, the success rates are highest when surgery is performed within the first 2–3 weeks after the initial appearance of signs of infection, likely due to glycocalyx maturation within the biofilm. Treatment success decreases sharply in implant retention surgeries performed more than 10 weeks after fracture stabilization [10, 11].

Modifiable patient factors have also been shown to influence the likelihood of infection eradication and the healing of both bone and soft tissues, setting the need for surgery in a balance with the benefit of preoperative patient optimization. For example, the probability of treatment failure increases 2.5-fold in patients with a body mass index over 30 [12], and smoking has been associated with a sharp reduction in treatment success rates [13]. Thus, to ensure optimal outcomes, it is critical to optimize patients preoperatively, including addressing factors that will negatively affect healing or the effectiveness of antimicrobial treatment, such as smoking cessation, limb revascularization, correction of nutritional alterations (obesity, malnutrition), metabolic control in diabetes mellitus, correction of vitamin D deficit, and decolonization of *Staphylococcus aureus* carriers, among others [12, 14].

Urgent surgery is justified in cases of severe sepsis (life- or limb-threatening), disease progression with rapid deterioration, or increasing fracture instability [9].

When Should the Patient Be Evaluated by a Multidisciplinary Team?

Based on the available evidence, all patients with an FRI should be treated by a multidisciplinary team composed of orthopedic and plastic surgeons, infectious disease physicians, microbiologists, and radiologists (occasionally other specialists too, such as vascular surgeons), because it leads to better outcomes [4, 14]. Interestingly, only a small proportion (< 15%) of published studies with FRI patients mention a multidisciplinary approach [15], a testament to the difficulty in overcoming the logistic challenges inherent to this approach. A team able to perform only some of the techniques to treat FRI will have a subconscious tendency to over-indicate these techniques, which is particularly undesirable in FRI, where choosing a simpler solution that provides a worse outcome is rarely worth the risk. This is because successive revision surgeries after failed treatment will grow in complexity, with increasing tissue loss after each debridement, reducing the possible reconstruction options. New technologies such as video consultations can be taken advantage of to consult with referral multidisciplinary teams early and thus improve outcomes.

Choice of a Single- vs. Multistage Strategy

The evidence to recommend a one- or two-stage approach is weak, and results have been found to be comparable [16–18]. Two-stage approaches are more common in the published literature, but one-stage treatments are increasingly performed, with similar success [19]. The choice depends on many factors, including the pathogen's antimicrobial resistance, availability of a biofilm-active treatment, size of the bone defect after debridement, quality of the soft tissue envelope, organizational factors, and surgeon experience.

Many prefer a two-stage approach, given the tendency of FRI to recur, to allow confirmation of infection eradication before definitive bone reconstruction [15, 20]. Moreover, many techniques (distraction osteogenesis, induced membrane) are multistage per se. Other factors that may favor a staged approach include concerns regarding the viability of the remaining bone, poor host fitness (discouraging a single long surgery), and the presence of difficult-to-treat pathogens [9]. Disadvantages of multiple-stage surgery are treatment costs and duration, and possibly a greater difficulty to achieve a complete functional recovery.

In staged approaches, the initial surgical stage will mainly focus on thorough debridement and tissue sampling. Stable soft tissue coverage is key to minimizing the probability of reinfection, but bone stability and dead space may be managed with temporary means (external fixation and antibiotic-loaded spacers, respectively). After surgery, targeted antimicrobial therapy is delivered and the patient is monitored clinically and serologically [15, 20]. Although early protocols proposed a delay of 6–8 weeks between stages, there is no evidence to support this or any other recommendation regarding the optimal timing for a second stage [9, 21]. Many consider that there should be no clinical or laboratory signs of infection recurrence 2 weeks after antibiotic therapy cessation, as a minimum time frame to plan definitive bone reconstruction [21]. This is based on studies in PJI where inflammatory biomarkers (C-reactive protein, erythrocyte sedimentation rate, white blood cell count) have been found to take about 2 weeks to elevate after antibiotic cessation if infection persists, but there is no reliable biomarker to prove the eradication of infection before the second stage. Winkler et al. found that successful outcomes of PJI treatment remained high despite omission of the antibiotic-free interval before reimplantation [22]. Planning for the second stage should be individualized considering the pathogen, host, degree of infection control and soft tissue status, among other factors, and renewed debridement and tissue resampling is strongly recommended in the second stage.

A single stage can, in our opinion, safely be performed if adequate fracture alignment and stability are achievable, the bony and soft tissue defects can be reconstructed after performing a thorough debridement, the host has little or no comorbidities (R1–2), the vascularization of the FRI site is adequate, and the causative pathogen is known and not difficult-to-treat, with available anti-biofilm antimicrobials (Fig. 3.1). The suitability of a single-stage (vs. multistage) strategy should always be reevaluated intraoperatively, and patients should be informed before surgery of the possibility of requiring an intraoperative change of plans.

Several factors influence the vascularization of the FRI site, including the anatomical location (e.g., the upper limb is generally better vascularized than the lower limb, and its arteries tend to be less impacted by peripheral artery disease) and choice of technique (e.g., flaps including bone flaps favor a single stage, as their intrinsic vascularity transports antibiotics to the FRI site [23]). The need for soft tissue flaps for coverage should not discourage from single-staging, for similar reasons, with the simultaneous combination of orthopedic revision and soft tissue flaps reporting good results [24, 25]. However, there is no evidence to support the abovementioned or any other criteria to advise a single-stage treatment.

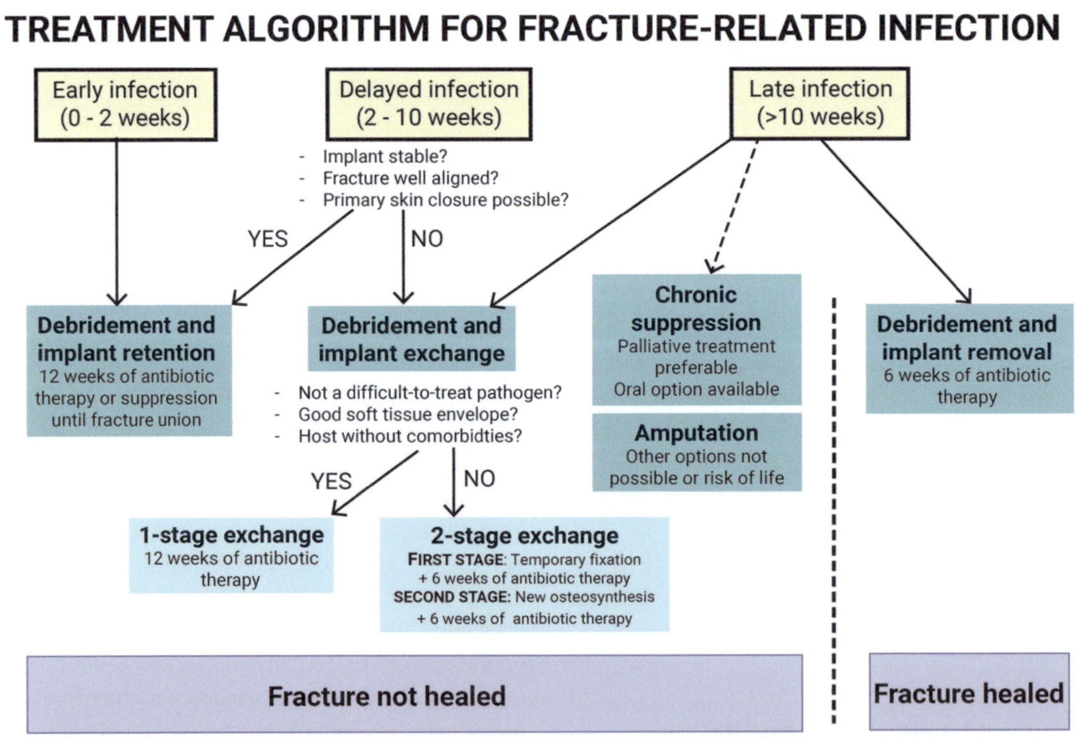

Fig. 3.1 Overview of the treatment algorithm for fracture-related infections. (Adapted from [1] Metsemakers WJ, Kuehl R, Moriarty TF, et al. (2018) Infection after fracture fixation: current surgical and microbiological concepts. Injury 49:511–522)

Preoperative Considerations of FRI Treatment

Except for a minority of selected patients best served with conservative treatments, FRI should be treated with a combination of surgery and targeted antimicrobial therapy.

Surgery should be performed as soon as possible on an optimized patient (early elective surgery). Both pre- and perioperative optimization and multidisciplinary team involvement are essential to obtaining good outcomes.

Evidence to recommend a one- vs. two-stage approach is weak. Two-stage approaches are more common in the published literature, but one-stage treatments are increasingly performed, with similar success. Factors that favor two stages include poor infection control, concerns regarding the viability of the remaining bone, high host comorbidity, and the presence of difficult-to-treat pathogens.

Intraoperative Considerations

Surgical Debridement, Irrigation, and Microbiological Sampling

Debridement is crucial in the management of FRI and the best predictor of success, because it is the part of the surgery in which the infection itself is addressed [1]. The main goal of debridement is to reduce the bacterial burden and eliminate as much biofilm as possible, in order to increase the efficacy of antimicrobials and reduce the risk of antimicrobial resistance development. This is carried out by excising all infected, poorly vascularized, or necrotic tissues, as well as foreign bodies such as previously implanted bone substitutes or non-incorporated grafts, and hardware (depending on whether the strategy involves implant retention, exchange or removal). Inadequate debridement has been associated with high recurrence rates and has been pointed out as the leading cause for treatment failure [26]. Therefore, it is fundamental that concerns regarding the reconstruction of the resulting bone or soft tissue defect do not compromise the quality of debridement [14, 27]. A useful strategy is to have one surgeon in charge of the debridement and another responsible for the subsequent reconstruction [14].

There is insufficient evidence to support the use of one debridement method over another or a specific margin, the only requirement is that only healthy viable tissue is kept [17, 28]. This includes removal of any visible pus and resecting nonviable bone and sequestra until healthy bleeding is encountered. Osteotomes or a high-speed burr should be used to remove any sclerotic or necrotic bone until capillary bleeding into the operative field ("paprika sign") is observed. The intramedullary canal, if involved, should be reamed if possible.

The skin incision should be carefully planned to facilitate closure or eventual soft tissue coverage, and any infected soft tissue should be removed, including sinus tracts. Preoperative diagnostic imaging can establish the relationship between sinus tracts and neurovascular structures, which should be preserved.

Tissue sampling for microbiological and histopathological analysis should also be performed at this stage. A minimum of five deep tissue samples should be obtained for microbiology, ideally from the bone-implant interface or adjacent to the fracture, using separate sterile instruments and a no touch technique, directly from the patient to the container. Swabs or samples from the sinus tract should be avoided [29]. Onsea et al. found that reamed bone obtained through the reamer-irrigator-aspirator system had a high diagnostic yield for infections involving the medullary canal [30]. For further details on appropriate sampling, refer to Chap. 2.

After debridement and sampling, the operative field should be washed with several liters of normal saline. Studies from open fractures showed that irrigation should be performed at low pressure to avoid bacterial seeding and that addition of antiseptics is not superior to saline [31, 32]. The optimal amount of fluid is unknown, and irrigation should be continued until the wound is macroscopically clean.

Management of Fracture Stability

Once debridement, sampling and irrigation have been performed, a new phase in the surgical strategy commences, including fracture stabilization, dead space management and soft tissue coverage. To plan for this latter part of the surgery, it is important to assess the quality of the soft tissues and the integrity of the bone, as these are vital for treatment success [9]. As the extent and characteristics of the defect (bone and/or soft tissue) are usually not known with precision until after completing debridement, extensive preoperative planning is required, as well as the ability to change plans quickly in view of intraoperative findings.

Bone stability and fracture union are essential for both limb function and infection eradication [6, 33]. Many options exist for fracture fixation in the setting of FRI, and data comparing the different methods is scarce [9]. The choice of fixation depends on many factors including the chronology of the infection, the type, and location of the infected hardware, fracture characteristics (configuration, location, healing progression, alignment and stability), pathogen(s) likely involved, and host type, among others. The different possibilities for management of bone stability and hardware will be discussed at length in the next chapters, Chaps. 4, 5, 6, 7, and 8. In this chapter, only a short overview will be provided.

In the setting of an FRI, any implants present can be removed, exchanged, or retained (Fig. 3.1). For healed fractures (F1), implant removal without functional loss is possible if bony stability is maintained after debridement, and infection can be controlled in a high number of patients even after a short antibiotic course [34]. For nonunited fractures however, or in case of loss of continuity of bone after debridement (F2–4), stabilization is needed and can be achieved through retention or exchange of the implanted hardware.

In acute or early FRIs, biofilm is less mature, the fracture has good healing potential still, and oftentimes, implant removal would complicate fracture management, particularly in complex periarticular fractures. Thus, these fractures are often best managed with implant retention, equivalent to a DAIR (debridement, antibiotic and implant retention) strategy in PJI. A systematic review found high success rates in early and delayed infections (less than 10 weeks after implantation), with remission of infection in over 80% of patients, but poorer outcomes beyond that period (67% success rate) [10]. Fracture union can be achieved as long as the osteosynthesis construct remains stable, and suppression until bony union is a valid alternative, allowing for a less complex implant removal once the fracture has healed in case of persistent signs of infection vs. revision of internal fixation. Rightmire et al. achieved a 68% union rate with suppressive treatment [13]. Implants were removed after union in 40% of the patients. Of the patients that had achieved union with suppressive therapy, recurrent infection appeared in 36% of patients with retained hardware and 16% in those in whom internal fixation had been removed, highlighting the fact that, though bony union is possible, it will not necessarily heal the infection. Berkes et al. similarly found a 71% union rate, but treatment failed significantly more in open fractures (58% union rate) and those stabilized with intramedullary nails (46% union rate) [35]. Remission of infection with retention of intramedullary nails was only achieved in 42% in another series, particularly in infections treated beyond 2 months after implantation [36]. The presence of an intramedullary nail had an odds ratio of failure of 4.0 (1.1–13.8) in a further series of 141 patients with early FRI treated with DAIR (24% recurrence rate vs. 13% recurrence rate overall) [37]. It would hence seem reasonable to recommend nail exchange in FRI stabilized with intramedullary nails, given the difficulty of debriding the medullary canal surrounding the nail and the ease of exchange (in comparison with revision of other implants), but a systematic review of 28 studies with 171 FRIs following intramedullary nailing of long bones was unable to find any differences between treatment strategies for infections up to 9 months after implantation [38]. Tsang et al.

achieved fracture union in 95% of cases with chronic suppression and retention of intramedullary nails where the fixation was stable with adequate alignment, the soft tissue coverage was adequate, and progression of bony healing was observed on follow-up X-rays. They also reported remission of infection in 98% of patients after definite eradication surgery including nail removal after union. Of concern, however, is that pathogens were isolated during eradication surgery after union in 75% of cases, and 13% presented multidrug resistance [39]. To sum up, implant retention can be successful, but it is not benign, and there is conflicting, low-quality evidence regarding which patients benefit best from it, with most recommendations being based on expert consensus. The reader is referred to Chap. 4 for further information on criteria for implant retention.

Implant exchange is indicated in late infections, FRIs with poor bone healing potential (F3), and if the retention strategy has failed or is unadvisable, such as cases with weeks-long exposed hardware or compromised host physiology, difficult-to-treat pathogens, or if no biofilm-active antimicrobial options are available. In these situations, after extensive debridement and removal of hardware, re-osteosynthesis can be performed in the same surgery or in a separate stage, particularly if adverse factors concur. The choice of a one- vs. two-stage fixation strategy depends on the pathogen's antimicrobial resistance and availability of anti-biofilm treatment, the size of the bony defect after debridement, soft tissue envelope, organizational factors and surgeon experience, among others. Results from both approaches have been found to be comparable [16].

Any hardware in the FRI site is susceptible to colonization by residual infection, as some pathogens will be present even after the best debridement due to bacterial persistence in canaliculi, osteoblasts, and other cells. The alternative is prolonged external fixation. However, prolonged external fixation puts a great physical and psychological strain on patients, so mixed protocols are often used [15]. Traditionally, an approach combining minimal internal fixation with supportive external fixation has been popular, but increased focus on construct stability has led several teams to defy this approach, especially as novel antibiotic carriers with better elution profiles have improved the local administration of high-dose antimicrobials [9]. The upper limb is more amenable to the exclusive use of internal fixation, as less hardware is necessary (no weight-bearing) and the soft tissue envelope is usually of greater quality [40]. In the lower limb, criteria have been proposed for internal fixation after a first stage of debridement and local antibiotic therapy: small defects (<2–4 cm), good bone stock and soft tissue quality, absence of multiresistant microorganisms, and a host without systemic or local compromising factors [41, 42]. However, it is estimated that under 5% of cases fulfill these requirements, and there is neither evidence to support those specific criteria nor wide acceptance of them [43].

Dead Space Management

In the context of FRI, dead space refers to the void left after surgical excision of necrotic bone and soft tissue. This void has the potential to be filled with a hematoma, creating a milieu favorable to the proliferation of pathogens which can then lead to infection recurrence. Management of dead space is thus crucial for the success of FRI treatment, and has been associated with superior results compared to debridement alone [44]. Additionally, techniques to manage dead space often also allow for the administration of local antimicrobials, which has been associated to lower infection recurrence rates [45].

Dead space can be managed in numerous ways, including bone void fillers, acute shortening, the induced membrane technique, segmental bone transport, and bone flaps. A systematic review of 50 studies comprising 1530 patients found an overall FRI eradication rate of 83%, but the authors were unable to determine the superiority of any one treatment option over the rest due to the lack of clear classification systems, potential underreporting of adverse events, and heterogeneity of patient series [46]. Thus, the

Table 3.1 General characteristics of antibiotic-impregnated bone void fillers

Bone void filler	Advantages	Disadvantages
Antibiotic-impregnated non-vascularized bone graft	High antibiotic release Quickly degraded Easy to use	Unpredictable elution kinetics, >95% released in <5 days Infection risk Heterogeneous evidence for its use
Antibiotic-impregnated polymethylmethacrylate	High antibiotic release Provides mechanical stability Good level of evidence supporting its use	Not biodegradable, requires removal Unfavorable elution, can favor resistance
Antibiotic-impregnated calcium sulfate and phosphate	Highly degradable Osteoconductive	High seroma rate High variability of material Slow degradation of calcium phosphates
Bioactive glass	Antimicrobial mechanism (no resistance) Osteoconductive	Slow degradation Stiff Not all formulations are antimicrobial
Antibiotic-impregnated collagen sponges	High antibiotic release Quickly degraded Easy to use	Unpredictable elution kinetics, >95% released in <5 days Infection risk Scarce evidence for its use

Modified from Arts C. Clinical evidence of biomaterials in osteomyelitis treatment. Literature review and decision-making considerations. Presented at the 42nd Annual Meeting of the European Bone & Joint Infection Society; 2024 September 26–28; Barcelona, Spain

choice of treatment strategy will depend on the size and location of the void, availability of different bone void fillers, or microsurgery, whether the defect is contained or not, other aspects of the surgical strategy (e.g., the need to harvest a flap for other purposes, whether a second stage is planned), host status, and surgeon preference. The strategy for dead space management is interrelated with management of stability and soft tissue coverage, as certain techniques address two or all three of these items (e.g., muscle flaps can be used to obliterate space and cover wounds; acute shortening with or without re-lengthening obliterates dead space through limb compression). These compound strategies are discussed further in other chapters (Chaps. 5 and 9). The present section will be devoted to the use of bone void fillers, most often used in F1 cases of the FRI Classification and in staged surgeries.

There are few comparative studies, with no bone void filler demonstrating superiority over the rest. The ideal bone void filler should be osteoinductive, osteoconductive, noncytotoxic, would have a favorable antimicrobial elution profile, and would not require removal. So far, the perfect filler does not exist, and every filler has both advantages and disadvantages. Some bone void fillers are *biologic* (bone grafts, muscle flaps), whereas others are *synthetic* (antibiotic-loaded polymethylmethacrylate (PMMA) bone cement, bioglass, ceramics, etc.) (Table 3.1) [47, 48]. *Synthetic* bone void fillers' biodegradability, capacity for osteoconduction, mechanical properties, and antimicrobial release profile are affected by their composition, microstructure (porosity), anisotropy, surface characteristics, shape, and size, with no one filler having demonstrated clear superiority over another. Thus, the choice of bone void filler will depend mainly on the size and location of the defect, availability, and surgeon preference.

Non-vascularized autologous bone graft is the only osteogenic option among those listed, as well as osteoinductive through bone matrix growth factors. It provides an osteoconductive scaffold and can provide some mechanical stability, but lacks antimicrobial properties and has limited availability. Admixing of antibiotics to autologous bone graft has been used in two-stage approaches, with favorable outcomes [46, 49]. However, evidence from large clinical series is lacking and the optimal doses of antibiotics are unknown. Additionally, concerns exist regarding antimicrobials' local cytotoxic effects on osteoclasts and osteoblasts, so the routine combination of autologous bone graft with local antibiotics is not recommended [48]. Allograft avoids the donor-site morbidity associated with autografts, but lacks osteogenic potential and can act as a sequestrum in case of persistence of pathogens in the dead space. Admixing of antibiotics to allograft has shown promising results after revision surgery for PJI [50], but surgeons should be aware of its capacity to act as a foreign body once the antimicrobials have been released. For more information on the use of bone autografts, allografts, their admixing with antibiotics, and their indications, the reader is referred to Chap. 5.

Polymethylmethacrylate (PMMA) is the most used and studied compound [48]. It has been employed for decades as an antimicrobial carrier, spacer (e.g., in Masquelet's induced membrane technique), to coat implants, or applied in the form of beads at the site of infection, including soft tissues. PMMA is widely available, easy to shape, easily mixed with antibiotics for impregnation, and comes in a variety of prepared formats.

There are, however, several issues associated with PMMA. Its main disadvantage is its nonresorbability, which imposes the need for a second stage to remove the PMMA, coupled with unfavorable (i.e., low and variable) antimicrobial elution kinetics. It is estimated that less of 10% of the antibiotics in PMMA will be released, and antibiotic inhibitory concentrations are not reliably maintained after only 2 weeks [48]. The result is that after an initially high antibiotic release, it elutes antibiotics at subtherapeutic levels, thus potentially promoting antibiotic resistance [51]. Though some authors have reported favorable outcomes with retained PMMA [52], persistent bacteria have been shown to colonize and form biofilm on the porous surface of PMMA spacers. For example, in a series of retrieved PMMA beads following PJI revision, bacteria were present on gentamicin-loaded beads in 90% of patients, and 68% of the pathogens isolated were resistant to gentamicin [53]. Furthermore, although there is some evidence that dissolution of powdered antimicrobials in distilled water may improve antibiotic release, the optimal antibiotic state for impregnation and release is yet unknown, as is the ideal antimicrobial dosage. Some publications suggest that, based on animal studies, greater doses are likely to reduce infection recurrence rates, but the concomitant increased bone cell toxicity could lead to a simultaneous reduction in bone union rates [48].

Other issues associated to PMMA use as an antibiotic carrier include the fact that it can only be loaded with heat-stable antibiotics, as its polymerization process is highly exothermic (surface temperatures of over 100 °C have been reported), and that the addition of antibiotics to PMMA can affect its setting characteristics and compromise its strength. For instance, more porous PMMA mixed with greater doses of antibiotics improves antibiotic release but results in easier fragmentation.

These drawbacks have led to interest turning toward other antimicrobial carriers, which do not require a second stage, are capable of delivering a wider range of antimicrobial agents, and provide a better elution profile.

Biodegradable ceramics such as calcium sulfate or phosphate release antibiotics gradually as they are degraded, giving rise to a more stable and complete release than when PMMA is used, maintaining local antibiotic levels above the minimum inhibitory concentration for several weeks. They are osteoconductive, lack immunologic side effects, and promote bone regeneration, and have not been associated with the emergence of specific antimicrobial resistance [54]. Their resorbable nature allows for single-stage management with over 90% success rates [19, 55]. The main drawback of using them is wound drainage, which can appear in 10–33% of cases, potentially resembling purulence. This drainage increases the risk of wound healing problems, and can be challenging to distinguish from recurrent infection. The risk of postoperative wound drainage has been associated with greater volumes of calcium sulfate or phosphate used, combination with soft tissue flap surgery and thinner soft tissue coverage [56, 57]. Calcium sulfates are resorbed faster and thus carry a lower risk of biofilm formation on them, but lack mechanical stability and associate poor bone formation, resulting in a higher risk of refractures if used in isolation. Some commercial products combine calcium sulfates with calcium phosphates (e.g., hydroxyapatite, calcium triphosphate), which are biodegraded slower, to benefit from the advantages of both. These compounds seemingly result in less wound healing problems and lower rates of infection recurrence and refractures, but are potentially more susceptible to bacterial colonization.

Bioactive glass is a synthetic silicate material that possesses intrinsic antibacterial properties through a local increase in pH and osmotic pressure. This, together with the local release of sodium and calcium ions, leads to the precipitation of a carbonate-like layer on the glass resembling bone. Bioglass is thus considered to be osteoconductive. It is easy to handle, and published observational studies report promising results, with infection eradication rates of 80–90% [58, 59]. However, it also has been associated with wound drainage and should not be used in non-contained defects or left in contact with the skin.

Both biodegradable ceramics and bioactive glass have shown promising results in single-stage treatments of small, infected defects. However, the published clinical experience with these materials is still limited and heterogeneous, of a limited level of evidence and with many cointerventions, so further evaluation is warranted [48, 60].

Other proposed compounds include hydrogels and collagen-based polymers. Hydrogels (hydrated polymerized macromolecules) can carry antibiotics and resorb rapidly, leaving no surfaces on which biofilm may form, but releasing antibiotics during a short period of time only. They lack structural strength and have been seldom studied in the setting of FRI. Collagen-based polymers have been used for other pathologies and, though their use as antibiotic-loaded bone void fillers is possible, their biodegradation is faster than what would be desirable for infected nonunions, and the experience with them is scarce and dated [48].

Another area of great interest is the use of implants with antibacterial properties themselves. This can be achieved through the coating of implants in the operative theatre itself with PMMA, resorbable ceramics, or hydrogels [61–64], or by using implants coated in silver, gentamicin poly(d, l-lactide), or povidone-iodine. Currently, evidence on these implants is limited to case series, mainly in the setting of surgeries at high risk for infection (i.e., open fractures), rather than for the treatment of FRI itself [65, 66].

Adequate Soft Tissue Coverage

Up to 40% of FRI require some sort of intervention (local, pedicled, or free flaps) to ensure a healthy soft tissue envelope surrounding the FRI site [67]. Debated topics regarding coverage are its timing, the role of microbiological culture results as a prerequisite for soft tissue closure, the best type of flap, and the role of negative pressure wound therapy (NPWT).

In short, soft tissue coverage can be safely performed in a single stage, adequate surgical debridement being more important than proof of negative cultures at the time of coverage [25, 68, 69]. NPWT is commonly used as a bridging therapy to definitive coverage, but the available evidence has found worse outcomes in the form of higher infection recurrence and reoperation rates when NPWT was employed [69–71]. In a large multicenter retrospective FRI cohort, Sweere et al. found that the use of NPWT was associated with a 28% recurrence rate (vs. 12% in controls), and that longer duration of NPWT was associated with a higher risk of recurrence (OR 1.04, 95% CI 1.01–1.07) [70]. McNally et al. reported a greater rate of infection recurrence or unplanned reoperation when NPWT was used (HR 3.5, 95% CI 1.85–6.51) [72]. Therefore, NPWT should not be seen as a definitive type of treatment but rather as a wound dressing, and, if needed, be used for as few days as possible.

For more information on soft tissue coverage in FRI, refer to Chap. 9.

Surgery in FRI

The essential surgical steps FRI are:

1. Surgical debridement is the greatest predictor of success. Debridement involves excision of all necrotic, poorly vascularized, and infected tissue to reduce the biofilm burden. Only healthy tissue must be kept, and quality of debridement must not be compromised due to concerns regarding the ensuing reconstruction. After debridement, the field must be irrigated with low-pressure saline until it is macroscopically clean.
2. Tissue sampling is the cornerstone of microbiological diagnosis and targeted antimicrobial therapy, and must be performed appropriately. At least 5 deep tissue specimens must be obtained with a no-touch technique and different sterile instruments.
3. Management of stability is key both for infection eradication and a good functional outcome. The main options are for the hardware to be removed, retained, or exchanged.
4. Dead space management is important to prevent fluid build-up that could promote infection recurrence. It is often interrelated with management of stability and soft tissue coverage. No strategy has proven superiority over the rest.
5. A healthy soft tissue envelope is critical to support bone healing and prevent recurrence and reinfection (reliable coverage). Over a third of patients will require tissue transfer. The available evidence suggests that early coverage is best.

Antimicrobial Therapy

Antimicrobial therapy can be administered locally and systemically, and is further discussed in Chap. 10. A short overview will be provided here.

The use of local antimicrobials has been shown to be an important adjunct in the treatment of FRI [45], as they can reach concentrations much higher than the minimum inhibitory concentration at the site of infection for a variable period of time, depending on the carrier used [48]. The local combination of vancomycin and gentamycin is purportedly active against nearly 95% of usual pathogens causing FRI [73].

The principles of systemic antibiotic therapy resemble those for other device-associated infections, with microbiological identification being the cornerstone of tailored treatment [74]. Therefore, antibiotic therapy should be avoided prior to surgical debridement and tissue sampling to prevent false-negative culture results, unless the patient is septic. If the patient has received antibiotics, they should ideally be withheld for 2 weeks prior to surgery and intraoperative sampling. This is particularly relevant for surgical strategies that include retention of the infected device or a single-stage exchange, when optimized antimicrobial treatment is most important.

Empirical intravenous therapy should be started as soon as intraoperative tissue samples have been obtained, and should be adapted to local antimicrobial resistance patterns and patient-specific risk factors (e.g., prior isolates, hospitalizations, or antimicrobial therapy), ensuring coverage of Gram-positive cocci (including methicillin-resistant strains) and Gram-negative bacilli, including *Pseudomonas aeruginosa* [75, 76]. Once the causative pathogen has been identified and the antimicrobial susceptibility profile is available, antimicrobial therapy should be adjusted to the narrowest spectrum, maintaining intravenous administration until the patient is stable, drains have been removed, and the wound is dry—typically within the first 5 to 14 days. Subsequently, oral therapy may be initiated, provided that agents with good bioavailability, adequate bone penetration, and activity against stationary-phase bacteria are available (OVIVA [77]). In cases managed with DAIR or single-stage exchange, combination therapy with rifampin for staphylococcal infections and quinolones for Gram-negative infections should be used whenever possible [75].

Similarly to the lack of randomized controlled trials regarding surgical strategies, limited evidence exists on the duration of systemic antimicrobial therapy. At present, recommendations from an international expert consensus suggest that antimicrobial therapy should be continued for a total of 12 weeks in infection eradication strategies involving implant retention or single-stage exchange [75]. This duration is also considered in two-stage exchange procedures when the second stage is performed within a short time interval (i.e., 2 weeks), or when no antibiotic-free interval is given to ensure the sterility of the surgical site at the time of implantation of the new hardware. In classic two-stage exchange procedures, the duration of antimicrobial therapy may be shortened to 6 weeks, followed by a 2-week antibiotic-free interval before the placement of the new implant. In the second stage, empirical intravenous antimicrobial therapy should be administered until microbiological cultures are identified as negative. In healed fractures in which the osteosynthesis material is removed, a 6-week treatment duration is also recommended.

It is likely that the abovementioned durations of systemic therapy can be shortened without reducing the infection eradication rate, especially if combined with local antimicrobial therapy and/or implants are not retained, although the available evidence to support this is scarce and retrospective [34, 78]. Shorter courses of antimicrobial treatment can also be justified in cases of segmental bone resection without internal fixation (i.e. segmental bone transport with a circular frame). There has been considerable resistance to reducing the 12-week regimen when implants are retained, but a large trial is currently underway comparing short- and long-term antibiotic regimens in early and delayed FRIs with retained implants [79]. Biofilm-active agents are expected to play a particularly significant role in these scenarios.

In any case, each patient should receive an individualized treatment plan determined through a multidisciplinary approach, based on the type of infection, type of orthopedic device, surgical approach, causative microorganisms, and the availability of highly effective antimicrobials [4].

The Role of Suppression

Antimicrobial suppression can be indicated in patients categorized as Cierny–Mader type C hosts (R4–5 in the FRI Classification) without options for optimization and where the aggressiveness of treatment surpasses its potential benefit, to alleviate symptoms during exacerbations. It can also be used in early FRIs of unhealed fractures with retained implants but good bone healing potential, as bony union will convert the FRI to a more favorable scenario in which early implant removal with a short course of antimicrobials is likely to resolve the infection (F1).

Suppressive therapy should be active against pathogens isolated from deep tissue samples, have a low propensity to induce resistance, be orally bioavailable, and have minimal side effects and toxicity [39]. If these conditions cannot be fulfilled or if associated soft tissue conditions warrant the decision, amputation may be considered. For more information on these scenarios, refer to Chaps. 8 and 10.

Bacteriophage Therapy

There is growing concern regarding multiresistant pathogens, which increase the need for novel therapies to confront FRIs. Significant attention has been directed at bacteriophages over the past decade.

Bacteriophages are viruses that infect, replicate within, and ultimately lyse specific bacterial hosts [80]. The advantages of phage therapy are their ability to address sessile bacteria embedded in biofilm, to self-replicate, to act synergistically with antibiotics, and to resensitize bacterial isolates to antimicrobials [81]. Additionally, unlike many antibiotics, due to their host specificity, they cause minimal disruption of the commensal microbiota [81]. However, reliable safety and efficacy data are lacking, as most of the published evidence involves personalized therapies (often, in the setting of PJI) [80, 81]. Though several case reports exist documenting the potential of phage therapy administered through a drainage system in the setting of difficult-to-treat musculoskeletal infections, no guidelines exist regarding phage susceptibility testing or protocols for administration of phage therapy, with different studies publishing different routes of administration, frequencies of administration, treatment duration, and phage titers [81, 82]. In addition, phage surface antigens may elicit a neutralizing immune response that accelerates phage elimination from the patient's body.

Regulations would require prefabricated bacteriophage cocktails to be submitted to costly phase I–IV clinical trials, as with other pharmaceutical products [83]. So far, a study protocol has been published to standardize phage therapy and collect prospective data on patients [84], a necessary step to advance research in this subject.

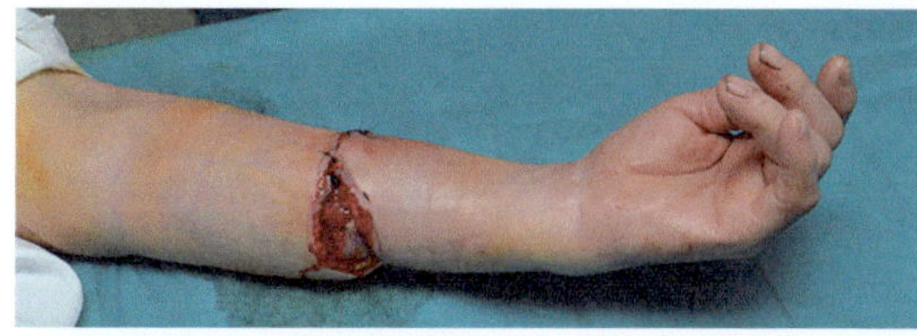

Fig. 3.2 Case 3.1, initial appearance of the traumatic injury in the operative theatre, before examination and debridement of the wound

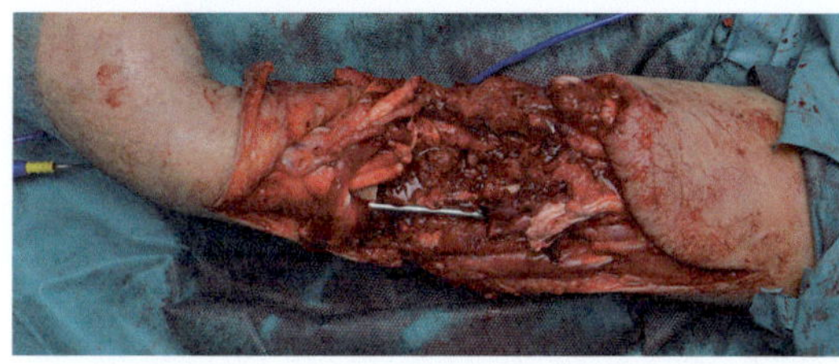

Fig. 3.3 Case 3.1, intraoperative photograph of the skeletal repair. The radius defect has been regularized and fixed with a dorsal 3.5 mm plate, prepared to receive a free fibula flap. The lacerated flexor and extensor tendons are yet to be repaired

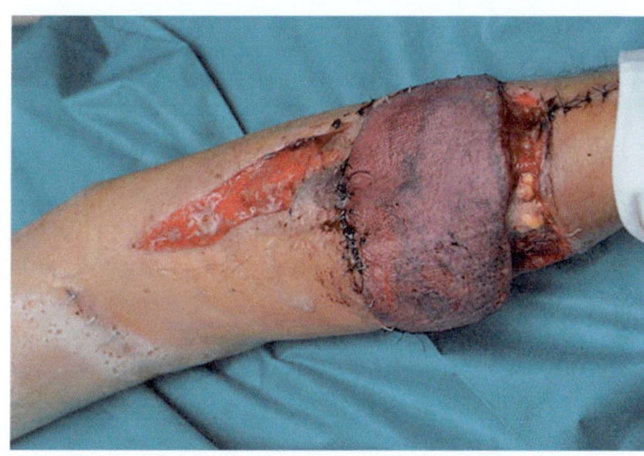

Fig. 3.4 Case 3.1, necrotic skin paddle of the fibula flap due to arterial thrombosis

Clinical Cases

Case 3.1

A 62-year-old male with an active lifestyle and no relevant medical history suffered a Gustilo IIIC open fracture of the left radius following an accident with a circular saw (Fig. 3.2). He had a 5 cm defect of the radial diaphysis, as well as injuries to multiple flexor tendons, the ulnar and median nerves, and the ulnar artery (Fig. 3.3). The fracture was reconstructed with a free fibula flap with a cutaneous island and a dorsal 3.5 mm plate. The flap suffered an early arterial microthrombosis which could not be salvaged (repeated thromboses despite re-dos of the anastomosis) (Fig. 3.4), so the devascularized bone was kept as an avascular graft and the wound was covered with a pedicled groin flap (Fig. 3.5).

Six months later, the patient presented at our outpatient clinic with several fistulae along the groin flap margins and a painful nonunion of the non-vascularized bone graft (F3 R1 I1, Fig. 3.6). He was taken into the operating room and, upon

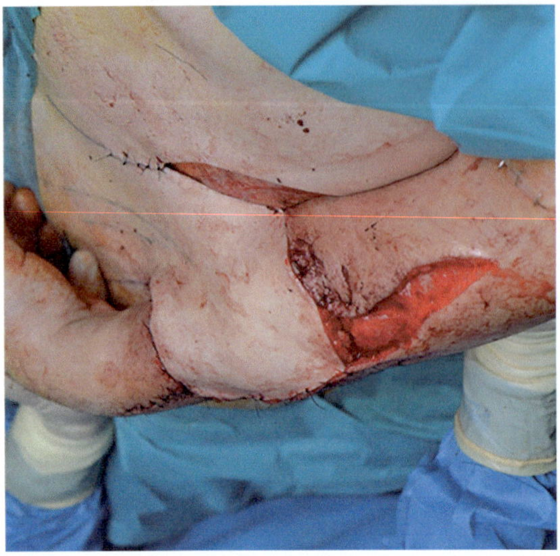

Fig. 3.5 Case 3.1, pedicled groin flap covering the soft tissue defect of the left forearm

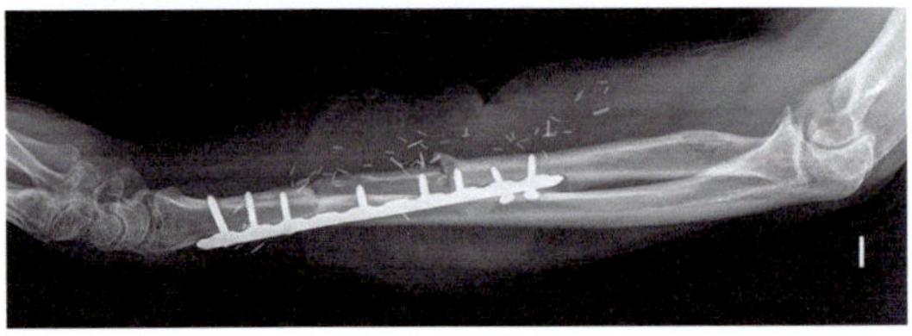

Fig. 3.6 Case 3.1, lateral conventional radiograph of the forearm 6 months after the injury, showing nonunion of the graft with peri-implant loosening and periosteal reaction at the fracture ends

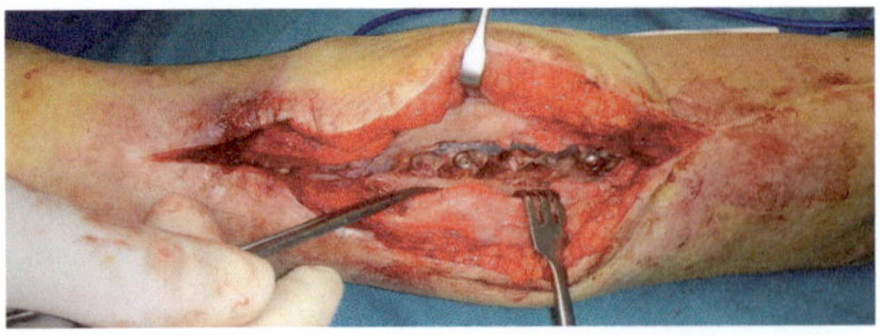

Fig. 3.7 Case 3.1, intraoperative photograph of the first surgical stage. The radius was approached dorsally by elevating the flap. Upon visualization of the internal fixation, macroscopic pus could be observed

approaching the fracture through a dorsal Henry approach, purulence was clearly visible in contact with the plate (Fig. 3.7). The plate and the bone graft were removed, debridement, irrigation and sampling were carried out, and an external fixator was implanted. Next, a PMMA spacer hand-mixed with high-dose vancomycin and gentamicin was placed into the defect for a Masquelet-induced membrane technique. A longitudinally slit chest tube was used to protect the volar soft tissue structures until the cement had cured, and then removed (Fig. 3.8).

Pseudomonas aeruginosa grew in all the cultures of intraoperative samples. Six weeks later, the membrane was incised, the PMMA spacer removed, and the defect filled with non-vascularized cancellous bone autograft (Fig. 3.9). The external fixator was also removed, and an intramedullary rod (Acumed, Hillsboro, Oregon, USA) was implanted (Fig. 3.10). The bone graft consolidated well, and at 1-year follow-up, the patient was able to painlessly practice sports and physical activities such as road cycling and had no signs of infection recurrence (Fig. 3.11).

Case 3.2

A 26-year-old male with liver steatosis and obesity had suffered a motorcycle accident 2 years prior to presentation, with a closed femur and open tibia fractures treated at another institution. The femoral fracture had healed but had several draining sinuses (F1 R2 I1), and the tibia had an infected nonunion of the proximal diaphysis, also with draining sinuses at the fracture site and proximal and distal interlocking screw sites (F3 R2 I3) (Figs. 3.12 and 3.13). He also had a fixed equinus deformity and a shortening of the right lower limb of approximately 3 cm.

Both fractures were treated with complete removal of the implanted hardware, debridement, and reaming of the medullary canal. Additionally, the tibial nonunion was compressed, allowing for adequate soft tissue closure (conversion to I2), and stabilized with a circular hexapod frame (Taylor Spatial Frame, Smith and Nephew, London, United Kingdom) (Fig. 3.14). *Klebsiella pneumoniae*, *Enterobacter cloacae,* and *Escherichia coli* grew in cultures of intraoperative samples. After completion of antibiotic treatment, further hexapod circular frames were applied for lengthening of the distal tibia through a percutaneous corticotomy and correction of the

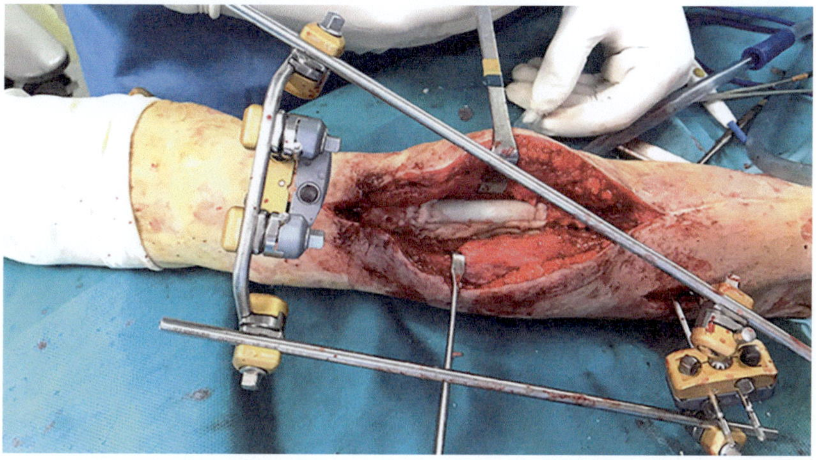

Fig. 3.8 Case 3.1, intraoperative photograph of the polymethylmethacrylate spacer filling the defect after debridement. The cement had been hand-mixed with high-dose vancomycin and gentamicin, and a longitudinally slit chest tube was used to protect the volar soft tissue structures until the cement had cured. The radius is stabilized with a Hoffmann II external fixator

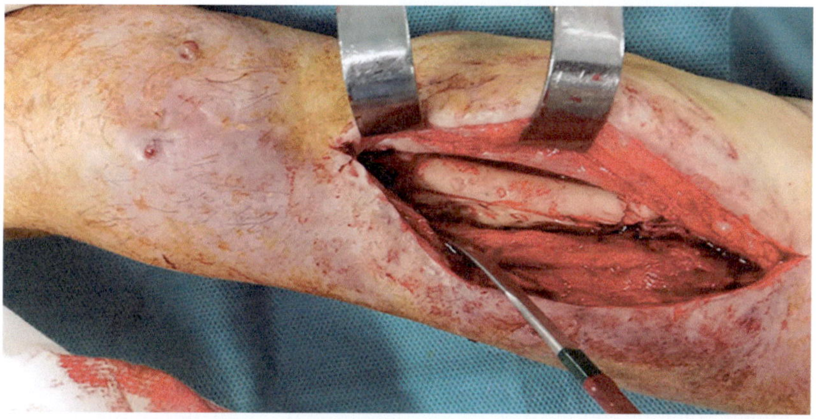

Fig. 3.9 Case 3.1, intraoperative photograph of the second stage of the induced membrane technique after Masquelet. The external fixator has been removed. The skin flap was elevated and the pseudo-capsule surrounding the spacer incised

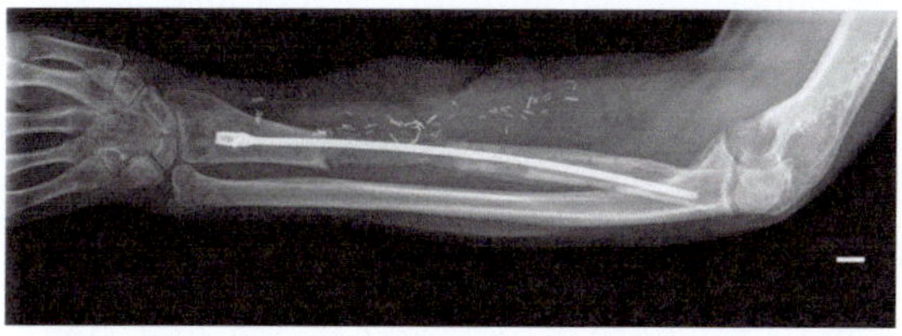

Fig. 3.10 Case 3.1, postoperative posterior-anterior conventional radiograph of the forearm after the second stage of surgery, showing internal fixation with an intramedullary nail of the radius (Acumed) and filling of the defect with non-vascularized cancellous autologous bone graft

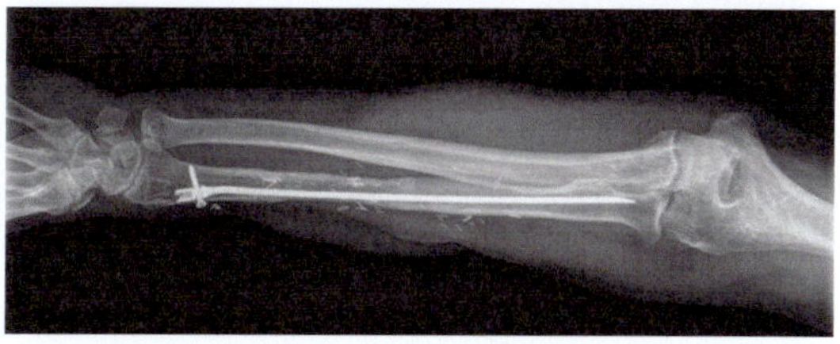

Fig. 3.11 Case 3.1, anterior-posterior conventional radiograph of the forearm 1 year after surgery. The graft has been incorporated well and the fracture has healed

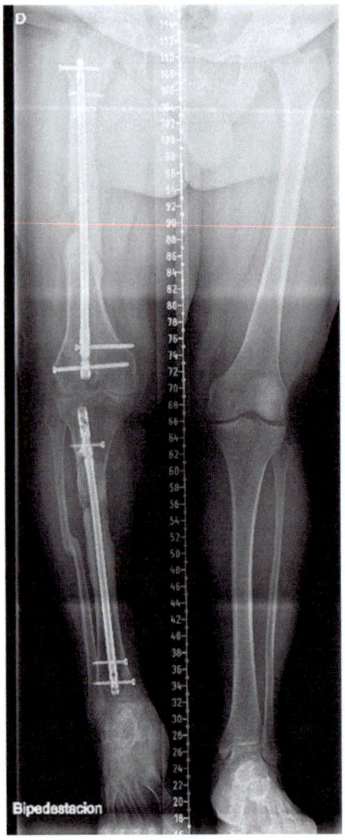

Fig. 3.12 Case 3.2, standing lower limb radiograph showing peri-implant radiolucency around the femoral nail and mobilization of the distal interlocking screws, as well as the tibial nonunion and limb-length discrepancy. The patient had a fixed equinus deformity

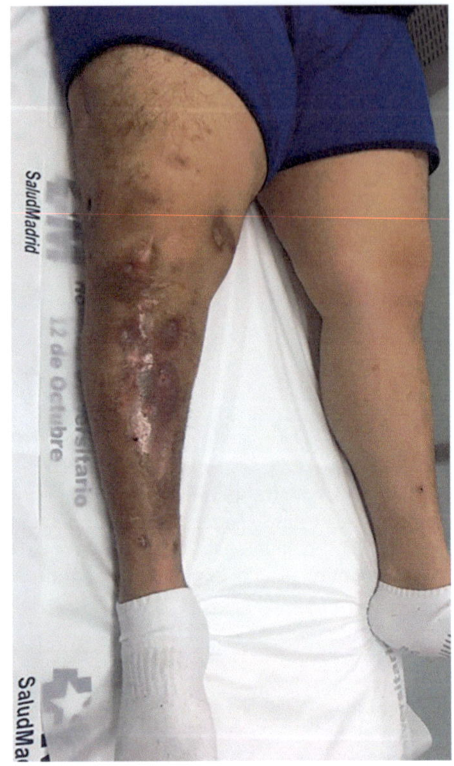

Fig. 3.13 Case 3.2, clinical image showing the post-traumatic scarring and fistulae, as well as the limb-length discrepancy

equinus deformity (Figs. 3.15 and 3.16). At the 2-year follow-up visit, the standing X-ray showed a united fracture and corrected limb length and alignment, and the patient had no signs of persistent infection (Fig. 3.17).

Case 3.3

A 37-year-old male suffered a segmental fracture of the left femur, injury of the superficial femoral artery and severe wounds on both lower limbs and his abdomen due to shrapnel in the context of an armed conflict (Fig. 3.18). The arterial injury was managed with a contralateral saphenous vein graft and the fracture fixed in a circular frame, but a persistent infection developed, the frame was removed, and serial debridements ensued, despite which the FRI persisted. Over a year (15 months) after the initial trauma, the patient was airlifted to Spain and transferred to our institution. At presentation, he had multiple fistulas following the trajectory of the superficial femoral artery ventrally, as well as the two nonunion sites. An abscess was visible adjacent to the superficial femoral artery (Figs. 3.19, see asterisk, and 3.20).

The patient rejected implantation of another circular frame for bone transport, so a two-stage strategy was devised. In the first stage, debridement including femoral canal reaming and removal of the infected superficial femoral artery graft was performed. The arterial defect was reconstructed using the ipsilateral saphenous vein, and a provisional lateral external fixator was implanted. Vancomycin-

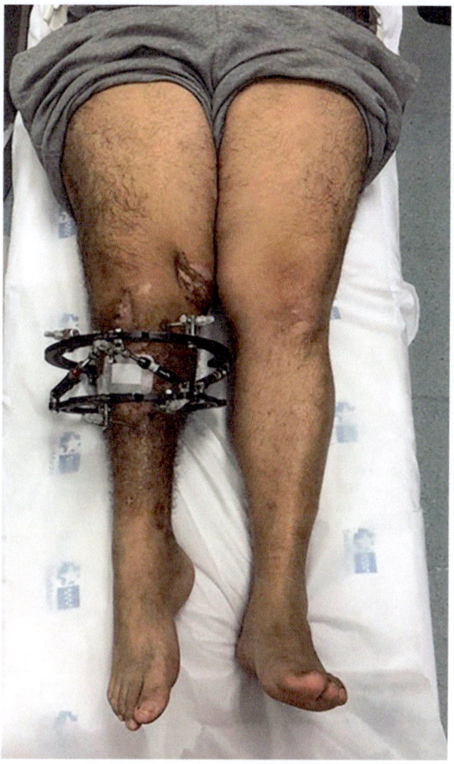

Fig. 3.14 Case 3.2, clinical image after the first stage of surgery. A hexapod circular frame has been applied to the proximal tibia, with acute shortening to address the skin defect after debridement. Note the increased limb-length discrepancy

and colistin-impregnated calcium sulfate beads were packed around the venous graft. Intraoperative cultures revealed multiresistant NDM-carbapenemase producing *Pseudomonas aeruginosa*. In the second stage 2 weeks later, the external fixator was exchanged for a 10-mm femoral nail (Metatan, Smith and Nephew, London, United Kingdom) coated with high-dose-vancomycin- and colistin-impregnated PMMA, fashioned intraoperatively using a 12-mm silicone tube as a mold (Figs. 3.21 and 3.22). The asterisk in Fig. 3.21 shows the silicone mold as it is incised longitudinally upon hardening of the cement. The final disposition is shown in Fig. 3.23, with the nail covered in a 1-mm layer of antibiotic-loaded bone cement and the calcium sulfate along the trajectory of the superficial femoral artery vascular graft (asterisks).

The patient was started on aztreonam, daptomycin, and colistin empirically. Following culture results, daptomycin was switched to ceftazidime/avibactam (aztreonam and colistin were maintained), for a total of 9 weeks of antibiotic treatment. At the 2-year follow-up, the patient did not have any signs or symptoms of infection.

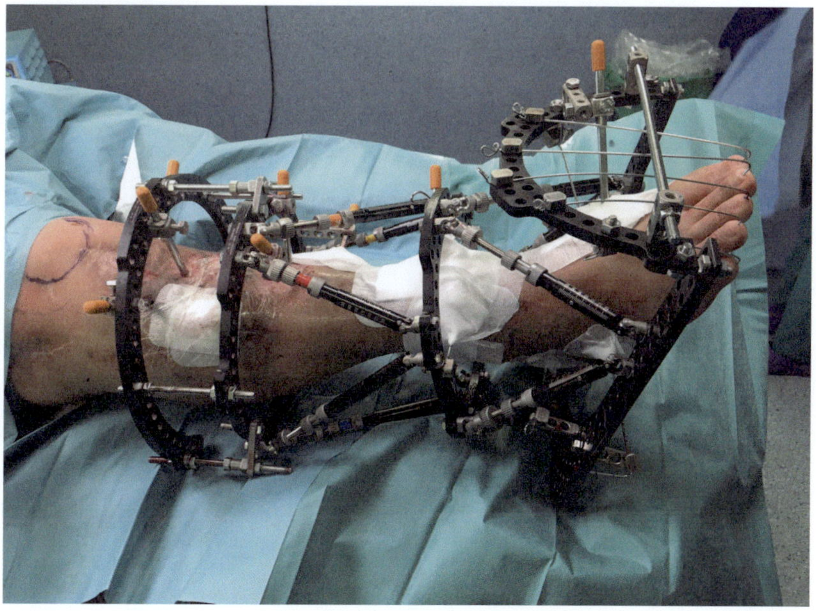

Fig. 3.15 Case 3.2, intraoperative photograph after the second surgery. The struts of the proximal tibial ring have been exchanged for a conventional Ilizarov system for added stability. The distal tibial hexapod frame is intended to provide lengthening through the distal tibial metaphysis, and another frame has been applied to the foot to correct the equinus deformity

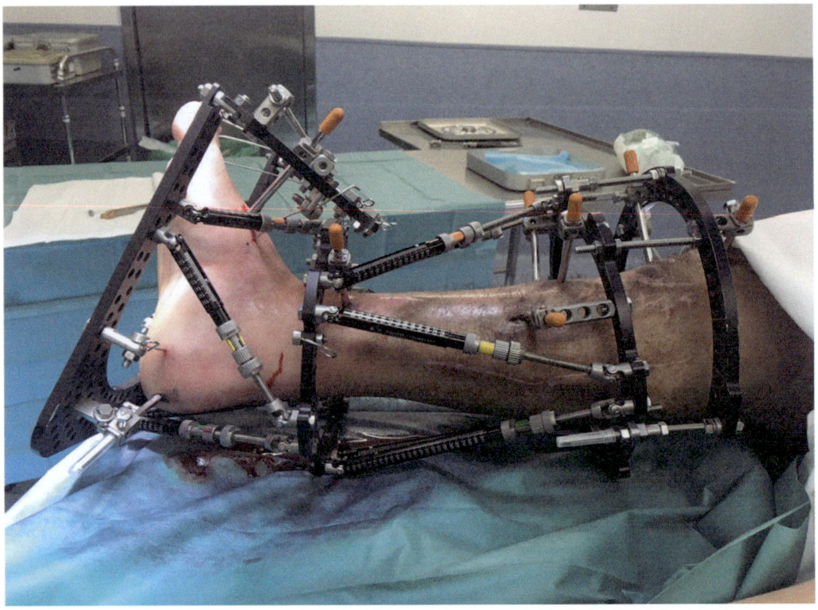

Fig. 3.16 Case 3.2, intraoperative photograph 3 months after Fig. 3.15, showing correction of the equinus deformity and lengthening of the distal tibia

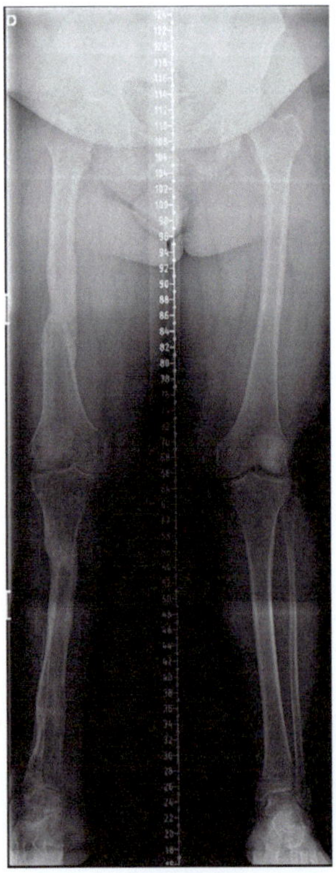

Fig. 3.17 Case 3.2, standing lower limb radiograph 2 years after commencing treatment, showing a united tibial fracture and corrected limb length and alignment

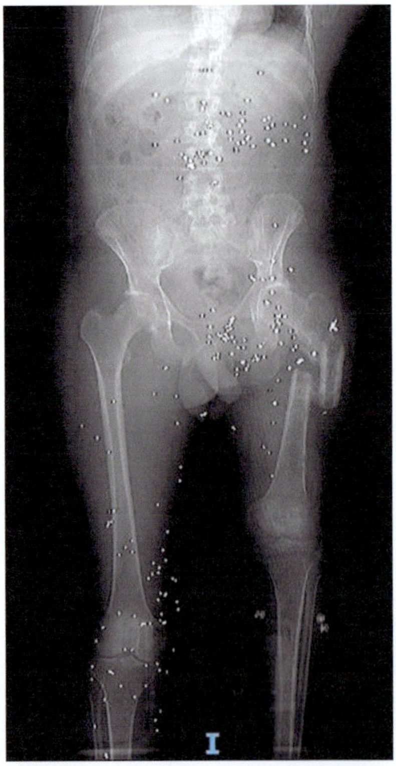

Fig. 3.18 Case 3.3, computed tomography scout view showing the segmental nonunion, as well as shrapnel in both lower limbs and the abdominopelvic region

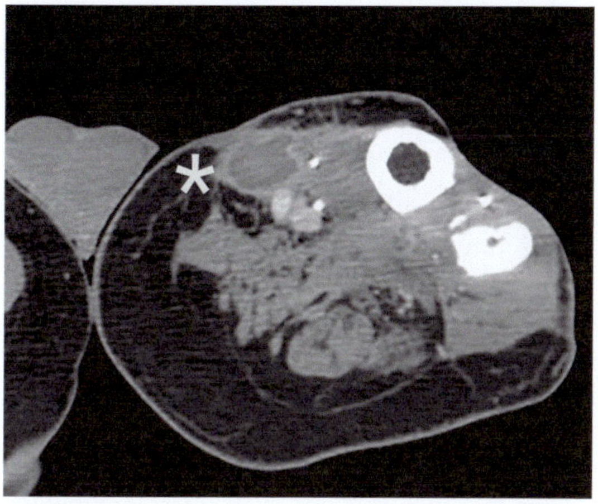

Fig. 3.19 Case 3.3, axial computed tomography image of the left proximal thigh. Note the abscess in the soft tissues adjacent to the superficial femoral artery with peripheral contrast enhancement (asterisk), the femoral fracture and shrapnel close to the bone and vascular structures

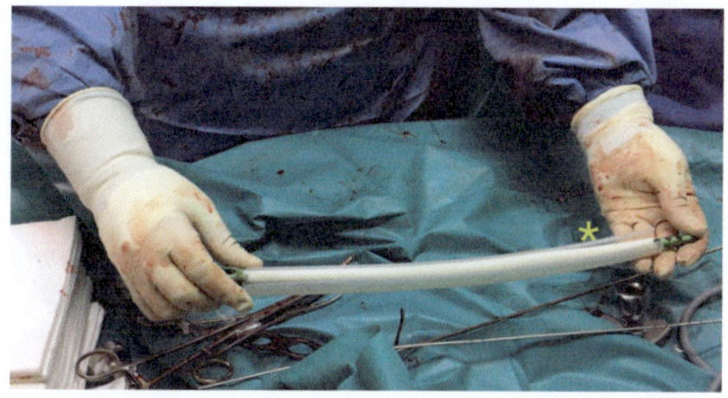

Fig. 3.21 Case 3.3, intraoperative photograph preparing an antibiotic-loaded cement-coated femoral nail. The 12-mm silicone sheath is longitudinally incised (asterisk), revealing the cement-covered nail inside

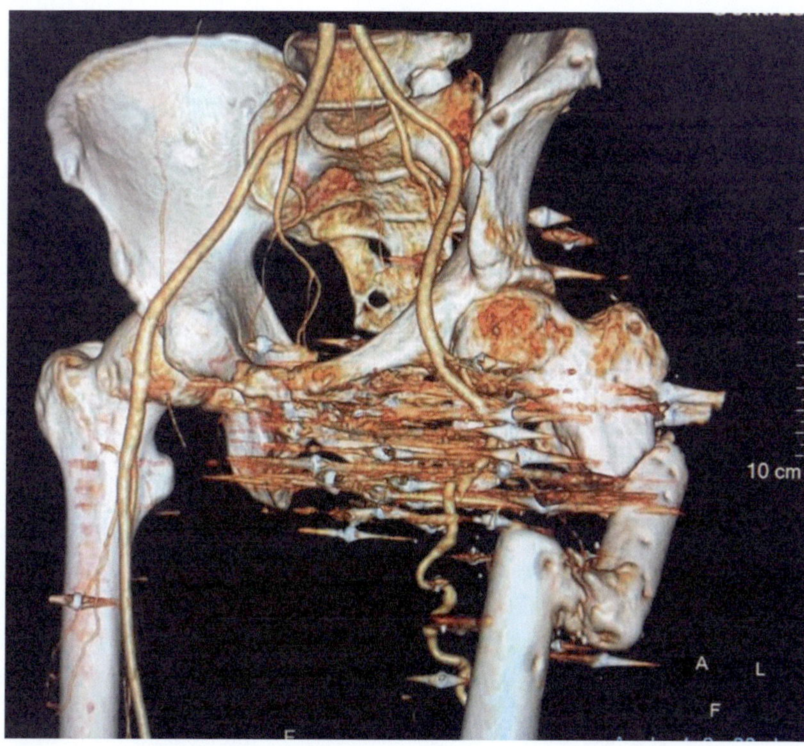

Fig. 3.20 Case 3.3, volumetric three-dimensional computed tomography reconstruction. The segmental nonunion can be observed, as well as multiple old pin tracts and abundant shrapnel in the anterior compartment

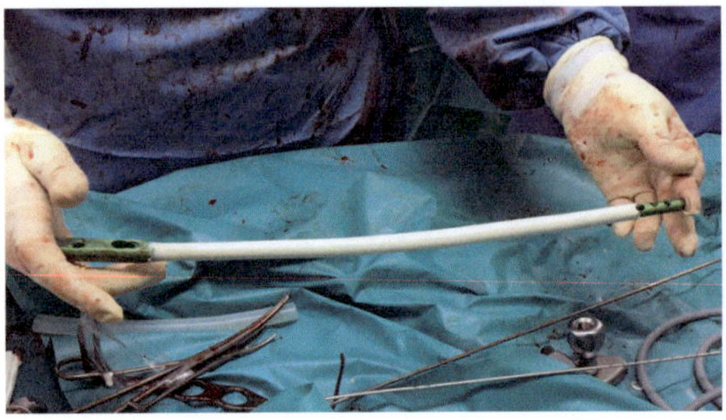

Fig. 3.22 Case 3.3, intraoperative photograph of the antibiotic-loaded cement coated femoral reconstruction nail. Note the locking screw holes remain free to allow for interlocking of the nail

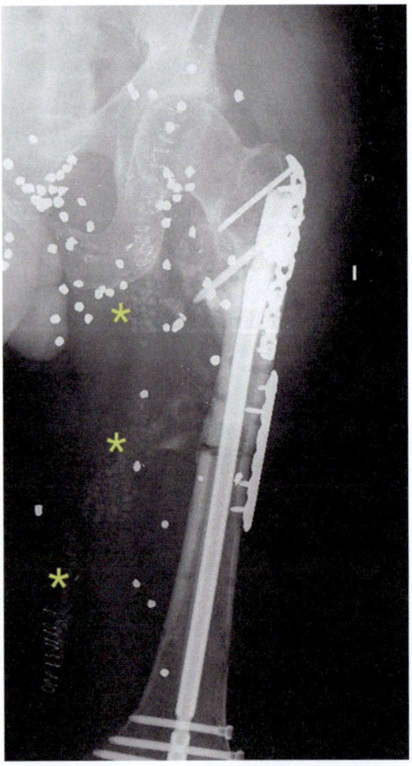

Fig. 3.23 Case 3.3, postoperative radiograph after internal fixation with the cement-coated nail. Resorbable calcium sulfate mixed with antibiotics can be observed along the path of the superficial femoral artery graft (asterisks)

Conclusions

Eradication of FRI requires a combination of surgery and targeted antimicrobial therapy. The cornerstones of treatment are (1) surgical debridement and irrigation, (2) tissue sampling, (3) fracture stabilization, (4) dead space management, (5) soft tissue coverage, and (6) appropriate antimicrobial therapy.

Surgery should be performed as soon as possible on an optimized patient (early elective surgery).

Multidisciplinary teams provide better outcomes. It is in the patient's best interest to involve them early.

One- and two-stage approaches have similar results in published studies. Criteria have been proposed to aid with this decision, but there is no evidence to support any of the proposed criteria. Factors that favor two stages include poor infection control, concerns regarding the viability of the remaining bone, a comorbid host, and the presence of difficult-to-treat pathogens. In the published literature, a two-stage approach is more common, but single-stage approaches are increasing.

Debridement is crucial in the management of FRI and the best predictor of success. It is critical that its quality is not compromised due to concerns regarding the reconstruction of the resulting bone and/or soft tissue defect. The available evidence does not support the use of one debridement method over another, or a specific margin, the only requirement is that only healthy viable tissue is kept.

After debridement, the operative field should be irrigated with low-pressure saline until the wound is macroscopically clean.

Stability is indispensable for a biomechanical environment that favors both bone healing and eradication of infection.

The strategy for dead space management is interrelated with management of stability and soft tissue coverage. No bone void filler has demonstrated superiority over the rest. The most often used filler is antibiotic-impregnated PMMA, but its non-resorbability and unfavorable antimicrobial elution kinetics increase the risk of antibiotic resistance. The main alternative is ceramics (calcium sulfates and phosphates) and bioactive glass, both of which are associated with prolonged wound drainage.

Over one third of FRIs cannot be closed directly and require soft tissue coverage techniques. NPWT is associated with worse outcomes and should be used for as few days as possible.

Antimicrobial therapy includes local antimicrobials, which can reach concentrations much higher than the minimum inhibitory concentration at the site of infection, and systemic antibiotic therapy. Microbiological identification is the cornerstone of tailored treatment, so antibiotic therapy should be avoided prior to sampling, or, at least, withheld for the 2 weeks before the surgery.

References

1. Depypere M, Morgenstern M, Kuehl R, Senneville E, Moriarty TF, Obremskey WT, Zimmerli W, Trampuz A, Lagrou K, Metsemakers W-J. Pathogenesis and management of fracture-related infection. Clin Microbiol Infect. 2020;26:572–8.
2. Metsemakers WJ, Kuehl R, Moriarty TF, Richards RG, Verhofstad MHJ, Borens O, Kates S, Morgenstern M. Infection after fracture fixation: current surgical and microbiological concepts. Injury. 2018;49:511–22.
3. Metsemakers WJ, Morgenstern M, McNally MA, et al. Fracture-related infection: a consensus on definition from an international expert group. Injury. 2018;49:505–10.
4. Rupp M, Walter N, Popp D, et al. Multidisciplinary treatment of fracture-related infection has a positive impact on clinical outcome-a retrospective case control study at a tertiary referral center. Antibiotics (Basel). 2023;12:230.
5. Alt V, McNally M, Wouthuyzen-Bakker M, Metsemakers W-J, Marais L, Zalavras C, Morgenstern M. The FRI classification – a new classification of fracture-related infections. Injury. 2024;55:111831.
6. Morgenstern M, Clauss M, Sendi P, Cadosch D, Osinga R, Metsemakers W-J. Treatment of fracture-related infections. In: Pape H-C, Borrelli Jr J, Moore EE, Pfeifer R, Stahel PF, editors. Textbook of polytrauma management: a multidisciplinary approach. Cham: Springer; 2022. p. 573–81.
7. Barla JD. Fracture-related infections. In: Slullitel P, Rossi L, Camino-Willhuber G, editors. Orthopaedics and trauma: current concepts and best practices. Cham: Springer; 2024. p. 805–10.
8. Giordano V, Giannoudis PV. Biofilm formation, antibiotic resistance, and infection (BARI): the triangle of death. J Clin Med. 2024;13:5779.
9. Marais LC, Zalavras CG, Moriarty FT, Kühl R, Metsemakers W-J, Morgenstern M. The surgical management of fracture-related infection. Surgical strategy selection and the need for early surgical intervention. J Orthop. 2024;50:36–41.
10. Morgenstern M, Kuehl R, Zalavras CG, McNally M, Zimmerli W, Burch MA, Vandendriessche T, Obremskey WT, Verhofstad MHJ, Metsemakers WJ. The influence of duration of infection on outcome of debridement and implant retention in fracture-related infection. Bone Joint J. 2021;103-B:213–21.
11. Trampuz A, Zimmerli W. Diagnosis and treatment of infections associated with fracture-fixation devices. Injury. 2006;37(Suppl 2):S59–66.
12. Lu V, Zhang J, Patel R, Zhou AK, Thahir A, Krkovic M. Fracture related infections and their risk factors for treatment failure-a major trauma centre perspective. Diagnostics (Basel). 2022;12:1289.
13. Rightmire E, Zurakowski D, Vrahas M. Acute infections after fracture repair: management with hardware in place. Clin Orthop Relat Res. 2008;466:466.
14. Metsemakers W-J, Morgenstern M, Senneville E, et al. General treatment principles for fracture-related infection: recommendations from an international expert group. Arch Orthop Trauma Surg. 2020;140:1013–27.
15. Bezstarosti H, Van Lieshout EMM, Voskamp LW, Kortram K, Obremskey W, McNally MA, Metsemakers WJ, Verhofstad MHJ. Insights into treatment and outcome of fracture-related infection: a systematic literature review. Arch Orthop Trauma Surg. 2019;139:61–72.
16. Nasser AAH, Fenton P, Bose D. Single stage versus two-stage orthoplastic management of bone infection. Injury. 2022;53:984–91.
17. Iliadis AD, Shivji F, Debuka E, Trompeter A, Narayan B, Heidari N. Current concepts in the prevention, diagnosis and treatment of fracture-related infection (FRI). Eur J Orthop Surg Traumatol. 2021;31:957–66.
18. Struijs PAA, Poolman RW, Bhandari M. Infected nonunion of the long bones. J Orthop Trauma. 2007;21:507–11.
19. McNally MA, Ferguson JY, Scarborough M, Ramsden A, Stubbs DA, Atkins BL. Mid- to long-term results of single-stage surgery for patients with chronic osteomyelitis using a bioabsorbable gentamicin-loaded ceramic carrier. Bone Joint J. 2022;104-B:1095–100.
20. Nauth A, Schemitsch E, Norris B, Nollin Z, Watson JT. Critical-size bone defects: is there a consen-

sus for diagnosis and treatment? J Orthop Trauma. 2018;32(Suppl 1):S7–S11.
21. Hohmann E, Glatt V, Tetsworth K. What is the optimal timing for bone grafting during staged management of infected non-unions of the tibia? A systematic review and best evidence synthesis. Injury. 2020;51:2793–803.
22. Winkler T, Stuhlert MGW, Lieb E, Müller M, von Roth P, Preininger B, Trampuz A, Perka CF. Outcome of short versus long interval in two-stage exchange for periprosthetic joint infection: a prospective cohort study. Arch Orthop Trauma Surg. 2019;139:295–303.
23. Tu Y-K, Yen C-Y. Role of vascularized bone grafts in lower extremity osteomyelitis. Orthop Clin North Am. 2007;38:37–49. vi
24. Piccato A, Crosio A, Antonini A, Battiston B, Titolo P, Tos P, Ciclamini D. Single-stage versus two-stage bone flap reconstruction in chronic osteomyelitis: multicenter outcomes comparison. Microsurgery. 2024;44:e31139.
25. Mifsud M, Ferguson JY, Stubbs DA, Ramsden AJ, McNally MA. Simultaneous debridement, Ilizarov reconstruction and free muscle flaps in the management of complex tibial infection. J Bone Jt Infect. 2020;6:63–72.
26. Conterno LO, Turchi MD. Antibiotics for treating chronic osteomyelitis in adults. Cochrane Database Syst Rev. 2013;2013:CD004439.
27. Mouzopoulos G, Kanakaris NK, Kontakis G, Obakponovwe O, Townsend R, Giannoudis PV. Management of bone infections in adults: the surgeon's and microbiologist's perspectives. Injury. 2011;42(Suppl 5):S18–23.
28. He S-Y, Yu B, Jiang N. Current concepts of fracture-related infection. Int J Clin Pract. 2023;2023:4839701.
29. Hellebrekers P, Rentenaar RJ, McNally MA, Hietbrink F, Houwert RM, Leenen LPH, Govaert GAM. Getting it right first time: the importance of a structured tissue sampling protocol for diagnosing fracture-related infections. Injury. 2019;50:1649–55.
30. Onsea J, Pallay J, Depypere M, et al. Intramedullary tissue cultures from the reamer-irrigator-aspirator system for diagnosing fracture-related infection. J Orthop Res. 2021;39:281–90.
31. FLOW Investigators, Bhandari M, Jeray KJ, et al. A trial of wound irrigation in the initial management of open fracture wounds. N Engl J Med. 2015;373:2629–41.
32. Gupta R, Sharma AR, Singhal A, Shail S, Masih GD. Concepts in wound irrigation of open fractures: where we came from, and where are we now? J Clin Orthop Trauma. 2021;23:101638.
33. Foster AL, Moriarty TF, Zalavras C, et al. The influence of biomechanical stability on bone healing and fracture-related infection: the legacy of Stephan Perren. Injury. 2021;52:43–52.
34. Lawrenz JM, Frangiamore SJ, Rane AA, Cantrell WA, Vallier HA. Treatment approach for infection of healed fractures after internal fixation. J Orthop Trauma. 2017;31:e358–63.
35. Berkes M, Obremskey WT, Scannell B, Ellington JK, Hymes RA, Bosse M, Southeast Fracture Consortium. Maintenance of hardware after early postoperative infection following fracture internal fixation. J Bone Joint Surg Am. 2010;92:823–8.
36. Oliveira PR, Leonhardt MC, Panico CT, Silva JB, Carvalho VC, Kojima KE, Silva JS, Lima ALL. Infection after intramedullary nailing of femoral and tibial diaphyseal fractures. Injury. 2023;54(Suppl 6):110821.
37. Buijs MAS, van den Kieboom J, Sliepen J, Wever KLH, van Breugel JM, Hietbrink F, Ijpma FFA, Govaert GAM. Outcome and risk factors for recurrence of early onset fracture-related infections treated with debridement, antibiotics and implant retention: results of a large retrospective multicentre cohort study. Injury. 2022;53:3930–7.
38. Makridis KG, Tosounidis T, Giannoudis PV. Management of infection after intramedullary nailing of long bone fractures: treatment protocols and outcomes. Open Orthop J. 2013;7:219–26.
39. Tsang S-TJ, van Rensburg AJ, Ferreira N. Is there a role for suppression of infection in managing fracture-related infection following intra-medullary nailing? Injury. 2024;55:111602.
40. del Piñal F, Innocenti M. Evolving concepts in the management of the bone gap in the upper limb. Long and small defects. J Plast Reconstr Aesthet Surg. 2007;60:776–92.
41. Bakshi AS, Singh A, Kaur H, Kaur G, Singh J. A comparative study of treatment with external fixator versus antibiotic coated intramedullary nail in infected non-union long bones. Cureus. 2022;14:e29659.
42. McNally M, Ferguson J, Mifsud M, Stubbs D. Internal fixation and local antibiotics for infected nonunions: technique and outcome at over one year. Orthop Proc. 2018;100-B:13. https://doi.org/10.1302/1358-992X.2018.8.013.
43. Chan JKK, Ferguson JY, Scarborough M, McNally MA, Ramsden AJ. Management of post-traumatic osteomyelitis in the lower limb: current state of the art. Indian J Plast Surg. 2019;52:62–72.
44. Pincher B, Fenton C, Jeyapalan R, Barlow G, Sharma HK. A systematic review of the single-stage treatment of chronic osteomyelitis. J Orthop Surg Res. 2019;14:393.
45. Sliepen J, Corrigan RA, Dudareva M, Wouthuyzen-Bakker M, Rentenaar RJ, Atkins BL, Govaert GAM, McNally MA, Ijpma FFA. Does the use of local antibiotics affect clinical outcome of patients with fracture-related infection? Antibiotics (Basel). 2022;11:1330.
46. Bezstarosti H, Metsemakers WJ, van Lieshout EMM, Voskamp LW, Kortram K, McNally MA, Marais LC, Verhofstad MHJ. Management of critical-sized bone defects in the treatment of fracture-related infection: a systematic review and pooled analysis. Arch Orthop Trauma Surg. 2021;141:1215–30.
47. Epstein G, Ferreira N. Dead space management strategies in the treatment of chronic osteomyelitis: a

retrospective review. Eur J Orthop Surg Traumatol. 2023;33:565–70.
48. Metsemakers W-J, Fragomen AT, Moriarty TF, Morgenstern M, Egol KA, Zalavras C, Obremskey WT, Raschke M, McNally MA, Fracture-Related Infection (FRI) Consensus Group. Evidence-based recommendations for local antimicrobial strategies and dead space management in fracture-related infection. J Orthop Trauma. 2020;34:18–29.
49. Chen C-E, Ko J-Y, Pan C-C. Results of vancomycin-impregnated cancellous bone grafting for infected tibial nonunion. Arch Orthop Trauma Surg. 2005;125:369–75.
50. Winkler H, Kaudela K, Stoiber A, Menschik F. Bone grafts impregnated with antibiotics as a tool for treating infected implants in orthopedic surgery – one stage revision results. Cell Tissue Bank. 2006;7:319–23.
51. Neut D, van de Belt H, van Horn JR, van der Mei HC, Busscher HJ. Residual gentamicin-release from antibiotic-loaded polymethylmethacrylate beads after 5 years of implantation. Biomaterials. 2003;24:1829–31.
52. Ganta A, Merrell LA, Adams J, Konda SR, Egol KA. Retention of antibiotic cement delivery implants in orthopedic infection associated with united fractures does not increase recurrence risk. J Orthop Trauma. 2024;38:190–5.
53. Neut D, van de Belt H, Stokroos I, van Horn JR, van der Mei HC, Busscher HJ. Biomaterial-associated infection of gentamicin-loaded PMMA beads in orthopaedic revision surgery. J Antimicrob Chemother. 2001;47:885–91.
54. Young BC, Dudareva M, Vicentine MP, Hotchen AJ, Ferguson J, McNally M. Microbial persistence, replacement and local antimicrobial therapy in recurrent bone and joint infection. Antibiotics (Basel). 2023;12:708.
55. Jacob CC, Daw JH, Santiago-Torres J. The efficacy of antibiotic-impregnated calcium sulfate (AICS) in the treatment of infected non-union and fracture-related infection: a systematic review. J Bone Jt Infect. 2023;8:91–7.
56. Du B, Su Y, Li D, Ji S, Lu Y, Xu Y, Yang Y, Zhang K, Li Z, Ma T. Analysis of risk factors for serous exudation of biodegradable material calcium sulfate in the treatment of fracture-related infections. Front Bioeng Biotechnol. 2023;11:1189085.
57. Shi X, Wu Y, Ni H, Li M, Zhang C, Qi B, Wei M, Wang T, Xu Y. Antibiotic-loaded calcium sulfate in clinical treatment of chronic osteomyelitis: a systematic review and meta-analysis. J Orthop Surg Res. 2022;17:104.
58. Lindfors N, Geurts J, Drago L, et al. Antibacterial bioactive glass, S53P4, for chronic bone infections – a multinational study. Adv Exp Med Biol. 2017;971:81–92.
59. Malat TA, Glombitza M, Dahmen J, Hax P-M, Steinhausen E. The use of bioactive glass S53P4 as bone graft substitute in the treatment of chronic osteomyelitis and infected non-unions - a retrospective study of 50 patients. Z Orthop Unfall. 2018;156:152–9.
60. Prada C, Bengoa F, Bhandari M. The management of fracture related infections: what practices can be supported by high-level evidence? J Orthop Surg (Hong Kong). 2022;30:10225536221119580.
61. Eikani C, Hoyt A, Cho E, Levack AE. The state of local antibiotic use in orthopedic trauma. Orthop Clin North Am. 2024;55:207–16.
62. Conway JD, Elhessy AH, Galiboglu S, Patel N, Gesheff MG. Efficacy of infection eradication in antibiotic cement-coated intramedullary nails for fracture-related infections, nonunions, and fusions. Antibiotics (Basel). 2022;11:709.
63. Elhessy AH, Rivera JC, Shu HT, Andrews T-J, Herzenberg JE, Conway JD. Intramedullary canal injection of vancomycin- and tobramycin-loaded calcium sulfate: a novel technique for the treatment of chronic intramedullary osteomyelitis. Strategies Trauma Limb Reconstr. 2022;17:123–30.
64. De Meo D, Martini P, Pennarola MF, Guarascio G, Rivano Capparuccia M, Iaiani G, Candela V, Gumina S, Villani C. Hydrogel coating versus calcium sulphate beads as a local antibiotic carrier for debridement procedures in acute periprosthetic joint infection: a preliminary study. Gels. 2023;9:758.
65. Savvidou OD, Kaspiris A, Trikoupis I, Kakouratos G, Goumenos S, Melissaridou D, Papagelopoulos PJ. Efficacy of antimicrobial coated orthopaedic implants on the prevention of periprosthetic infections: a systematic review and meta-analysis. J Bone Jt Infect. 2020;5:212–22.
66. Alt V. Antimicrobial coated implants in trauma and orthopaedics-A clinical review and risk-benefit analysis. Injury. 2017;48:599–607.
67. Müller SLC, Morgenstern M, Kuehl R, Muri T, Kalbermatten DF, Clauss M, Schaefer DJ, Sendi P, Osinga R. Soft-tissue reconstruction in lower-leg fracture-related infections: an orthoplastic outcome and risk factor analysis. Injury. 2021;52:3489–97.
68. Alt V, Rupp M, Kerschbaum M, Prantl L, Geis S. Treatment strategies for fracture-related infections with concurrent soft tissue damage. Unfallchirurgie (Heidelb). 2024;127:103–9.
69. Marais LC, Hungerer S, Eckardt H, Zalavras C, Obremskey WT, Ramsden A, McNally MA, Morgenstern M, Metsemakers W-J, Group the FC. Key aspects of soft tissue management in fracture-related infection: recommendations from an international expert group. Arch Orthop Trauma Surg. 2023;144:259.
70. Sweere V, Sliepen J, Haidari S, Depypere M, Mertens M, Ijpma F, Metsemakers W-J, Govaert G. Use of negative pressure wound therapy in patients with fracture-related infection more than doubles the risk of recurrence. Injury. 2022;53:3938–44.
71. Hellebrekers P, Leenen LPH, Hoekstra M, Hietbrink F. Effect of a standardized treatment regime for infection after osteosynthesis. J Orthop Surg Res. 2017;12:41.

72. McNally M, Corrigan R, Sliepen J, Dudareva M, Rentenaar R, Ijpma F, Atkins BL, Wouthuyzen-Bakker M, Govaert G. What factors affect outcome in the treatment of fracture-related infection? Antibiotics (Basel). 2022;11:946.
73. Baertl S, Walter N, Engelstaedter U, Ehrenschwender M, Hitzenbichler F, Alt V, Rupp M. What is the most effective empirical antibiotic treatment for early, delayed, and late fracture-related infections? Antibiotics (Basel). 2022;11:287.
74. Sendi P, Zimmerli W. Antimicrobial treatment concepts for orthopaedic device-related infection. Clin Microbiol Infect. 2012;18:1176–84.
75. Depypere M, Kuehl R, Metsemakers W-J, Senneville E, McNally MA, Obremskey WT, Zimmerli W, Atkins BL, Trampuz A, Fracture-Related Infection (FRI) Consensus Group. Recommendations for systemic antimicrobial therapy in fracture-related infection: a consensus from an international expert group. J Orthop Trauma. 2020;34:30–41.
76. Depypere M, Sliepen J, Onsea J, Debaveye Y, Govaert GAM, Ijpma FFA, Zimmerli W, Metsemakers W-J. The microbiological etiology of fracture-related infection. Front Cell Infect Microbiol. 2022;12:934485.
77. Li H-K, Rombach I, Zambellas R, et al. Oral versus intravenous antibiotics for bone and joint infection. N Engl J Med. 2019;380:425–36.
78. Seidelman J, Ritter AS, Poehlein E, et al. Multisite study of the management of musculoskeletal infection after trauma: the MMUSKIT study. Open Forum Infect Dis. 2024;11:ofae262.
79. Garrigós C, Rosso-Fernández CM, Borreguero I, Rodríguez P, García-Albea R, Bravo-Ferrer JM, Rodríguez-Baño J, Del Toro MD, DURATIOM team. Efficacy and safety of different antimicrobial DURATions for the treatment of infections associated with Osteosynthesis material implanted after long bone fractures (DURATIOM): protocol for a randomized, pragmatic trial. PLoS One. 2023;18:e0286094.
80. Metsemakers W-J, Fragomen AT, Moriarty TF, Morgenstern M, Egol KA, Zalavras C, Obremskey WT, Raschke M, McNally MA. Evidence-based recommendations for local antimicrobial strategies and dead space management in fracture-related infection. J Orthop Trauma. 2020;34:18–29.
81. Walter N, Bärtl S, Alt V, Rupp M. Recent advancements and future directions in fracture related infections: a scoping review. Injury. 2024;55:111902.
82. Walter N, Mirzaei M, Deng L, Willy C, Alt V, Rupp M. The potential of bacteriophage therapy as an alternative treatment approach for antibiotic-resistant infections. Med Princ Pract. 2024;33:1–9.
83. Ferry T, Onsea J, Roussel-Gaillard T, Batailler C, Moriarty TF, Metsemakers W-J. Bacteriophage therapy in musculoskeletal infections: from basic science to clinical application. EFORT Open Rev. 2024;9:339–48.
84. Onsea J, Uyttebroek S, Chen B, et al. Bacteriophage therapy for difficult-to-treat infections: the implementation of a multidisciplinary phage task force (The PHAGEFORCE study protocol). Viruses. 2021;13:1543.

4 Fracture-Related Infection in Healed Fractures (F1), Fractures with Good Bone Healing Potential (F2), and Fractures with Poor Bone Healing Potential (F3)

Jose Baeza-Oliete, Amparo Ortega-Yago, and Nieves Vanaclocha

Introduction

Fracture-related infection (FRI) is one of the most devastating complications that can happen after a fracture, significantly hindering the healing process and the patient's recovery. It is infrequent after low-energy closed fractures (1%), but can arise in as many as 30% of complex open fractures [1, 2].

For successful management, the general principles discussed in Chaps. 3 and 10 should be observed. As pointed out therein, surgical treatment is based on sampling, debridement, and irrigation, as well as management of stability, dead space, and soft tissues, in combination with postoperative targeted antibiotic therapy [2, 3]. The cornerstone is debridement, which includes resecting all the necrotic and infected tissue (bone and soft tissues) and extraction of foreign bodies (e.g., broken screws, sutures). The quality of the debridement is the best predictor of outcome and should not be limited by concerns regarding the consequent bone and/or soft tissue defects [2, 4]. This is one of the reasons why multidisciplinary approaches, including consultants of orthopedic surgery, plastic surgery, infectious diseases, radiology, and others, result in better outcomes [3, 5, 6]. Specifically, early orthoplastic approaches result in less amputations and less revision surgeries [7, 8].

In this chapter, we will focus on the surgical management of FRI in healed fractures and in unhealed fractures with good and poor bone healing potential (F1–3 in the FRI classification). Critical bone defects and unreconstructible bone defects are addressed in Chaps. 5, 7, and 8, to which the reader is referred for further information on FRI management in these scenarios.

Note that preoperative patient optimization (smoking cessation, glycemic control, adequate nutrition, etc.) as well as optimal soft tissue management are essential to achieve both infection eradication and bone healing [7, 9, 10]. They are addressed in Chaps. 3 and 10, to which the reader is referred for further information on them.

J. Baeza-Oliete (✉) · A. Ortega-Yago
Department of Traumatology and Orthopedics, University and Polytechnic Hospital La Fe, Valencia, Spain

N. Vanaclocha
Orthoplastics Unit and Department of Plastic and Reconstructive Surgery, University and Polytechnic Hospital La Fe, Valencia, Spain

N. Vanaclocha (ed.), *Treatment of Fracture-Related Infection*,
https://doi.org/10.1007/978-3-031-92452-1_4

Planning Treatment in FRI

To plan treatment in FRI, answer the following questions:

- Is the fracture consolidated? Is there a stable callus formation?
- How is the fixation? Is it stable, and is the fracture reduction satisfactory?
- Which bone is affected? Is the fracture diaphyseal, metaphyseal or epiphyseal?
- Are there any implants inside, and what kind (plate, nail, external fixation)?
- Are there any other foreign bodies (e.g. bone graft, cement) to be removed?
- What is the status of the soft tissues surrounding the fracture?
- Are there any related systemic host factors that might affect the outcome?
- Have cultures been obtained previously? Were there any difficult-to-treat microorganisms identified by previous cultures?

Fracture-Related Infection in Healed Fractures (F1)

F1 cases include those in which the FRI was diagnosed on a consolidated fracture, those with a previously known FRI in which the fracture healed during antibiotic suppression, and those with recurring FRI on a healed fracture after implant removal [11].

If there are implants present, they can be safely removed without loss of stability (and thus, loss of limb function) [11, 12]. This usually suffices for infection eradication [13].

Both if there were implants that have been removed or if there were no implants to remove, assess dead space after debridement. Effective dead space management (e.g., by filling medullary cavities with antibiotic-loaded resorbable carriers) is essential to prevent fluid accumulation and minimize the risk of infection recurrence. Dead space management often goes hand in hand with achieving adequate soft tissue coverage, which, as previously pointed out, is crucial to preventing infection recurrence [1, 11]. The reader is referred to Chaps. 3 and 9 for more information on management of dead space and soft tissues.

The degree of bone healing can be difficult to assess preoperatively, largely due to artifacts on the computed tomography (CT) images caused by the metal hardware. Often, there will be preoperative doubts whether the bone has united enough for stability to be kept after hardware removal. Even if imaging tests suggest consolidation of three out of four cortices, sometimes intraoperative evaluation reveals instability after hardware removal and debridement. It is thus wise to have a plan in place for each scenario (bone stability versus instability after implant removal and debridement).

Fracture-Related Infection in Fractures with Good Bone Healing Potential (F2)

When Can a Fracture Be Considered to Have Good Healing Potential?

This is the most crucial point in treating FRI in unhealed fractures [11]. An infected fracture can be considered to have good healing potential when conditions are optimal for bone union [3, 11]:

- Favorable biology (viable bone ends) and biomechanics (stable osteosynthetic construct and satisfactory reduction, i.e., good alignment and bone contact). This corresponds to F2 in the FRI Classification.
- High likelihood of bacterial load reduction after debridement to levels that will not interfere with fracture healing (i.e., adequate debridement is deemed possible).
- A healthy soft tissue envelope and reliable wound coverage are either present or will be achieved surgically early (I1–4).

Most often, it will only be possible to assess these conditions intraoperatively.

When Is Implant Retention Advisable?

Evidence to guide implant retention or removal is weak [1, 14]. Regardless of the approach, fracture stability must be warranted for both bone healing and adequate infection control [3, 15].

Debridement, antibiotics, and implant retention (DAIR) approaches have lower success rates than implant exchange, but can achieve FRI resolution in >70% of well-selected patients [13, 16]. DAIR success depends strongly on the quality of the debridement and the presence of the above-mentioned optimal conditions for bone healing [1, 11]. Note that a healthy soft tissue envelope is indispensable for implant retention success, due to its contribution to both bone healing and fighting infection. Thus, in I3–4 cases, early (ideally simultaneous) flap coverage must be performed. The consequence of this is that if the intention is for the implant to be retained, it is wise to arrange for a surgeon capable of performing flaps to be present in the surgery in anticipation of a flap being potentially needed, as opposed to involving said surgeon(s) postoperatively only once the team realizes that there is a post-debridement soft tissue defect to be managed, which inevitably delays coverage.

It is also worth highlighting that retention of intramedullary nails has been associated with a higher rate of treatment failure [17]. This is probably because if an intramedullary nail is retained, most of its large surface area will remain inaccessible in the intramedullary canal and so effective debridement is unlikely to be possible. As a result, *nail exchange is strongly recommended* even when conditions are otherwise optimal for bone union [1, 2].

Attention must be drawn to the fact that smokers have found to have a risk of DAIR failure over 3.5 times higher in comparison with nonsmokers [18].

Also of note, even when all conditions are optimal, DAIR has a relatively high rate of infection recurrence (20–30%) [13, 16]. This is because metabolically inactive sessile bacteria in residual biofilm will remain adhered to implants and, once antibiotic therapy is stopped, will transition into metabolically active phenotypes to originate a recurrence. It is challenging to predict which of these theoretically optimal patients will fail based on the available evidence. Longer duration of infection has been associated with a higher failure rate in DAIR cases [19, 20]. However, though a weeks-based time criterion has traditionally been used to help determine whether an implant is best retained or not, specific time cut-offs are arbitrary, and the current evidence suggests that time is unrelated to postoperative outcome [13, 20]. Consequently, this criterion should not be used to decide on a treatment strategy. Infection by a difficult-to-treat microbe was also considered to favor implant exchange or removal, but the causative pathogen is most often known *postoperatively*, so generally the decision regarding implant retention must be taken without that piece of information [11, 14].

To sum up, the patients most benefited by a DAIR approach are F2 cases in whom adequate debridement is possible (this excludes intramedullary nails), a healthy soft tissue envelope is either present or will be achieved with early surgery (it will contribute to both bone healing and fighting infection), and the host is an R1 in the FRI Classification (absence of relevant systemic factors that negatively impact healing) (Table 4.1). In such cases, the risks associated with implant exchange (loss of reduction, further bone loss) are likely to outweigh its benefits.

Many teams remove the internal fixation implants as soon as the fracture has consolidated for the theoretical reduction in the risk of infection recurrence that it entails. However, there is currently insufficient evidence to support this practice routinely [21].

Implant Exchange

In F2 cases where adequate debridement is not possible if the implant is retained (e.g., intramedullary nails), or there are host factors or comorbidities that negatively impact healing, implant exchange is the wiser option. There are two main options: exchange for another nail or plate, or conversion to external fixation. There is no clear

Table 4.1 Summary of the main fixation strategies in F1–3 cases (note that care must be individualized for each patient, and strategies differing from these can also be appropriate)

	F1	F2	F3
I1–2	R1–4 remove implant if present + direct wound closure	R1–2 DAIR vs.[a] exchange for new plate/nail (I2: Consider preventive flap) R3 exchange for new nail/plate (I2: Consider prophylactic flap) vs.[b] external fixation R4 external fixation	R1–2 exchange for new nail/plate ± shortening vs.[b] bone void filler R3 exchange for new nail/plate ± shortening R4 acute shortening + external fixation
I3–4	R1–3 remove implant if present + flap R4 remove implant if present + flap vs.[c] wound care + antibiotic suppression	R1–2 DAIR vs.[a] exchange for plate/nail, + flap R3 exchange for a nail/plate vs.[b] external fixation, + flap R4 external fixation + flap vs.[c] wound care + antibiotic suppression	R1–2 exchange for new nail/plate + flap ± shortening vs.[b] bone void filler R3 exchange for a nail/plate ± shortening + tissue transfer R4 acute shortening + external fixation + tissue transfer
I5	R1–2 amputation R3–4 amputation vs.[c] antibiotic suppression + wound care		

DAIR debridement, antibiotics, and implant retention
[a]Depends on whether adequate debridement is possible while retaining the implant
[b]Depends mostly on degree of infection control and location of the FRI
[c]Depends on multiple factors including life expectancy and possibility of good limb functionality with an external prosthesis, refer to Chap. 8 for more information

evidence favoring one over the other [6], the choice depending on multiple factors including the degree of infection control, the quality of the soft tissue envelope, and host status [13, 19].

The patients most benefited by exchange for another nail or plate are F2 R1–2 I1–4 cases in whom adequate debridement has been possible. The risk of infection recurrence with this "new metal" approach has been reported to be around 10% lower than with DAIR, with no significant differences in rates of bone union [13].

If a new nail is being implanted, where possible, antibiotic-loaded cement-coated nails are preferred [2, 19]. Though commercialized antimicrobial coatings specific for intramedullary nails exist, most teams use one of the multiple methods described to hand-make them (mostly with polymethylmethacrylate, PMMA, off-label), which are considerably cheaper [21, 22]. Heterogeneity in the distribution of antibiotics in the PMMA and in the thickness of the nail coating along the nail have been pointed out as issues, but antibiotic-loaded cement-coated nails remain a good option [21]. Most often, these nails are used as a bridge therapy to be followed by definitive internal fixation as they confer less stability than regular intramedullary nails (they must be thinner to make space for the cement).

The alternative is external fixation, which can be used for definitive stabilization or followed by definitive internal fixation once the infection is considered eradicated. The rates of fracture consolidation with definitive external fixation appear to be no different in comparison to osteosynthesized FRIs, albeit more reoperations appear to be required to secure union if external fixators are used [23]. However, external fixators are significantly more uncomfortable for the patient, and anatomic reduction may be challenging (or sometimes, not even possible) to achieve with them. Thus, they are often reserved for cases of poor infection control or R4-type hosts (comorbidities with established end-organ damage which predispose to a poor outcome), especially if the soft tissue envelope is in a poor condition [11].

Fracture-Related Infection in Fractures with Poor Bone Healing Potential (F3)

Infected fractures with poor bone healing potential (F3) do not present favorable biological and/or biomechanical conditions for bone union. Thus, DAIR is not advised, and *implant exchange or conversion to external fixation* are recommended [11, 15]. The typical scenario of an F3-type FRI is an infected nonunion with nonviable bone ends, fixation unstable and/or reduction unaceptable but without major bone loss (a critical infected bone defect would correspond to an F4 type in the FRI classification).

After debridement, a small, noncritical bone defect may arise. Often, it can be managed with acute shortening satisfactorily [11]. When not, non-vascularized cancellous bone autograft (with or without antibiotics, used according to Masquelet's induced membrane technique or not) is an option. The reader is referred to Chap. 5 for more information on the use and indications of bone grafts and acute shortening.

Regarding fixation in F3 cases, R1–2 hosts with I1–4 soft tissues in whom adequate debridement has been possible are generally good candidates for implantation of a new nail or plate (in combination with early flap coverage, where appropriate) [13]. As previously pointed out, anticipating the potential need for a flap (and planning the surgery accordingly) is key to avoiding the new nail or plate being exposed for days or even weeks until soft tissue coverage can be procured, with the risk of reinfection that this entails.

R4-type hosts and patients with poor infection control or instability usually benefit best from external fixation [11, 13]. External fixation can also be considered in patients with critical soft tissue situations, which can range from an I2 situation at the distal tibia to a variety of I3 or I4 cases, especially if soft tissue coverage will be delayed, to avoid exposed internal fixation devices.

Clinical Cases

Case 4.1

A 44-year-old healthy male suffered multiple fractures due to a car accident, including a Gustilo–Anderson type IIIC open fracture of the left distal femur and a type II open fracture of the left tibial shaft, along with a peroneal nerve injury. The femoral fracture was plated (Fig. 4.1),

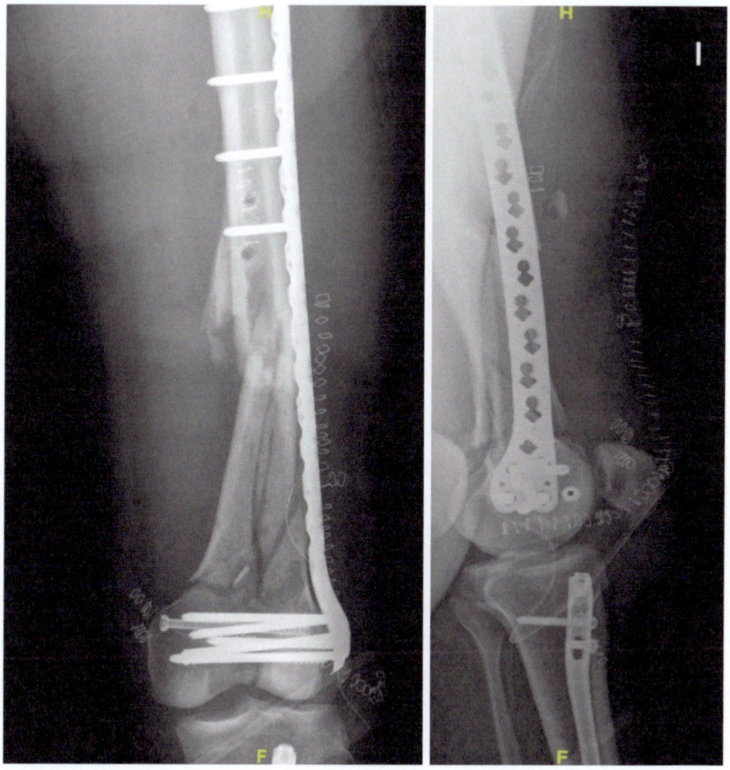

Fig. 4.1 Case 4.1, X-rays on the first postoperative day after osteosynthesis of the comminuted, Gustilo–Anderson type IIIC open fracture of the left distal femur

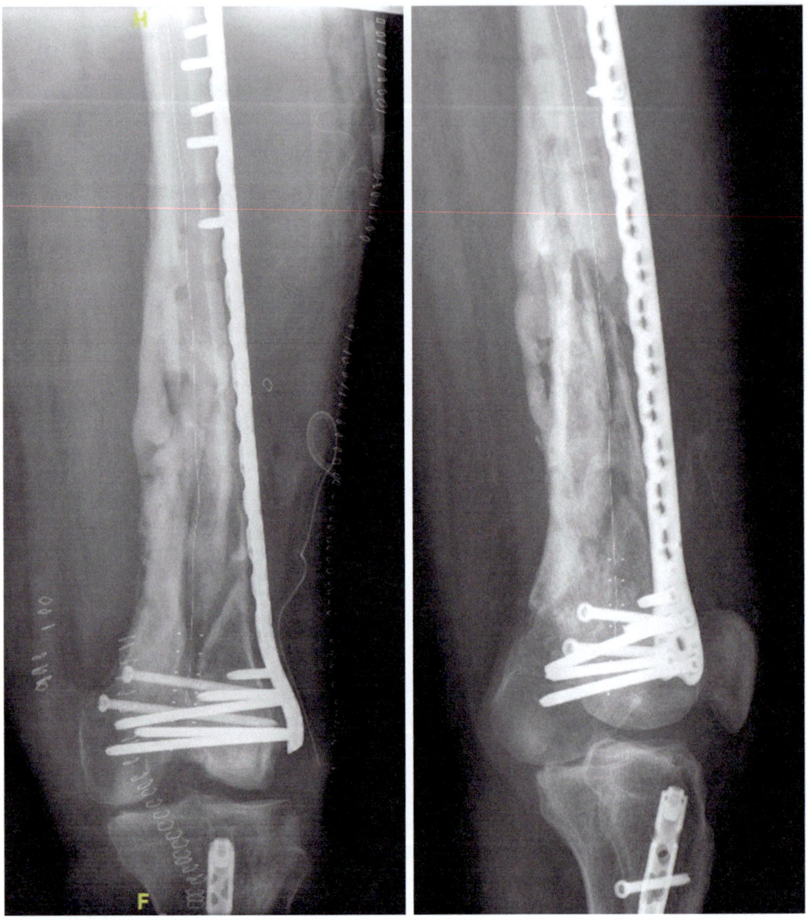

Fig. 4.2 Case 4.1, X-rays on the third postoperative day after debridement and exchange of the infected femoral plate for a new plate and a carbon fiber nail (radiolucent)

the tibial fracture was nailed. On the sixth postoperative day, he developed a fever and knee swelling, which persisted for another week (F2 R1 I1), so 2 weeks after the osteosynthesis surgery, a DAIR was undertaken. *Enterobacter cloacae* grew on intraoperative cultures. Ongoing low-grade fever led the team to perform a second debridement 3 days after the first debridement. Following this second debridement, the patient had a favorable recovery, and he was discharged. However, nonunion and knee stiffness ensued (F3 R1 I1), so 10 months after DAIR the team performed a new debridement and exchanged the femoral plate for a new plate plus a carbon fiber nail to better monitor the nonunion (Fig. 4.2). A Judet quadricepsplasty, achieving 50° of knee flexion, was also performed. The patient had early and persistent drainage through the surgical wound, so he was taken back to the operating room 5 days later for debridement, lavage, and implantation of antibiotic-loaded calcium sulfate beads on the debrided site.

The patient was then referred to our institution. He had an active fistula in the posterior thigh and significant knee stiffness. The CT scan showed bone sequestra and osteolysis (Fig. 4.3), as well as continuity of the posterior, medial cortex, and part of anterior cortex (F3 R1 I2). After evaluation from our Bone Infections Committee, we obtained new cultures, thoroughly debrided the site (the posterior cortex was healthy, so we were able to preserve it) and implanted a gentamicin-, vancomycin- and ceftazidime-loaded cement-coated nail to aid femoral stabilization. Intraoperative cultures were positive for *Enterococcus faecalis*, so the patient received daptomycin and meropenem for 12 weeks. At the 2-year follow-up visit (Fig. 4.4), there was no recurrence of the infection, and knee flexion reached 90°. He currently walks with a cane due to the peroneal nerve lesion sequelae.

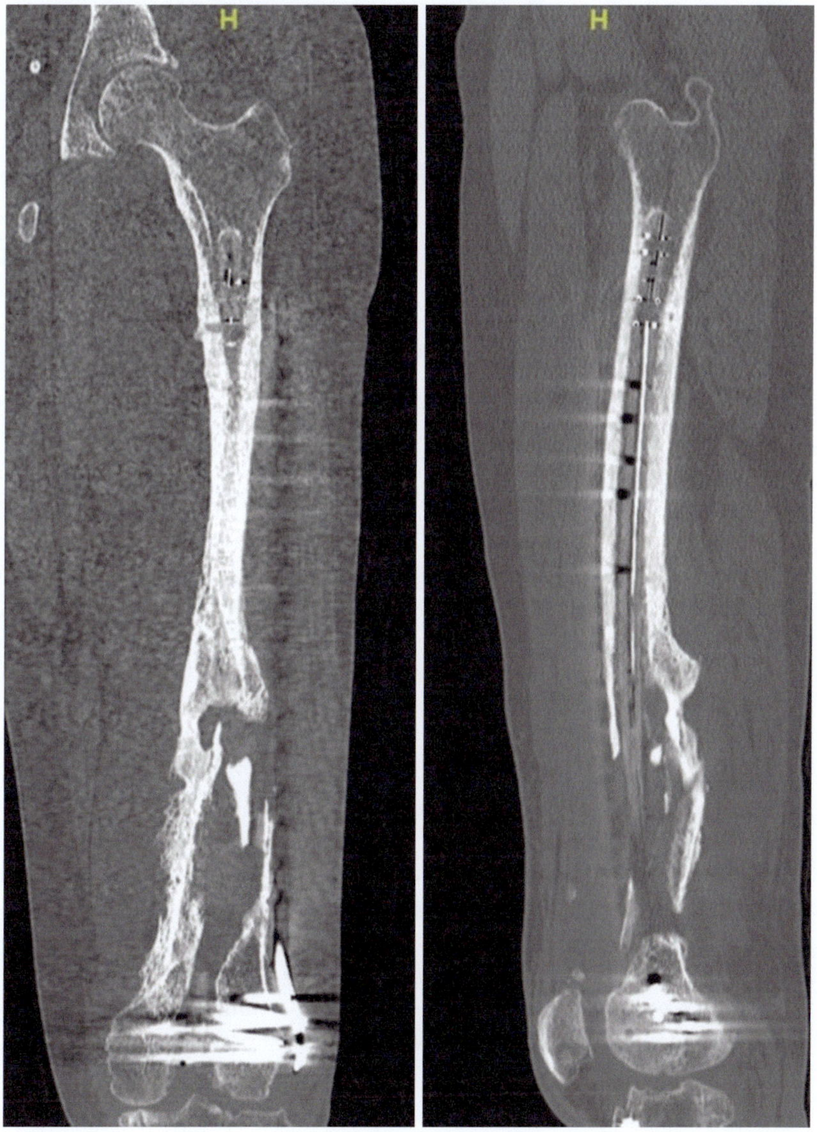

Fig. 4.3 Case 4.1, computed tomography images showing a bone sequestrum and osteolysis

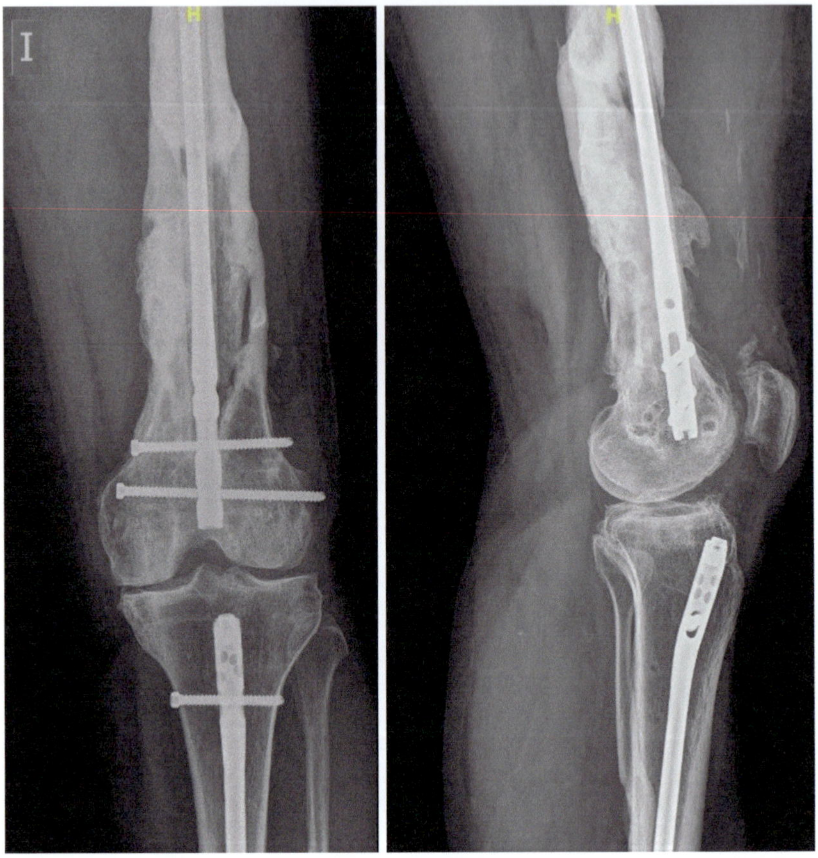

Fig. 4.4 Case 4.1, X-rays at 2 years after the last surgery. The patient has a healed, stable femur, and the infection has not recurred

Case 4.2

A 48-year-old male without any relevant medical history suffered a pilon fracture of the left ankle after a bicycle fall. He underwent reduction and osteosynthesis with tibial and peroneal plates, but had a torpid postoperative recovery and developed tibiotalar osteoarthritis, due to which a tibiotalar arthrodesis was performed.

Five years after arthrodesis, he developed a fistula with purulent drainage at the medial maleollus, due to which he was referred to our institution (Fig. 4.5). The CT scan showed lack of union and failure of the arthrodesis (Fig. 4.6) (F3 R1 I2). After evaluation from our Bone Infections Committee, we removed the hardware, debrided thoroughly, obtained samples, irrigated, and implanted vancomycin- and gentamycin-impregnated calcium sulfate into the 2.5 cm defect that had resulted (Fig. 4.7) (F3 R1 I2). A circular external fixator was also implanted for stabilization and eventual shortening and re-lengthening. Methicillin-sensitive *Staphylococcus epidermidis* grew on intraoperative cultures, and the patient received antibiotics for 12 weeks. He had an uneventful recovery, and shortening was performed, but the patient adapted well to the dysmetria and declined re-lengthening. At the 5-year follow-up visit, the patient has had no recurrences of the infection, wears a specialized platform shoe but otherwise walks without aids and painlessly (Figs. 4.8 and 4.9).

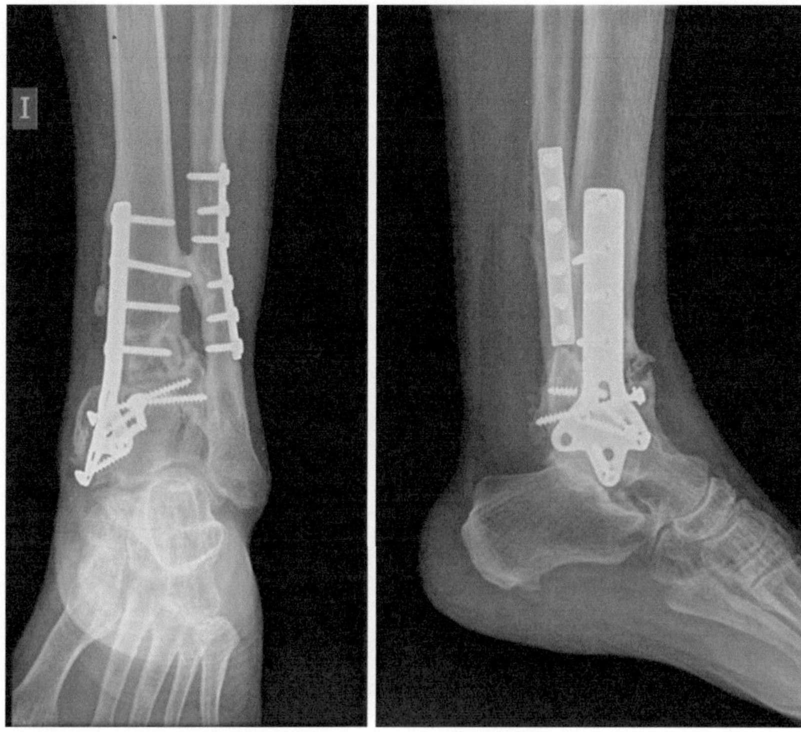

Fig. 4.5 Case 4.2, X-rays 5 years after ankle arthrodesis showing tibiotalar nonunion

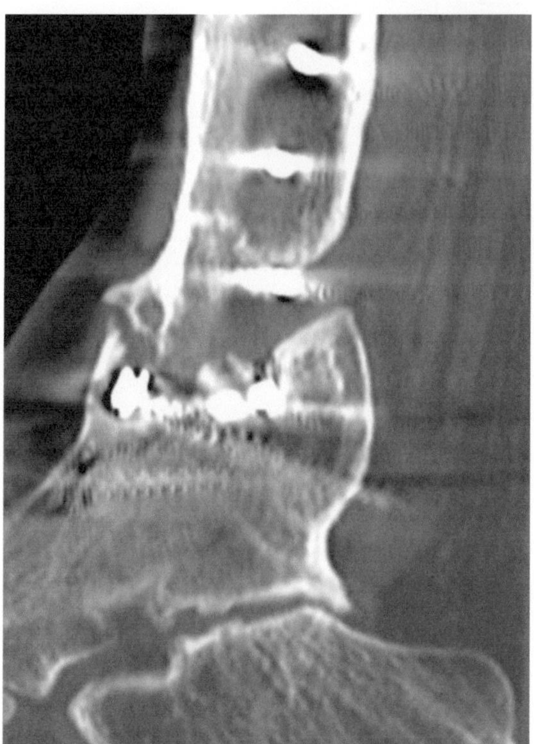

Fig. 4.6 Case 4.2, computed tomography imagen 5 years after ankle arthrodesis showing tibiotalar nonunion and bone sclerosis

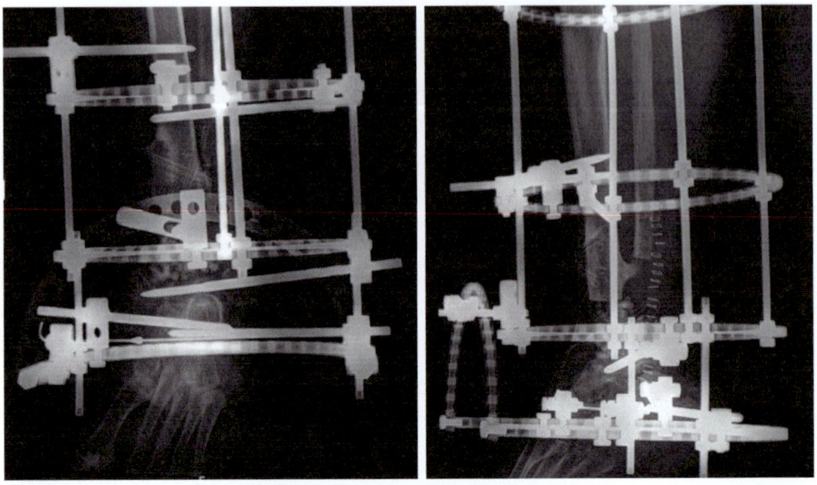

Fig. 4.7 Case 4.2, X-rays on the first postoperative day after debridement, implantation of vancomycin- and gentamycin-impregnated calcium sulfate into the 2.5 cm post-debridement defect and stabilization with a circular external fixator

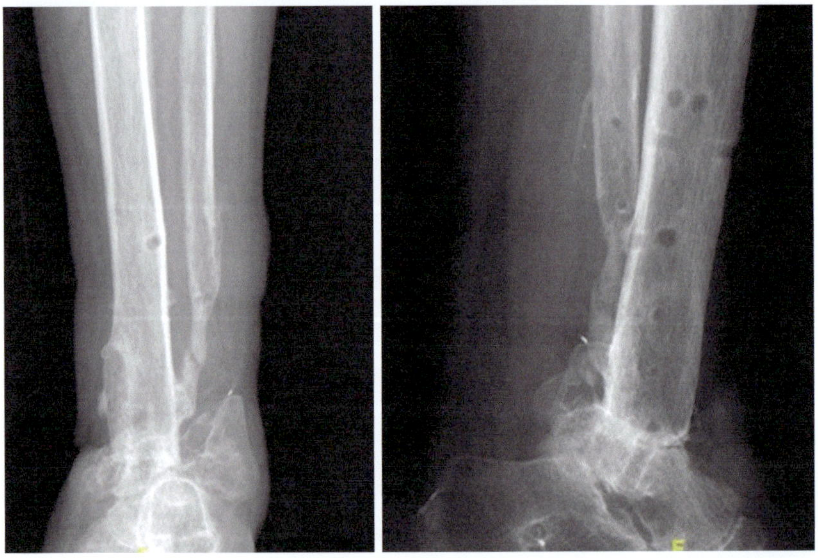

Fig. 4.8 Case 4.2, X-rays on the 5-year follow-up visit showing bone union

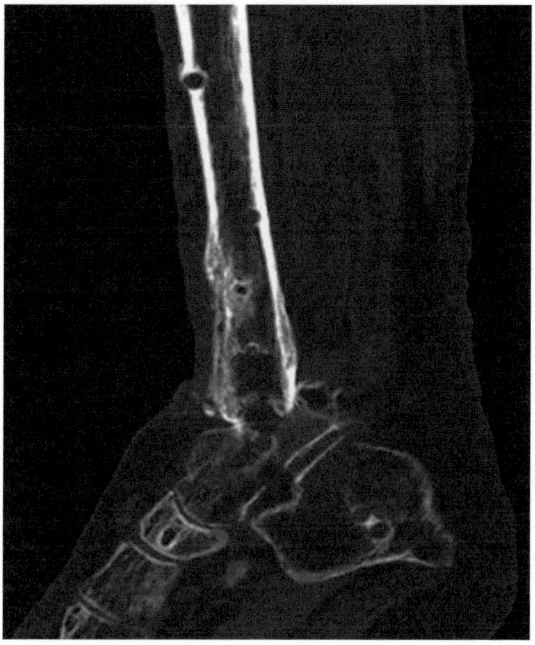

Fig. 4.9 Case 4.2, computed tomography image on the 5-year follow-up visit showing bone union, and no signs of infection recurrence

Conclusions

FRI treatment is challenging. Thorough debridement is its cornerstone. Assessing the healing potential and soft tissue status as well as optimizing systemic host pathologies is critical.

If a fracture has consolidated (F1), dead space management is key. Any implants present should be removed. After hardware removal and targeted antibiotic therapy, the infection usually heals.

The patients that benefit the most from DAIR are R1-type hosts with optimal conditions for bone union: favorable biology (viable bone ends) and biomechanics (stable osteosynthetic construct, satisfactory reduction), adequate debridement has been possible, and a healthy soft tissue envelope is either present or will be achieved surgically early (I1–4). If these conditions are not met, implant exchange or conversion to external fixation is a wiser option. Retention of intramedullary nails is associated to a high rate of treatment failure, probably due to most of their surface being inaccessible for debridement, so their exchange is recommended even when conditions are otherwise optimal for retention.

Even in optimal cases, around 1 in every 4 patients that undergo DAIR will suffer an infection recurrence (patients must be counselled accordingly).

In F3 cases (nonviable bone ends, instability, unacceptable reduction), DAIR is not advised.

Multiple treatment strategies exist for implant exchange in FRI, with no clear evidence favoring one over the other. The patients most benefited by exchange for another nail (preferably, coated by antibiotic-loaded cement) or plate are F2 R1 I1–4 cases in which adequate debridement would not have been possible with implant retention (e.g., intramedullary nails), and F3 R1–2 I1–4. The patients most benefited by external fixation are R4-type hosts or those with poor infection control or instability. It can also be considered in patients with critical soft tissue situations.

References

1. Morgenstern M, Clauss M, Sendi P, Cadosch D, Osinga R, Metsemakers W-J. Treatment of fracture-related infections. In: Textbook of polytrauma management: a multidisciplinary approach. 3rd ed. Berlin: Springer; 2022. p. 573–81.
2. Barla JD. Fracture-related infections. In: Orthopaedics and trauma. Berlin: Springer; 2024. p. 805–10.
3. Moriarty TF, Metsemakers W-J, Morgenstern M, Hofstee MI, Vallejo Diaz A, Cassat JE, Wildemann B, Depypere M, Schwarz EM, Richards RG. Fracture-related infection. Nat Rev Dis Primers. 2022;8:67.
4. Depypere M, Morgenstern M, Kuehl R, Senneville E, Moriarty TF, Obremskey WT, Zimmerli W, Trampuz A, Lagrou K, Metsemakers W-J. Pathogenesis and management of fracture-related infection. Clin Microbiol Infect. 2020;26:572–8.
5. Rupp M, Walter N, Popp D, et al. Multidisciplinary treatment of fracture-related infection has a positive impact on clinical outcome-a retrospective case control study at a tertiary referral center. Antibiotics (Basel). 2023;12:230.
6. Bezstarosti H, Van Lieshout EMM, Voskamp LW, Kortram K, Obremskey W, McNally MA, Metsemakers WJ, Verhofstad MHJ. Insights into treatment and outcome of fracture-related infection: a systematic literature review. Arch Orthop Trauma Surg. 2019;139:61–72.
7. Azoury SC, Stranix JT, Kovach SJ, Levin LS. Principles of orthoplastic surgery for lower

extremity reconstruction: why is this important? J Reconstr Microsurg. 2021;37:42–50.
8. Olesen UK, Pedersen NJ, Eckardt H, Lykke-Meyer L, Bonde CT, Singh UM, McNally M. The cost of infection in severe open tibial fractures treated with a free flap. Int Orthop. 2017;41:1049–55.
9. Iliadis AD, Shivji F, Debuka E, Trompeter A, Narayan B, Heidari N. Current concepts in the prevention, diagnosis and treatment of fracture-related infection (FRI). Eur J Orthop Surg Traumatol. 2021;31:957–66.
10. Marais LC, Hungerer S, Eckardt H, Zalavras C, Obremskey WT, Ramsden A, McNally MA, Morgenstern M, Metsemakers W-J, FRI Consensus Group. Key aspects of soft tissue management in fracture-related infection: recommendations from an international expert group. Arch Orthop Trauma Surg. 2024;144:259–68.
11. Alt V, McNally M, Wouthuyzen-Bakker M, Metsemakers W-J, Marais L, Zalavras C, Morgenstern M. The FRI classification – a new classification of fracture-related infections. Injury. 2024;55:111831.
12. Bezstarosti H, Metsemakers WJ, van Lieshout EMM, Voskamp LW, Kortram K, McNally MA, Marais LC, Verhofstad MHJ. Management of critical-sized bone defects in the treatment of fracture-related infection: a systematic review and pooled analysis. Arch Orthop Trauma Surg. 2021;141:1215–30.
13. McNally M, Corrigan R, Sliepen J, Dudareva M, Rentenaar R, Ijpma F, Atkins BL, Wouthuyzen-Bakker M, Govaert G. What factors affect outcome in the treatment of fracture-related infection? Antibiotics (Basel). 2022;11:946.
14. Viol A, Pradka SP, Baumeister SP, Wang D, Moyer KE, Zura RD, Olson SA, Zenn MR, Levin SL, Erdmann D. Soft-tissue defects and exposed hardware: a review of indications for soft-tissue reconstruction and hardware preservation. Plast Reconstr Surg. 2009;123:1256–63.
15. Foster AL, Moriarty TF, Zalavras C, et al. The influence of biomechanical stability on bone healing and fracture-related infection: the legacy of Stephan Perren. Injury. 2021;52:43–52.
16. Lu V, Zhang J, Patel R, Zhou AK, Thahir A, Krkovic M. Fracture related infections and their risk factors for treatment failure-a major trauma centre perspective. Diagnostics (Basel). 2022;12:1289.
17. Berkes M, Obremskey WT, Scannell B, Ellington JK, Hymes RA, Bosse M, Southeast Fracture Consortium. Maintenance of hardware after early postoperative infection following fracture internal fixation. J Bone Joint Surg Am. 2010;92:823–8.
18. Rightmire E, Zurakowski D, Vrahas M. Acute infections after fracture repair. Clin Orthop Relat Res. 2008;466:466–72.
19. Marais LC, Zalavras CG, Moriarty FT, Kühl R, Metsemakers W-J, Morgenstern M. The surgical management of fracture-related infection. Surgical strategy selection and the need for early surgical intervention. J Orthop. 2024;50:36–41.
20. Morgenstern M, Kuehl R, Zalavras CG, McNally M, Zimmerli W, Burch MA, Vandendriessche T, Obremskey WT, Verhofstad MHJ, Metsemakers WJ. The influence of duration of infection on outcome of debridement and implant retention in fracture-related infection. Bone Joint J. 2021;103-B:213–21.
21. Metsemakers W-J, Fragomen AT, Moriarty TF, Morgenstern M, Egol KA, Zalavras C, Obremskey WT, Raschke M, McNally MA. Evidence-based recommendations for local antimicrobial strategies and dead space management in fracture-related infection. J Orthop Trauma. 2020;34:18–29.
22. Walter N, Rupp M, Krückel J, Alt V. Individual and commercially available antimicrobial coatings for intramedullary nails for the treatment of infected long bone non-unions – a systematic review. Injury. 2022;53(Suppl 3):S74–80.
23. Frank F, Hotchen A, Valand P, Stubbs D, Ferguson J, McNally M. The management of unhealed fracture-related infections with a single-stage protocol and without bone graft. Orthopaedic Proceedings. 2024;106-B:10.

Management of Fracture-Related Infection in Critical Bone Defects

5

Nieves Vanaclocha, Alberto Pérez-García, and Javier Martínez

Introduction

Fracture-related infections (FRIs) are one of the most challenging complications that can arise after a fracture. Most often, they affect the long bones, particularly those of the lower limb [1]. Though some FRIs may be uncomplicated and easily resolved, patients with an infected critical bone defect (i.e., one that will not heal without surgery) face protracted treatments and a significant worsening of their quality of life for years, with a high number of revision surgeries, psychological stress, limited participation in social activities, and loss of income [2–5].

Evidence regarding the different treatment modalities for infected bone defects is scarce and usually comprises small observational studies, at best prospective and frequently retrospective, with very heterogeneous patient cohorts, management protocols, and outcome variables [5–7]. Often, the cohorts include and analyze jointly both infected and aseptic defects, the latter group having a very different biological situation and higher rates of treatment success than FRI cases, so the results from these studies have limited external validity for the FRI-only population. Underreporting of adverse effects has also been pointed out as an issue [6]. The recent focus on standardization in FRI is setting the scene for the generation of higher-quality evidence, and the situation is slowly changing. However, as of this writing there is very limited high-quality evidence to guide decision-making, and no gold standard for the treatment of infected bone defects [1, 5, 6].

This chapter will focus on the available options for bone reconstruction in infected critical bone defects. They can be broadly divided into those based on *local bone regeneration* and those based on *bone replacement*. Since there is currently no gold standard, the reconstructive strategy must be tailored to each patient (comorbidities, compliance, and preferences) and their defect (location, size and shape, condition of surrounding soft tissues), with the team's experience and preferences also playing a role [1, 6–8]. The road to recovery is long and difficult, so it is important to have thorough discussions with

N. Vanaclocha (✉)
Orthoplastics Unit and Department of Plastic and Reconstructive Surgery, University and Polytechnic Hospital La Fe, Valencia, Spain

A. Pérez-García
Orthoplastics Unit and Department of Plastic and Reconstructive Surgery, University and Polytechnic Hospital La Fe, Valencia, Spain

Department of Surgery, Universitat de València, Valencia, Spain

J. Martínez
Unidad de Patología Séptica y Reconstructiva del Aparato Locomotor, Cirugía Ortopédica y Traumatología, Hospital Clínico Universitario Virgen de La Arrixaca, Murcia, Spain

N. Vanaclocha (ed.), *Treatment of Fracture-Related Infection*,
https://doi.org/10.1007/978-3-031-92452-1_5

patients regarding all the options [9, 10]. In some cases, the benefits of limb salvage must be weighed against those of amputation (refer to Chap. 8 for more information on this matter).

Note that the general principles discussed in complementary chapters (Chaps. 3 and 10) must be adhered to for success. This includes preoperative patient optimization (addressing poor nutrition and obesity, comorbidities such as diabetes or peripheral arterial disease, smoking cessation, etc.), as it will increase the likelihood of infection eradication and improve tissue healing (both of soft tissues and of bone) [5, 11].

Bone Reconstruction Techniques Based on Local Bone Regeneration

These techniques depend on native bone ends for healing, so their outcomes will be better, the better the state of the bone ends. They comprise bone grafts, acute shortening and re-lengthening (ASRL), and bone transport.

Non-vascularized Bone Grafts

Non-vascularized bone grafts are osseous tissue that is harvested from a donor area in a way that its irrigation is not preserved. The resulting devascularized bone is then implanted into the post-debridement defect at the FRI site.

Non-vascularized bone autografts are taken from another site in the patient's body, typically the iliac crest, or from the femoral canal by reaming (note that reaming may affect viability of the grafted cells) [1, 12]. Generally, cancellous bone is preferred, for its purported lower risk of subsequent sequestra [6, 13]. Non-vascularized autogenous bone has mostly osteoconductive properties, because only the grafted cells in contact with the native bone ends and wound bed can survive. The rest of the autograft provides a scaffold to be slowly colonized by native bone cells, a process known as creeping substitution.

The main advantage of non-vascularized bone autografts in FRI is that the procedure is fast, easy, and the most available out of all the techniques to manage bone defects. Consequently, they are one of the most frequently performed procedures for small to moderate defects (<5 cm), usually in a staged approach [6, 14, 15].

However, the amount of non-vascularized bone autograft that can be harvested without significant morbidity is very limited, they barely provide any mechanical stability, and they are, by definition, not vascularized. Due to this lack of vascularization, only the cells closest to the native bone ends and wound bed can survive, and only *if* the adjacent native tissues are well vascularized, including healthy bone ends and a healthy soft tissue envelope. The rest of the grafted cells will die within hours of implantation. This, on one hand, provides necrotic tissue on which any remaining bacteria may feed, and on the other, is responsible for creeping substitution to be a slow, unreliable process, limited to the vicinity of the junction between the graft and the native bone ends [15, 16]. As a result, the larger the defect that non-vascularized bone grafts are used for, the higher the rate of resorption and infection recurrence [6, 7].

To decrease the rates of resorption and infection recurrence, the induced membrane technique was proposed by Masquelet et al. [17]. It involves first filling the defect with an antibiotic-impregnated spacer and allowing a capsule to grow around it for 4 to 8 weeks. Then, the capsule is carefully incised, and the spacer is substituted for non-vascularized bone autograft. The principle is that graft take will be boosted by isolating the graft from the surrounding hostile environment (potential residual infection, inflamed tissues) [14, 18]. Despite initial enthusiasm, it has been associated with the highest recurrence rate of the techniques discussed in this chapter (over 12%), and high rates of complications (up to 50%) and secondary surgeries to manage them, mostly regrafting due to graft resorption [6, 19, 20]. Consequently, this technique has proven unable to expand the indications of non-vascularized bone autografts. The poor quality of the bone regenerated with this technique is another drawback, and one of the culprits of the low predictability of its results.

Another variation of use is to admix antimicrobials with the bone autograft to deliver high doses of antimicrobials locally. Concerns regarding the known osteocyte and osteoblast toxicity of many antibiotics (including quinolones, which are widely used in FRI due to their anti-biofilm activity) has prevented widespread application of this practice [13, 21]. So far, a pooled analysis of techniques for the management of infected bone defects observed a slightly higher primary healing rate and slightly shorter time to union of cancellous bone autografts with antibiotics in comparison with cancellous bone autografts *without* antibiotics, similar rates of infection recurrence, but many more surgical revisions (over double) when antibiotics were added [6]. Given the scarce experience with this treatment modality and unknown optimal antimicrobial dosing for local application, it is currently not recommended to routinely add antibiotics to bone autografts [21].

In yet another attempt at improving outcomes with non-vascularized bone grafts, some teams added bone morphogenetic proteins (BMPs). The role of BMPs in FRI is still unclear [1, 22, 23]. The first few case series with bone autografts with BMP-2 or BMP-7 showed promising results, but enthusiasm waned as further investigations reported complications [2, 22]. These complications appear to be dose-dependent (supraphysiological doses of BMPs are used), and derive at least partially from their uncontrolled delivery, which results in leaching into surrounding tissues where effects such as ectopic bone formation or nerve damage are produced [2, 22]. There has been improvement on these issues with delivery methods that are more precise in terms of dosage and location, such as incorporation into a collagen-hydroxyapatite composite or reverse dynamization [22]. In any case, further studies are needed to elucidate the potential of BMPs in the treatment of infected bone defects, including what added value they provide.

To sum up, the patients that most benefit from non-vascularized bone autografts are those with small defects, a healthy soft tissue envelope and good infection control [7, 16].

The size up to which it is acceptable to graft is a matter of controversy. Given the very limited amount of non-vascularized autologous bone that can be harvested without significant morbidity, and the increasing rate of resorption and infection recurrence with increasing graft size, most teams limit their non-vascularized bone autograft use to small- to moderately sized defects (5–7 cm at most) [6, 7]. Additionally, there is no evidence to guide how many times it is reasonable to re-graft (vs. changing the technique) in FRI. Given that each revision surgery will be significantly more complex and that graft failure reflects unsupportive native tissues (which *worsen* with each subsequent surgery), the authors of this chapter believe that one failed grafting in an FRI patient should elicit change to a different reconstruction technique.

Bone allografts are harvested from a deceased donor. Their use has traditionally not been recommended in FRI cases due to high rates of infection recurrence, nonunion, and late fractures in these patients [13, 15, 21]. However, there is renewed interest in them as potential carriers of local antibiotics, for they can store much larger amounts of antimicrobials (antibiotics, porphyrins, etc.) than polymethylmethacrylate (PMMA) and other carriers, with promising results in the few published case series (almost all, non-FRI patients) that exist [13, 21]. In FRI, it is of particular importance that once the antimicrobial is released, the allograft will act as a foreign body, susceptible to colonization by any remaining bacteria. Additionally, as with autografts, there are concerns regarding the negative effects of local antibiotics on bone allograft incorporation, and the published research has heterogenous protocols without comparative data [13, 21]. The scarce available literature does not answer many important questions for practical application: what kind of allograft (fresh-frozen or freeze-dried, demineralized or not) best carries antimicrobials, which impregnation method (manual mixing, soaking, iontophoresis, etc.) results in the most desirable pharmacokinetic profile, and what is the optimal antibiotic/bone graft ratio? So far, the use of antibiotic-impregnated bone allografts in FRI patients is experimental.

Techniques Based on Distraction Osteogenesis

ASRL and bone transport are techniques based on distraction osteogenesis, generally at rates of

0.50–1 mm/day (note that the higher the rate of distraction, the higher the risk of angular deviations [12]).

These techniques are multistage. The multiple trips to the operating room (OR) are more inconvenient for patients, but allow for the team to wait until the infection is considered eradicated to start definitive bone reconstruction through distraction [12, 24].

The main advantages of this group of techniques are their lack of dependence on donor bone availability (and the restrictions on the size of bone that can be reconstructed that this entails, unlike non-vascularized bone grafts or bone flaps) and that they allow almost immediate loading, weight-bearing being critical to diminish the risks of prolonged immobilization, including osteopenia, sarcopenia, and joint stiffness [16, 24]. They also keep the amount of foreign material at the FRI site to a minimum, something desirable from a microbiological point of view as any hardware in the FRI site will be susceptible to colonization by remaining pathogens. Another significant advantage is that the surgical procedures associated to bone transport and ASRL are usually less technically demanding, faster and less invasive than bone flap surgeries, so techniques based on distraction osteogenesis can be performed on more comorbid hosts. Other advantages include the morbidity being limited to the FRI site (unlike non-vascularized bone grafts and bone flaps, which involve other anatomical areas), and that these techniques allow correction of any associated deformities or limb-length discrepancies, if they are present.

The main drawback associated with these techniques is the prolonged external fixation that they require (over 6 months in almost all cases, and often over a year) [7, 16, 25]. It is assessed using standard indices such as the Bone Healing Index (total treatment time, starting from the day of the corticotomy, divided by amount of bone lengthening achieved), which represents the time required to regenerate 1 cm of bone, and the External Fixation Index (time the patient has the external fixator on divided by the amount of bone lengthening achieved), which represents the time that the external fixator will remain implanted per cm of defect managed. In infected bone defects, reported bone healing indexes are approximately 1.5 months/cm, and external fixation indexes around 2 months/cm [25, 26]. The bigger the bone defect, the longer the external fixation time, which, without a good physical rehabilitation program, then results in a higher risk of complications such as stiffness and decreased range of motion of nearby joints, as well as a higher physical and emotional toll on patients [27].

Other disadvantages of techniques based on distraction osteogenesis include the need for specialized equipment and slower bone union than with techniques based on bone replacement, because techniques based on local bone regeneration depend on local bone and soft tissues, which are scarred from the trauma and prolonged inflammation [7, 25].

Complications are not common in experienced teams with rigorous techniques, and are usually resolved with either conservative treatment or outpatient secondary surgery. They include docking site nonunion, pin tract infections (almost always minor, not requiring removal), pin or wire loosening or breakage, axial deviations, and refractures [7, 25]. Specifically, docking site nonunion remains one of the most frequent and critical complications in distraction osteogenesis (bone ends of mismatching sizes tend to unite tenuously [12]), with reported incidence rates ranging from negligible to as high as 83% across different series [26, 28]. This had led several specialized centers to adopt systematic bone grafting protocols at the docking site, using predefined criteria that include the degree of cortical bone coaptation, the condition of the surrounding soft tissue envelope, host status, and the projected duration of regenerate maturation. In short, most patients undergoing bone transport require a planned secondary procedure to optimize union at the docking interface, and grafting has become an integral and anticipated component of the reconstructive algorithm in complex infected bone defects.

Note that pain is not rare but usually indicative of a complication, its management being key to both rule out a complication (e.g., minor peri-pin

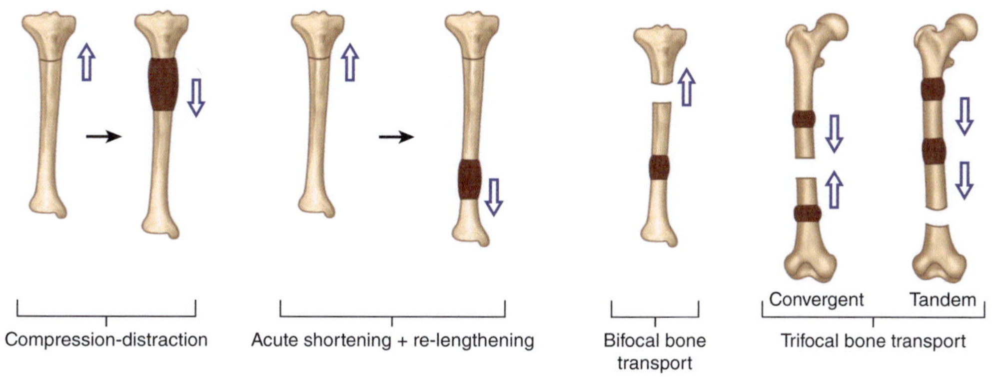

Fig. 5.1 Types of distraction in FRI. Left: ASRL. Bifocal bone transport. Trifocal convergent bone transport. Trifocal tandem bone transport

inflammation due to improper cleaning) and because the patient must be able to walk painlessly to benefit the most from these techniques and to encourage vascular growth to the limb, which aids healing [12].

Due to these strengths and weaknesses, ASRL and bone transport are most useful for lower limb defects, where they will enable early weight-bearing. They are less well-suited for upper limb defects or metaphyseal defects [15, 29]: in the upper limb, preservation of nearby joint motion is more important (and more limiting, if reduced) than ability to load axially early, especially in the forearm. The forearm, as well as functioning as a joint, has a high density of noble structures (e.g., tendons, nerves) that make external fixator implantation challenging and can suffer attritional damage if they are adjacent to a pin or wire (they will rub against it with muscle activity). In metaphyseal defects, epiphyseal osteolysis complicates the implantation of a stable pin for external fixation in that area, joint complications are more frequent than with shaft defects, and the multiple debridements needed with these techniques can compromise the joint and lead to arthrodesis. The new fixation systems, which allow good stability even with very small bone segments, are likely to cater to these kinds of defects better and diminish these problems.

Acute shortening involves shortening of the limb to bring the bone fragments into contact with each other. Small shortenings are generally well-tolerated, especially in the upper limb, and re-lengthening is rarely necessary, significantly simplifying and shortening treatment.

When re-lengthening is needed (ASRL), a percutaneous corticotomy is performed to allow distraction to achieve isometry (unifocal distraction, see Fig. 5.1). The corticotomy can be performed in the same stage as the shortening or in a second stage once the infection is considered eradicated. Most often, the corticotomy will be performed at a healthy site away from the nonunion (as opposed to distracting the FRI site, *compression-distraction*).

The main advantages of acute shortening, with or without re-lengthening, are [30]:

- Simple and fast technique.
- Provides immediate stability.
- Aids in managing dead space (collapse of the bone defect) and any soft tissue defect present (a skin graft often suffices for coverage after acute shortening).
- For ASRL, treatment time may be slightly shorter (0.63 days less per 1 cm of length gained [30]) in comparison with bone transport.

However, the bigger the shortened defect, the higher the risk of acute neurovascular kinking, which can result in soft tissue compromise (preoperative planning accounting for transverse incisions or Z-plasties being essential) or even nerve palsies, and the greater the changes to muscle resting length, which entail less muscular efficiency and higher risk of biomechanical joint alterations, such as foot drop [16, 30, 31]. As a result, though success in much bigger defects has been reported, most teams will restrict their use of acute shortening (with or without later re-lengthening) to 3–4 cm [30, 31]. Other drawbacks include the need to shorten the non-involved bone to achieve compression at the fracture site in locations with two parallel bones (e.g., leg, forearm, with some teams favoring a short transport in those locations to avoid this), the risk of limited distraction due to neurovascular pedicle contracture, and ASRL's higher dependency on bone grafting in comparison with bone transport [30, 31]. In lower limb FRIs, the patient will have to wear a specialized platform shoe (some patients adapt to this well and prefer the dysmetria to re-lengthening).

All things considered, as acute shortening simultaneously addresses stability, dead space, and the soft tissues, it is especially suitable for FRI patients with small defects that will not need re-lengthening and when a shortening osteotomy of the parallel non-involved bone is not necessary (e.g., concomitant fibular fracture). In patients in whom re-lengthening would be needed, those with moderately sized defects (up to about 4 cm) in the lower limb are often good candidates for ASRL, as early weight-bearing will be enabled.

For bone transport, first, a corticotomy is performed and a callus allowed to form (7–21 days, "latency period," depending on the way in which the corticotomy is performed). Next, the corticotomized fragment is translated along the transport segment towards the docking point through the external fixator ("activation period" or "distraction phase"). Finally, the translated fragment must unite at the docking point ("consolidation period"). Bone union and complication rates are no different than those with ASRL, but unlike ASRL, limb length must not be shortened [30].

Any preexisting misalignments should be corrected before initiating transport (especially in cases of monolateral fixation), and close monitoring is recommended to prevent and promptly correct axial deviations, joint deformities, or wire rupture [27, 31].

Table 5.1 Strengths and weaknesses of circular frames and monolateral external fixators for bone transport in infected nonunions

	Circular frame	Monolateral frame
Strengths	More stable (more uniform weight distribution around a central axis), better fixation of cancellous bone Allows deformity correction in all three planes simultaneous to distraction Provides better control of the transported segment	Easier to implant Easier soft tissue access, if needed (e.g., for a microvascular anastomosis)
Weaknesses	Implantation technically more challenging and time-consuming for surgeon Many surgeons have little or no experience with them	Less stable Higher risk of refracture after frame removal Harder to correct deformities and compensate for technical mistakes

There is controversy as to whether circular or monolateral fixators are best to perform bone transport. They each have strengths and weaknesses (Table 5.1), and both can be used successfully [7, 32].

The main advantages of bone transport are its applicability to bone defects of any size (albeit with significantly higher complication rates for defects >10 cm long [27]) and its ability to restore limb-length discrepancies. The main trade-offs are its complexity and prolonged external fixation time (roughly 2 months for every centimeter of bone defect to be reconstructed in experienced hands), demanding highly of both the patient and the team [2, 7, 25]. Additionally, unlike ASRL, it does not manage dead space or the soft tissue envelope, so these issues will have to be addressed elsewhere (refer to Chap. 3 for information on bone void fillers and to Chap. 9 for information on management of the soft tissues).

Some teams have proposed strategies to reduce external fixation time. The main one is trifocal bone transport, where *two* fragments are transported (thus also referred to as double-level transport) [12, 23]. Faster consolidation rates than those with bifocal bone transport are reported, with a similar rates of complications controlling for defect size [27, 33]. There is a concentric variant for diaphyseal defects (*convergent bone transport*), where a proximal fragment and a distal fragment advance toward each other, and an eccentric variant for metaphyseal defects (*tandem transport*), where both fragments are either proximal or distal and they advance in the same direction toward the other bone end (Fig. 5.1). Alternatively, there are a few published series of FRI patients who underwent hybrid bone transport over a nail [34, 35] or plate [36], which were implanted once the infection had been considered eradicated and before starting distraction, or even transport over a magnetically driven intramedullary bone transport nail, with improved patient comfort [37, 38]. The results reported in all these case series were good, but the clinical experience with these techniques in FRI patients is scarce and risk of recurrence is a concern, so caution is advised. It is possible that their adoption increases in the future as further evidence of their safety from an infectious point of view becomes available.

To reduce the high rates of nonunion at the docking site [7, 27], and thus reduce the number of secondary procedures, the most important and best-studied strategy is early grafting of the docking site. Other alternatives, supported only by a few case series, include the accordion maneuver (a cycle of alternating distraction and compression [39]), secondary intramedullary nailing, and low-intensity pulsed ultrasound [12, 23].

The patients with infected bone defects that benefit from bone transport the most are those which have bone deformities and/or malalignments, or in the rare event of a bifocal fracture, especially in the lower limb as these patients will benefit from early weight-bearing [12, 31]. Though there are no formal limits on the size of the defect to which bone transport can be applied, it is mostly used for infected defects between 4 and 10 cm owing to the external fixation time that they require and the availability of better-suited techniques for both smaller and larger defects [10, 31].

Techniques Based on Local Bone Regeneration

These techniques depend on native bone ends for healing, so their outcomes will be better, the better the state of the bone ends.

The patients that most benefit from non-vascularized bone autografts are those with small bone defects with good coverage and infection control. Creeping substitution is a slow, unreliable process, so regrafting is common.

Techniques based on distraction osteogenesis allow almost immediate loading, so they will be of greatest value in the lower limb, where they will enable early weight-bearing.

- Acute shortening manages simultaneously stability, dead space, and the soft tissues (wound closure is simplified). It is especially suitable for FRI patients with small defects that will not need re-lengthening and a shortening osteotomy of the parallel non-involved bone is not necessary. ASRL is a good option for patients with infected bone defects up to 3–4 cm.
- Bone transport is especially suitable for patients with bone deformities or malalignments. Due to the prolonged external fixation time associated with this technique, it is mostly used for defects between 4 and 10 cm.

Bone Reconstruction Techniques Based on Bone Replacement

This Group of Techniques Is Comprised by Bone Flaps Bone flaps are the only treatment modality that does not depend on native bone ends for union so long as the debridement has been adequate, as healthy vascularized bone from another anatomical area is imported to the FRI site. In short, since healing depends on healthy vascularized bone, bone flaps have the shortest time to union, lowest complication rate and lowest number of surgical revisions out of all the available techniques [6], at the cost of donor-site morbidity and prolonged protected axial load. Bone flaps are discussed at length in Chap. 6, but an overview will be provided here.

The main characteristic of bone flaps is their *intrinsic blood supply*, which is responsible for most of their advantages, as this blood supply [6, 15, 29]:

- Transports systemic antibiotics and immune system cells to the FRI site, so bone flaps tolerate (and fight) residual infection well.
- Provides bone flaps with intrinsic ability for bone healing, resulting in high union rates and the fastest bone union out of all the available techniques.
- Allows bone flaps to retain their biomechanical properties, so they have none to minimal resorption and will hypertrophy as a response to the increased functional demands, gradually mimicking the host bone in shape and size.
- Allows reliable survival of bone flaps in hostile recipients, such as those with extensive scarring from high-energy trauma and/or previous surgeries (unlike bone grafts, which heavily depend on quality of the wound bed for survival).
- Enables incorporation of other tissues (skin, tendons, muscle, etc.) for simultaneous reconstruction of multiple structures, management of dead space, and/or the soft tissue envelope.
- Only a single stage is required.

However, bone flaps also have significant disadvantages, including prolonged protected weight-bearing (the time to union of a fibula flap is significantly longer than the equivalent bifocal fracture), donor-site morbidity, and greater technical difficulty and surgical times. Note that the longer surgical times impose a minimum fitness requirement for the hosts (in general, R3-type hosts or healthier, with more unfit hosts being seldom candidates for this kind of procedures).

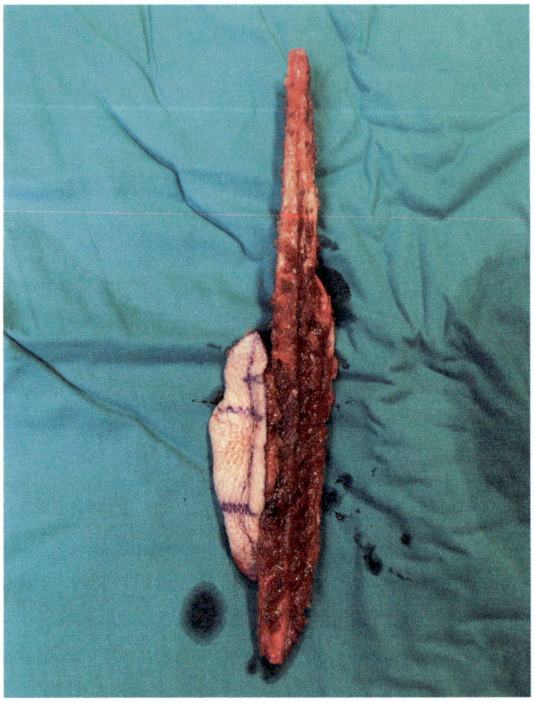

Fig. 5.2 Free osteocutaneous fibula flap. Note the flap pedicle on the border of the flap contralateral to the skin paddle

The most commonly used bone flap in the management of infected bone defects is the fibula flap (Fig. 5.2) [1, 6, 40]. This is because it can provide the most girth and length (up to 20 cm, or more in tall individuals) out of the bone flaps, it has a tubular shape (convenient for long bone defects) and is very versatile (it can be harvested with a skin island to provide reliable wound coverage or with soleus muscle for dead space management) [40–42]. The presence of both periosteal and endosteal circulation allows corticotomies to be performed and the fibula to be placed in an array of configurations, such as side-by-side, double-barrel, or encased in the medullary cavity of bones like the humerus or femur [15, 40, 43]. The main complication of the fibula flap is stress fracture, of which wide ranges have been reported (between 0% and 25%) [15, 42], probably owing to differences in fixation methods, weight-bearing protocols and the recipient bone's strain and location. Stress fractures usually happen within the first few months of weight-bearing, and can be treated nonsurgically if not displaced, on account of the flap's intrinsic healing capacity. Preventive measures include correct alignment and protected weight-bearing until adequate hypertrophy is obtained [42]. Other risks include microanastomotic thrombosis (<5% in experienced hands, with flap loss being rare) and nonunion (<8%) [6, 40]. Donor-site morbidity is not infrequent (about 10%) but is generally minor, including flexor hallucis longus contracture, transient numbness of the dorsum of the foot, and ankle pain [7, 40, 44].

The patients with infected critical bone defects most benefited by bone flaps are those with vascular compromise of the FRI site (they will benefit from the additional blood supply brought by the bone flap), such as after previous unsuccessful attempts with other techniques, and those with a soft tissue defect requiring tissue transfer (I3–4), as these patients will need a flap anyway [5, 15, 29]. Additionally, the larger the defect, the stronger the indication for a bone flap, because there will be less reconstructive alternatives available.

Techniques Based on Bone Replacement

Bone flaps replace the bone defect with healthy vascularized bone. Thus, they result in the shortest times to union, lowest complication rate and lowest number of surgical revisions. The tradeoffs are donor site morbidity and prolonged protected axial load.

The FRI patients that benefit the most from bone flaps are those with:

- Vascular compromise of the FRI site, e.g. previous unsuccessful attempts.
- Soft tissue defect requiring tissue transfer (I3–4).

Additionally, the larger the defect, the stronger the indication for a bone flap (there will be less alternatives for bone reconstruction).

Consider also that the higher degree of joint motion preservation in comparison with distraction osteogenesis techniques favors bone flaps for defects in the upper limb or in metaphyseal bone defects when the adjacent joint is still salvageable.

Clinical Cases

Case 5.1

A 47-year-old male, a diabetic smoker, had a medial opening wedge proximal tibial osteotomy performed at a different institution due to gonarthrosis. An intraoperative tibial plateau fracture was produced and fixed with a plate. A dehiscence exposing the plate ensued (F2 R2 I3). A debridement, antibiotics, and implant retention (DAIR) approach was carried out 4 weeks after the osteotomy, including the implantation of gentamicin-loaded calcium sulfate into the defect and a negative pressure wound therapy (NPWT) device. The patient was started on empirical intravenous vancomycin and gentamycin. Multiresistant *Staphylococcus haemolyticus* grew on cultures of intraoperative samples, so gentamycin was changed for amikacin (vancomycin was maintained). Purulent discharge persisted despite this treatment, so after 2 months the patient was referred to our institution (Fig. 5.3).

At our institution we first obtained samples, debrided the site, filled the 2 cm bone defect with vancomycin- and gentamycin-impregnated calcium sulphate and provided stable wound coverage with a medial gastrocnemius flap (Fig. 5.4, F4 R2 I3). The patient received empirical intravenous meropenem and daptomycin for 2 weeks, followed by oral levofloxacin and amoxicillin-clavulanic for 6 weeks (no microorganisms grew on intraoperative cultures). He had a good postoperative recovery, without pain or any signs of infection and quickly normalized serum biomarkers, so 1 month after the first stage we implanted a hexapod fixator and performed a corticotomy for ASRL. During the 1-month-long distraction, a pin broke. It was exchanged for a

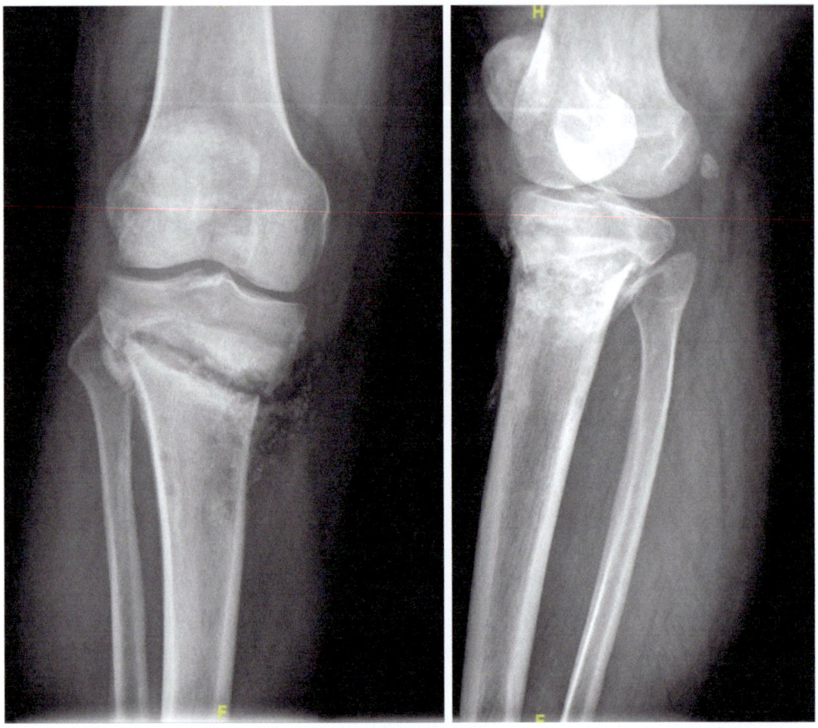

Fig. 5.3 Case 5.1, X-rays upon the patient's arrival to our institution, 4 months after osteosynthesis with a plate. A proximal tibia nonunion can be observed

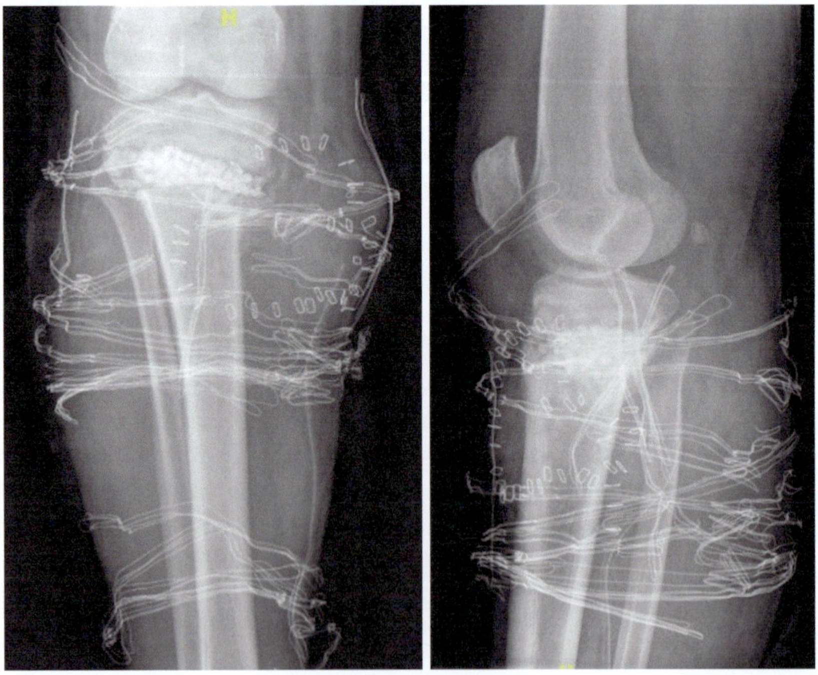

Fig. 5.4 Case 5.1, X-rays 1 day after sampling, debridement, implantation of vancomycin- and gentamycin-impregnated calcium sulfate into the tibial defect and coverage with a medial gastrocnemius flap

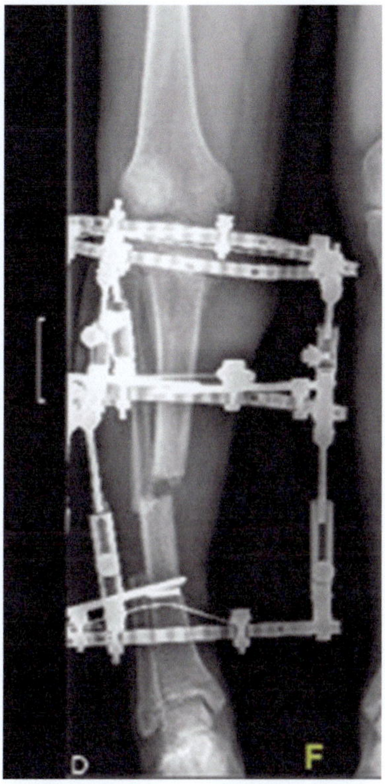

Fig. 5.5 Case 5.1, X-rays 3 weeks after starting distraction, when a broken pin was exchanged for a new one. Notice the 11° varus that had developed after pin breakage

new one, and the 11° varus that had developed after pin breakage was corrected (Fig. 5.5). Five months after circular fixator implantation, bone union was observed, and the fixator was removed. At the 1-year postoperative visit, the patient reported some difficulty in going up and down stairs but had no dysmetria and walked without aids (Fig. 5.6).

Case 5.2

A 54-year-old male, a smoker, suffered a comminute fracture of the right distal tibia after a 3-m fall (Fig. 5.7). He underwent surgery with a locked plate at a different institution (Fig. 5.8). Six months later, the patient presented with a swollen leg and a fistula with purulent discharge, without signs of bone union (F4 R2 I2), so he was taken back to the OR. He was sampled, debrided, the tibial hardware retained (the fibular osteosynthesis was removed) and the 2 cm tibial defect was filled with iliac bone autograft. The cultures from intraoperative samples did not exhibit bacterial growth. Initially, the postoperative recovery was satisfactory, without pain or signs of infection, and good bone healing progression on CT. However, at 6 months the patient developed a new fistula, and multiple screws had broken (Fig. 5.9, F4 R2 I3). He was started on empiric amoxicillin-clavulanic and was referred to our institution.

Our Bone Infections Committee recommended a free fibula flap, but the patient did not want morbidity on anatomical areas other than his right leg, so we offered him bone transport as a second choice, and he accepted. We first obtained samples, debrided thoroughly, implanted vancomycin- and gentamycin-impregnated calcium sulfate into the 7 cm defect, then performed a proximal tibial corticotomy and implanted a circular external fixator (Fig. 5.10). The patient was started on empiric intravenous daptomycin and piperacillin-tazobactam, which was switched to oral linezolid and rifampicin after *Staphylococcus pseudintermedius* and *Bacillus circulans* grew on cultures

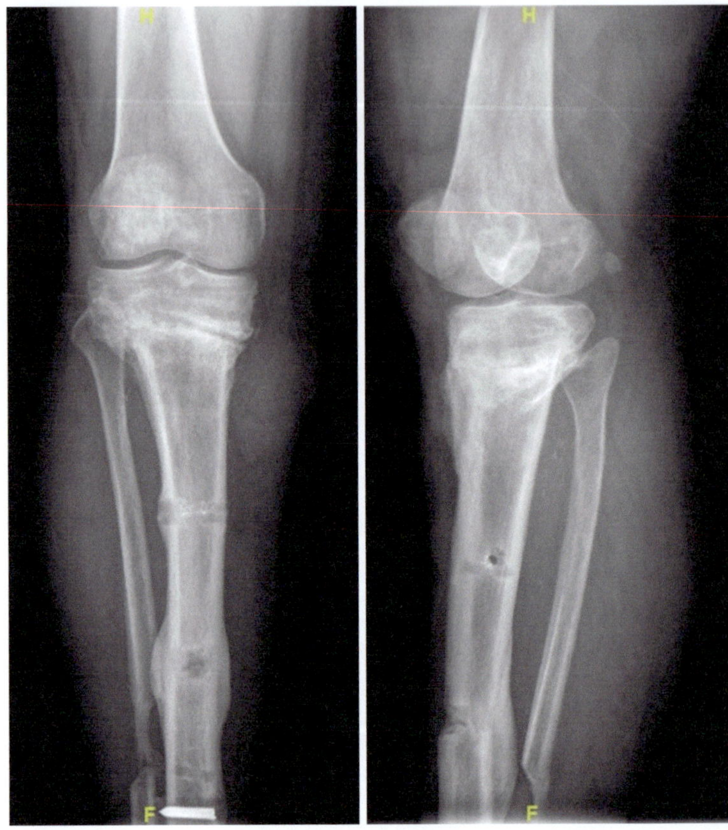

Fig. 5.6 Case 5.1, X-rays at 1 year postoperatively, showing good alignment and strengthening regenerate

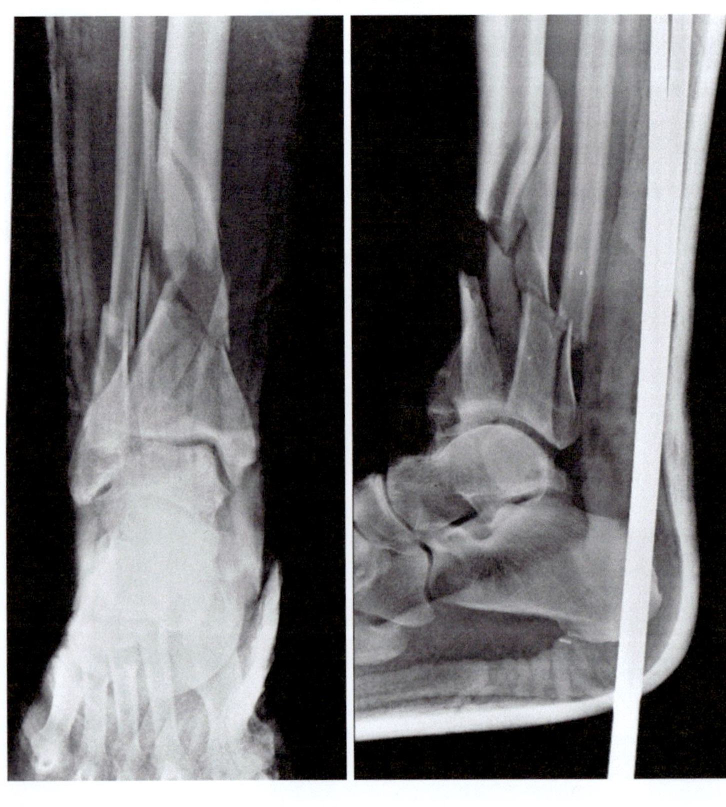

Fig. 5.7 Case 5.2, X-rays upon the patient's arrival to the emergency room, showing a comminute fracture of the right distal tibia

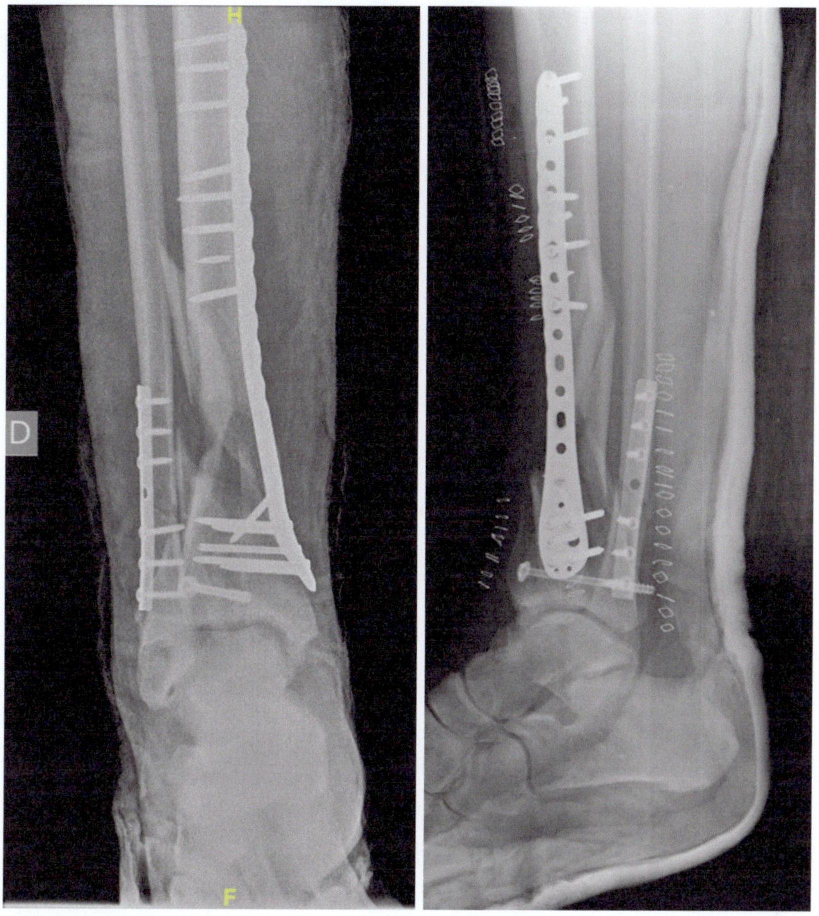

Fig. 5.8 Case 5.2, X-ray on the first postoperative day after tibial and fibula fractures reduction and plating

from intraoperative samples. Bone transport was carried out over 6 months without incidents, but the docking site did not show radiographic signs of bone union after 9 months (Fig. 5.11). We applied the accordion maneuver, but the nonunion at the docking site persisted, so we finally performed an ankle arthrodesis with a retrograde nail, augmented with a small amount of bone autograft. Union was observed a year after this last surgery, 6 years after the initial trauma (Fig. 5.12). At the last follow-up consultation, 9 years after the initial trauma, the patient walked painlessly without aids and was working.

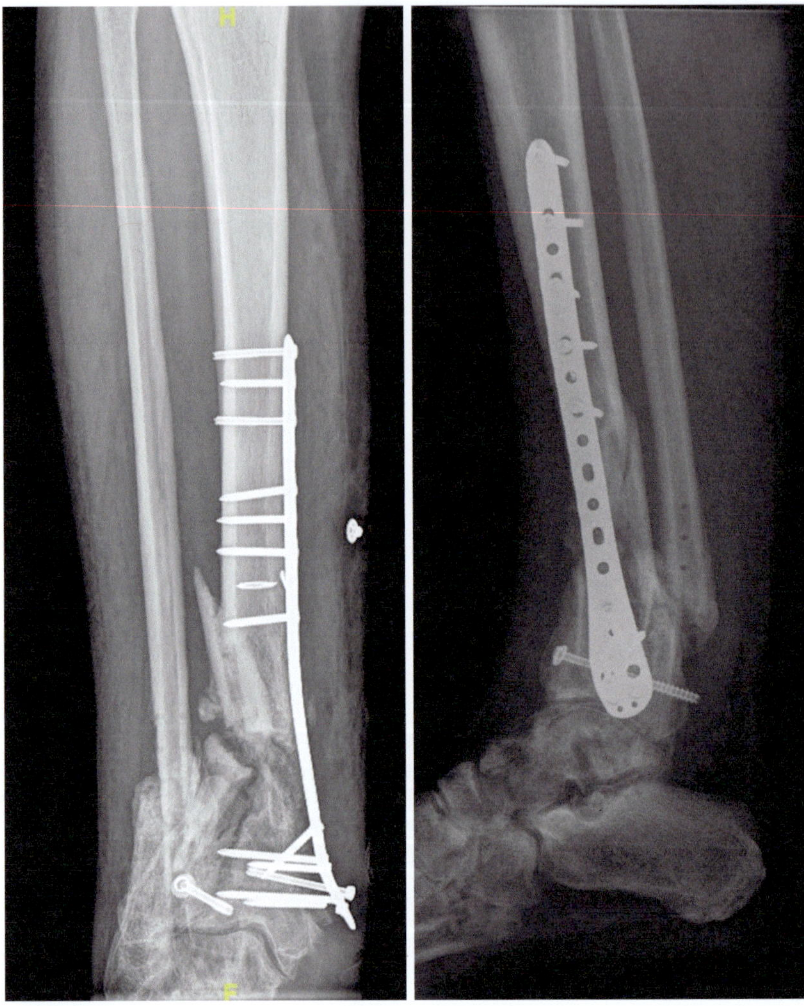

Fig. 5.9 Case 5.2, X-ray at 6 months after DAIR (debridement, antibiotics, and implant retention) and iliac crest autograft. Notice the multiple broken screws

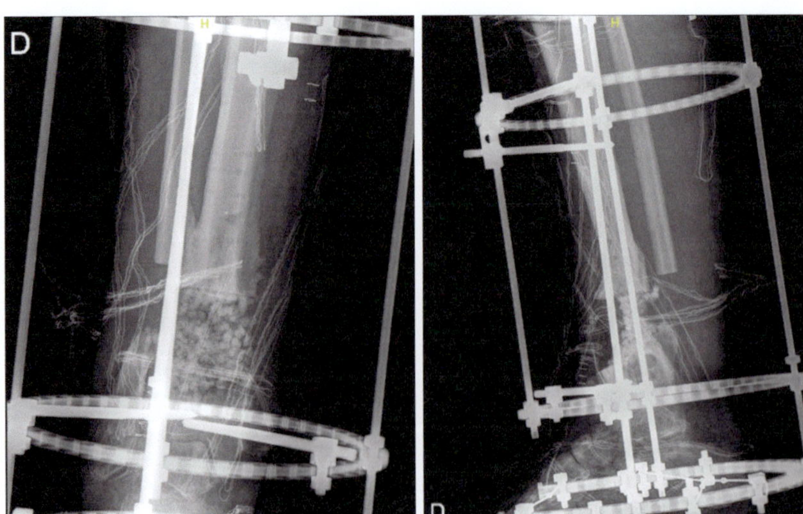

Fig. 5.10 Case 5.2, X-ray on the first postoperative day after sampling, debridement, placement of vancomycin- and gentamycin-impregnated calcium sulfate in the defect, proximal tibial corticotomy, and circular external fixator implantation for bone transport

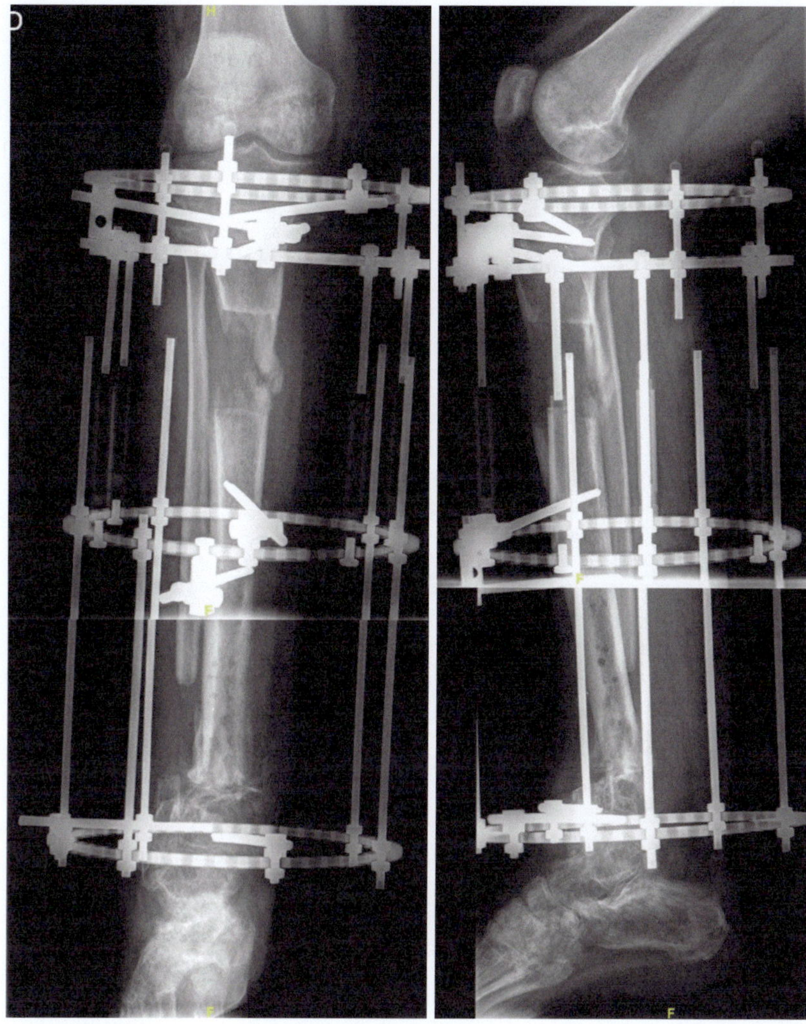

Fig. 5.11 Case 5.2, X-rays at 9 months after ending of the bone transport activation phase. The docking site has not yet consolidated

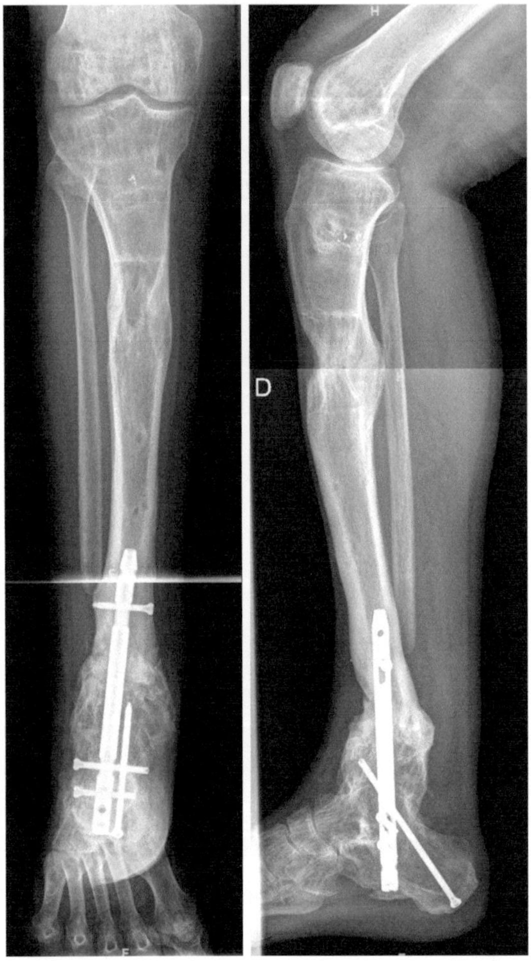

Fig. 5.12 Case 5.2, X-rays 1 year after ankle arthrodesis with a retrograde nail and a small amount of non-vascularized bone autograft. The nonunion site has healed

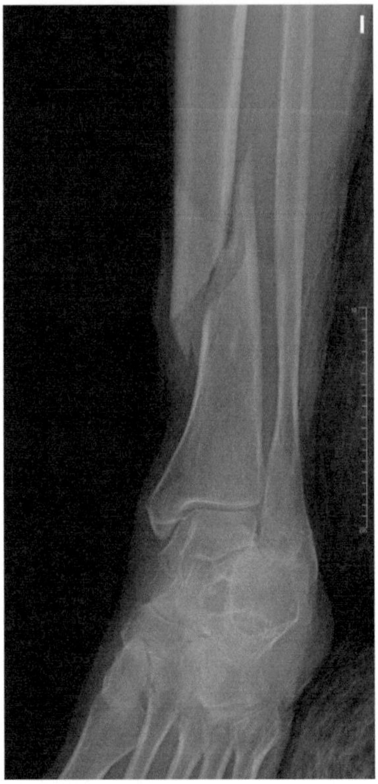

Fig. 5.13 Case 5.3, X-rays upon the patient's arrival to the emergency room, showing a left tibial diaphyseal fracture

Case 5.3

A 56-year-old female, an overweight smoker with chronic obstructive pulmonary disease, was admitted due to a left tibial diaphyseal fracture after a traffic accident (Fig. 5.13). She was treated with open reduction and internal fixation (Fig. 5.14), and quit smoking following her surgeon's recommendations. At 2 weeks postoperatively, the wound broke down, without exposing hardware, bone, or tendons, so it was treated conservatively with dressings and oral ciprofloxacin. At 3 months postoperatively, there were X-ray signs of partial consolidation, but the wound had worsened, exposing the tibialis anterior tendon (Fig. 5.15), so the patient was referred to our institution.

We obtained samples, removed the hardware, debrided thoroughly, filled the 8 cm segmental defect with a gentamicin- and vancomycin-impregnated PMMA spacer and implanted an external fixator (F4 R2 I4) (Fig. 5.16). The patient was started on intravenous daptomycin and piperacillin-tazobactam. After a week, we had culture results (ampicillin-resistant *Klebsiella oxytoca*) and the soft tissue conditions had improved, so we removed the PMMA spacer and reconstructed the bone defect with a free osteoseptocutaneous fibula flap (Fig. 5.17). At 2 weeks postoperatively, the patient's wounds had healed and she was discharged on oral ciprofloxacin. At 6 months postoperatively, there were X-ray signs of union at the ends of the fibula flap. At the three-year follow-up, the patient remained free of signs or symptoms of infection and walked painlessly without aids (Figs. 5.18 and 5.19).

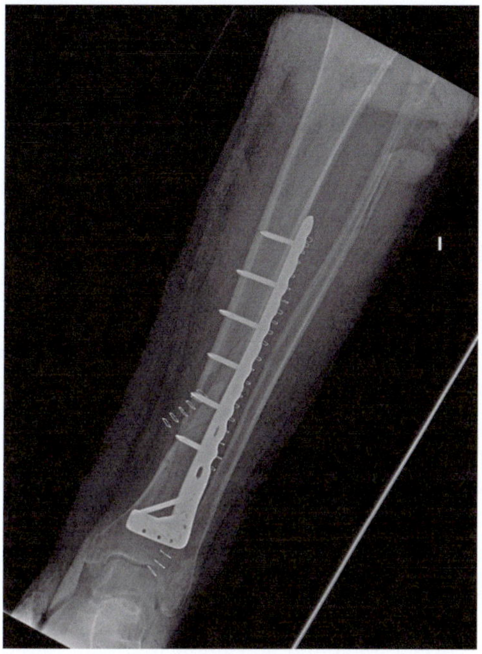

Fig. 5.14 Case 5.3, X-rays on the first postoperative day after reduction and osteosynthesis of the left tibial fracture

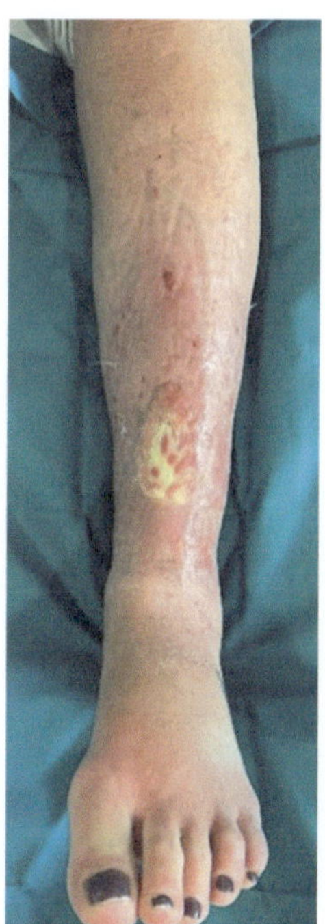

Fig. 5.15 Case 5.3, clinical appearance of the wound at 3 months postoperatively. The tibialis anterior tendon is exposed

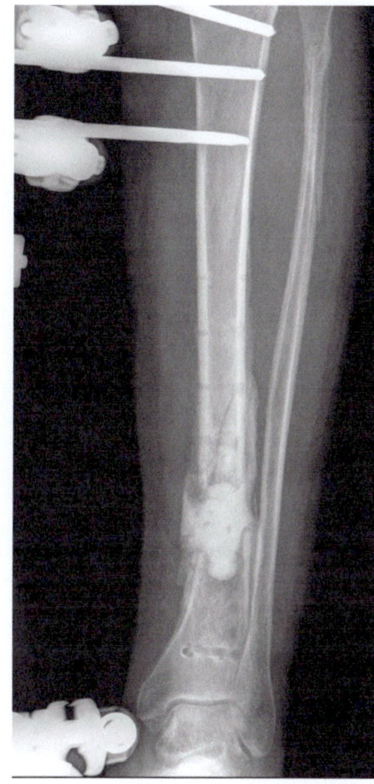

Fig. 5.16 Case 5.3, X-ray on the first postoperative day after sampling, debridement, antibiotic-loaded polymethylmethacrylate implantation, and external fixation

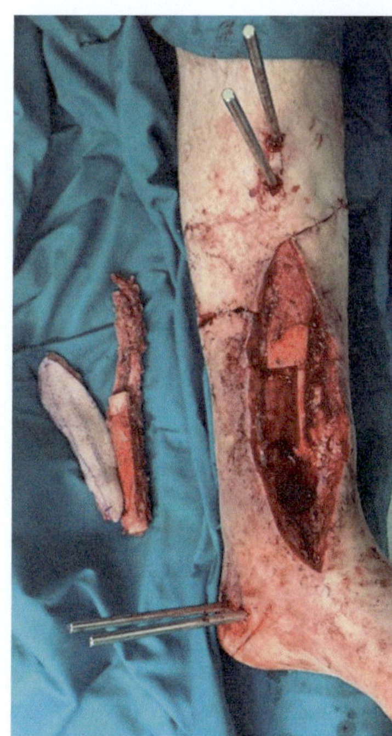

Fig. 5.17 Case 5.3, intraoperative picture showing the free fibula osteocutaneous flap

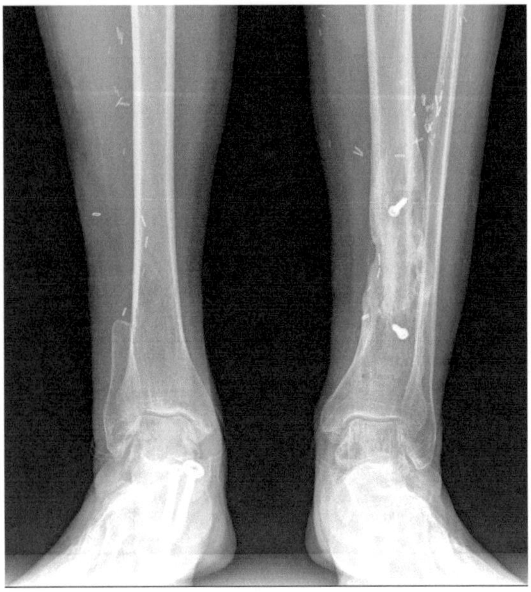

Fig. 5.18 Case 5.3, standing X-ray (anteroposterior view) 2 years after fibula flap transfer. Note the fibula flap's hypertrophy

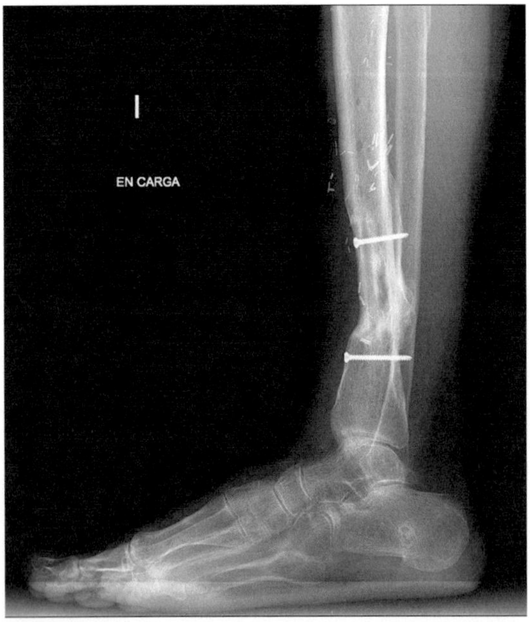

Fig. 5.19 Case 5.3, standing X-ray (lateral view of the left ankle) 2 years after fibula flap transfer. The screws, though excessively long, did not bother the patient so they were not removed

Conclusions

There is no gold standard for the treatment of infected bone defects. The reconstructive strategy will depend on the patient (their comorbidities, compliance, and preferences), their defect (location, size and shape, condition of surrounding soft tissues), and the team's experience and preferences.

Bone reconstruction techniques based on *local bone regeneration* depend on native bone ends for healing, so their outcomes will be better, the better the state of the bone ends. They comprise bone grafts and techniques based on osteogenesis distraction (ASRL and bone transport).

The patients that most benefit from bone autografts (in the context of Masquelet's induced membrane technique or not, with or without local antibiotics) are those with small defects, a healthy soft tissue envelope and good infection control. The larger the defect that bone autografts are used for, the higher the rate of resorption and infection recurrence.

Distraction osteogenesis techniques allow almost immediate loading, so they will be of greatest value in the lower limb, where they will enable early weight-bearing. Secondary procedures are the norm, not the exception (the most common one is docking-site grafting). Acute shortening manages simultaneously stability, dead space, and the soft tissues, so it is especially suitable for FRI patients with defects that will not need re-lengthening. ASRL is a good option for patients with infected bone defects up to 3–4 cm (some patients adapt to the specialized platform shoe well and decline re-lengthening). Bone transport is mostly used for infected bone defects of the lower limb between 4 and 10 cm, and is especially useful in patients with bone deformities and malalignments.

Bone reconstruction techniques based on *bone replacement* are bone flaps. They have the shortest time to union and lowest complication rate out of all the available techniques, at the cost of donor-site morbidity and prolonged protected axial load. The patients best benefited by bone flaps are those with vascular compromise of the FRI site (e.g., previous unsuccessful attempts), precarious soft tissue coverage (I3–4), an upper limb defect, or a metaphyseal bone defect. Additionally, the larger the defect, the stronger the indication for a bone flap (there will be less available techniques).

References

1. Bezstarosti H, Van Lieshout EMM, Voskamp LW, Kortram K, Obremskey W, McNally MA, Metsemakers WJ, Verhofstad MHJ. Insights into treatment and outcome of fracture-related infection: a systematic literature review. Arch Orthop Trauma Surg. 2019;139:61–72.
2. Nauth A, Schemitsch E, Norris B, Nollin Z, Watson JT. Critical-size bone defects: is there a consensus for diagnosis and treatment? J Orthop Trauma. 2018;32(Suppl 1):S7–S11.
3. Tetsworth KD, Burnand HG, Hohmann E, Glatt V. Classification of bone defects: an extension of the orthopaedic trauma association open fracture classification. J Orthop Trauma. 2021;35:71–6.
4. Barla JD. Fracture-related infections. In: Orthopaedics and trauma. Berlin: Springer Nature; 2024. p. 805–10.
5. Marais LC, Zalavras CG, Moriarty FT, Kühl R, Metsemakers W-J, Morgenstern M. The surgical management of fracture-related infection. Surgical strategy selection and the need for early surgical intervention. J Orthop. 2024;50:36–41.
6. Bezstarosti H, Metsemakers WJ, van Lieshout EMM, Voskamp LW, Kortram K, McNally MA, Marais LC, Verhofstad MHJ. Management of critical-sized bone defects in the treatment of fracture-related infection: a systematic review and pooled analysis. Arch Orthop Trauma Surg. 2021;141:1215–30.
7. Kadhim M, Holmes L, Gesheff MG, Conway JD. Treatment options for nonunion with segmental bone defects: systematic review and quantitative evidence synthesis. J Orthop Trauma. 2017;31:111–9.
8. Prada C, Bengoa F, Bhandari M. The management of fracture related infections: what practices can be supported by high-level evidence? J Orthop Surg (Hong Kong). 2022;30:10225536221119580.
9. Metsemakers W-J, Morgenstern M, Senneville E, et al. General treatment principles for fracture-related infection: recommendations from an international expert group. Arch Orthop Trauma Surg. 2020;140:1013–27.
10. Azoury SC, Stranix JT, Kovach SJ, Levin LS. Principles of orthoplastic surgery for lower extremity reconstruction: why is this important? J Reconstr Microsurg. 2021;37:42–50.
11. Lu V, Zhang J, Patel R, Zhou AK, Thahir A, Krkovic M. Fracture related infections and their risk factors for treatment failure-a major trauma Centre perspective. Diagnostics (Basel). 2022;12:1289.
12. Chaudhary MM. Infected nonunion of tibia. Indian J Orthop. 2017;51:256–68.
13. Anagnostakos K, Schröder K. Antibiotic-impregnated bone grafts in orthopaedic and trauma surgery: a systematic review of the literature. Int J Biomater. 2012;2012:538061.
14. He S-Y, Yu B, Jiang N. Current concepts of fracture-related infection. Int J Clin Pract. 2023;2023:4839701.
15. del Piñal F, Innocenti M. Evolving concepts in the management of the bone gap in the upper limb. Long and small defects. J Plast Reconstr Aesthet Surg. 2007;60:776–92.
16. Panteli M, Giannoudis PV. Chronic osteomyelitis: what the surgeon needs to know. EFORT Open Rev. 2016;1:128–35.
17. Masquelet AC, Fitoussi F, Begue T, Muller GP. Reconstruction of the long bones by the induced membrane and spongy autograft. Ann Chir Plast Esthet. 2000;45:346–53.
18. Tsang S-TJ, Ferreira N, Simpson AHRW. The reconstruction of critical bone loss. Bone Joint Res. 2022;11:409–12.
19. Wang J, Yin Q, Gu S, Wu Y, Rui Y. Induced membrane technique in the treatment of infectious bone defect: a clinical analysis. Orthop Traumatol Surg Res. 2019;105:535–9.
20. Morelli I, Drago L, George DA, Gallazzi E, Scarponi S, Romanò CL. Masquelet technique: myth or reality? A systematic review and meta-analysis. Injury. 2016;47(Suppl 6):S68–76.
21. Metsemakers W-J, Fragomen AT, Moriarty TF, Morgenstern M, Egol KA, Zalavras C, Obremskey WT, Raschke M, McNally MA. Evidence-based recommendations for local antimicrobial strategies and dead space Management in Fracture-Related Infection. J Orthop Trauma. 2020;34:18–29.
22. Wildemann B, Ignatius A, Leung F, Taitsman LA, Smith RM, Pesántez R, Stoddart MJ, Richards RG, Jupiter JB. Non-union bone fractures. Nat Rev Dis Primers. 2021;7:57.
23. Emara KM, Ghafar KAA, Al Kersh MA. Methods to shorten the duration of an external fixator in the management of tibial infections. World J Orthop. 2011;2:85–92.
24. Chan JKK, Ferguson JY, Scarborough M, McNally MA, Ramsden AJ. Management of post-traumatic osteomyelitis in the lower limb: current state of the art. Indian J Plast Surg. 2019;52:62–72.
25. Yin P, Ji Q, Li T, et al. A systematic review and meta-analysis of Ilizarov methods in the treatment of infected nonunion of tibia and femur. PLoS One. 2015;10:e0141973.
26. Salcedo Cánovas C, Martínez Ros J, Ondoño Navarro A, Molina González J, Hernández Torres A, Moral Escudero E, Medina Quirós M. Infected bone defects in the lower limb. Management by means of a two-

stage distraction osteogenesis protocol. Eur J Orthop Surg Traumatol. 2021;31:1375–86.
27. Kukreja K, Reyaz S, Kumar MN. Outcome of bone transport using Ilizarov external fixator in infected non-union of tibia with large bone defects: comparison of those with 5–10 cm bone defect with those having ≥ 11 cm bone defect. Indian J Orthop. 2024;58:345–53.
28. Tetsworth K, Paley D, Sen C, Jaffe M, Maar DC, Glatt V, Hohmann E, Herzenberg JE. Bone transport versus acute shortening for the management of infected tibial non-unions with bone defects. Injury. 2017;48:2276–84.
29. Ren G-H, Li R, Hu Y, Chen Y, Chen C, Yu B. Treatment options for infected bone defects in the lower extremities: free vascularized fibular graft or Ilizarov bone transport? J Orthop Surg Res. 2020;15:439.
30. Wen H, Zhu S, Li C, Xu Y. Bone transport versus acute shortening for the management of infected tibial bone defects: a meta-analysis. BMC Musculoskelet Disord. 2020;21:80.
31. Rigal S, Merloz P, Le Nen D, Mathevon H, Masquelet A-C, French Society of Orthopaedic Surgery and Traumatology (SoFCOT). Bone transport techniques in posttraumatic bone defects. Orthop Traumatol Surg Res. 2012;98:103–8.
32. Tennyson M, Krzak AM, Krkovic M, Abdulkarim A. Cambridge protocol for management of segmental bone loss. J Orthop Case Rep. 2021;11:45–50.
33. Liu K, Zhang H, Maimaiti X, Yusufu A. Bifocal versus trifocal bone transport for the management of tibial bone defects caused by fracture-related infection: a meta-analysis. J Orthop Surg Res. 2023;18:140.
34. Kocaoglu M, Eralp L, Rashid HU, Sen C, Bilsel K. Reconstruction of segmental bone defects due to chronic osteomyelitis with use of an external fixator and an intramedullary nail. J Bone Joint Surg Am. 2006;88:2137–45.
35. Maimaiti X, Liu K, Yusufu A, Xie Z. Treatment of tibial bone defects caused by infection: a retrospective comparative study of bone transport using a combined technique of unilateral external fixation over an intramedullary nail versus circular external fixation over an intramedullary nail. BMC Musculoskelet Disord. 2024;25:284.
36. Huang Q, Xu YB, Ren C, et al. Bone transport combined with bone graft and internal fixation versus simple bone transport in the treatment of large bone defects of lower limbs after trauma. BMC Musculoskelet Disord. 2022;23:157.
37. Blair JA, Puneky GA, Swaminathan N, Klahs KJ, Davis JM. Tibial bone transport with a single implant all-internal bone transport nail. J Orthop Trauma. 2023;37:e294–300.
38. Stoneback JW, Erdman MK, Marecek GS. Management of segmental tibial bone defects with a motorized intramedullary bone transport nail: a case review with follow-up. J Orthop Trauma. 2021;35:S13–8.
39. Makhdom AM, Cartaleanu AS, Rendon JS, Villemure I, Hamdy RC. The accordion maneuver: a noninvasive strategy for absent or delayed callus formation in cases of limb lengthening. Adv Orthop. 2015;2015:912790.
40. Shin EH, Shin AY. Vascularized bone grafts in orthopaedic surgery. JBJS Rev. 2017;5:e1.
41. Al Deek NF, Kao H-K, Wei F-C. The fibula osteoseptocutaneous flap: concise review, goal-oriented surgical technique, and tips and tricks. Plast Reconstr Surg. 2018;142:913e–23e.
42. Beris AE, Lykissas MG, Korompilias AV, Vekris MD, Mitsionis GI, Malizos KN, Soucacos PN. Vascularized fibula transfer for lower limb reconstruction. Microsurgery. 2011;31:205–11.
43. Tu Y-K, Yen C-Y. Role of vascularized bone grafts in lower extremity osteomyelitis. Orthop Clin North Am. 2007;38(37–49):vi.
44. Ling XF, Peng X. What is the price to pay for a free fibula flap? A systematic review of donor-site morbidity following free fibula flap surgery. Plast Reconstr Surg. 2012;129:657–74.

Transfer of Vascularized Bone in Fracture-Related Infection

6

Fernando Holc, Pedro Bronenberg Victorica, Nieves Vanaclocha, and Jorge Guillermo Boretto

Introduction

Fracture-related infections (FRIs) are a major challenge in orthopedic surgery. Their management is especially complex when they are associated with critical-size bone defects, that is, those that do not heal without intervention [1, 2].

Several techniques are available to address infected bone defects. The choice of surgical technique is based on several factors, including the defect's characteristics (location, size, and shape), the condition of the surrounding soft tissues, the patient's comorbidities and treatment compliance, as well as the surgeon's experience and preferences [3–5]. For more information on technique selection, refer to complementary Chap. 5.

One of the available techniques is bone flaps. In this chapter, we will focus on how bone flaps differ from other alternatives in FRI treatment, which patients benefit the most from them, which bone flaps are most frequently used in the context of FRI, and what their possible complications are.

How Do Bone Flaps Differ from Other Alternatives in FRI Treatment?

The techniques to address infected critical bone defects can be broadly divided into two groups: those based on local bone regeneration and those based on bone replacement.

Techniques based on local bone regeneration are faster and less invasive than bone flaps but rely on local bone and soft tissues (usually scarred from the trauma and prolonged inflammation) for healing. Thus, they have better outcomes, the better the state of the local tissues. They include non-vascularized bone grafts (in the context of Masquelet's induced membrane technique or not, with or without antibiotics) and techniques based on osteogenic distraction (acute shortening and re-lengthening, and bone transport).

The patients that most benefit from non-vascularized bone autografts are those with small defects with good soft tissue coverage and infection control (the larger the defect, the higher the rate of resorption and infection recurrence). Creeping substitution is slow and unreliable, so results of bone grafting are unpredictable, and regrafting is often necessary.

F. Holc · P. Bronenberg Victorica · J. G. Boretto (✉)
Hand and Upper Extremity Department, Instituto de Ortopedia y Traumatología "Prof. Dr. Carlos Ottolenghi". Hospital Italiano de Buenos Aires, Ciudad Autónoma de Buenos Aires, Argentina
e-mail: jorge.boretto@hospitalitaliano.org.ar

N. Vanaclocha
Orthoplastics Unit and Department of Plastic and Reconstructive Surgery, University and Polytechnic Hospital La Fe, Valencia, Spain

N. Vanaclocha (ed.), *Treatment of Fracture-Related Infection*,
https://doi.org/10.1007/978-3-031-92452-1_6

Techniques based on osteogenic distraction allow early weight-bearing, but need prolonged external fixation and associate a high number of secondary procedures. The bigger the defect to be reconstructed, the longer the external fixation time and so the greater the involvement of nearby joints (namely, joint stiffness).

Techniques based on bone replacement involve the provision of non-native, healthy bone that speeds consolidation, at the cost of donor site morbidity and prolonged protected axial load. This group comprises *bone flaps*, also referred to as "vascularized bone grafts." In this publication, we will only use the term "bone flaps" to avoid confusion with non-vascularized bone grafts, which (unlike flaps) are avascular. As we will see, this difference in vascularity is responsible for most of the advantages and drawbacks of flaps.

A bone flap is a segment of living bone that remains attached to its vascular pedicle and is transferred from its original location to a new location [6]. The pedicle can be divided and re-anastomosed to recipient vessels elsewhere (*free flap*, which can be transferred to anywhere in the body as long as there are available recipient vessels) or left attached to its original donor vessels (*pedicled flap*, which can move only as far as the pedicle will stretch without vasospasm and consequent ischemia) [7]. The choice between using a pedicled or a free bone flap depends mainly on the availability of an appropriate pedicled flap (proximity of potential donor sites, sufficient reach of the pedicle (length and arc of rotation), feasibility of harvesting as much bone from the donor as the recipient needs), as free flaps involve microsurgery, which is much more technically demanding [8]. In FRI, nearby bone is seldom usable as a flap because of its involvement in either the initial trauma or the subsequent infection, so most often, free flaps will be needed.

The flap pedicle contains vessels that supply blood to the bone through transosseous and/or periosteal vessels [9]. This *intrinsic blood supply* allows the transplanted bone to remain alive at its new location, regardless of the conditions of the local tissues, and is responsible for most of the advantages of bone flaps in the FRI scenario:

- It aids infection eradication by allowing immune cells and antibiotics to reach the FRI site [10]. Patients treated with bone flaps had the lowest infection recurrence rates in a meta-analysis comparing outcomes after (nonvascularized) bone grafts, induced membrane technique, bone transport, and bone flaps [11].
- It enables primary bone healing through the action of live osteoblasts, even in the most challenging scenarios [13]. The union rates reported for infected bone defects treated with bone flaps are over 80%, with faster mean times to union (just under 5 months) than the rest of the techniques (infection being a risk factor for delayed bone healing [14, 15]) [9, 16–18].
- It allows bone flaps to retain their biomechanical properties. As well as the abovementioned improved bone healing, bone flaps hypertrophy in response to mechanical loading, and have scarce bone resorption (since the osseous tissue in bone flaps is alive, bone flaps do not undergo creeping substitution) [6, 7, 12].
- The same pedicle can nurture both bone and other tissular components such as skin and/or muscles (composite flaps), which can be used to manage soft tissue defects and/or dead space simultaneously.

In other words, the main advantage of bone flaps is their reliability. That is, they survive reliably in hostile environments, fight infection, and lead to predictable union if the principles of FRI management have been observed [19]. Other advantages include their versatility (they can include corticocancellous bone, periosteum, epiphysis, and joint), and the fact that they only require a single surgical procedure [8].

However, there are also significant drawbacks to bone flap use. They include donor-site morbidity, which is frequently not insignificant (see section *What Are the Complications of Bone Flaps?* below), as well as longer surgical times and a higher technical demand. Free bone flaps require high technical expertise, a qualified team, and rigorous postoperative follow-up, as well as being particularly challenging in the setting of FRI (recipient dissection is difficult and cumbersome, the recipients are usually far away from the FRI site, vasospasm is common, etc.). Consequently, in many institutions, this type of procedure is not available.

Which Patients Benefit the Most from Treatment with Bone Flaps?

As previously pointed out, bone flaps entail donor-site morbidity, which must be weighed against the advantages of using a bone flap. The FRI patients that will benefit the most from bone flaps are those which have poor vascularity of FRI site (inadequate blood supply to the defect), such as after previous unsuccessful attempts with other techniques, or the need for concomitant soft tissue coverage with a flap (these patients will need a flap anyway) [6, 20–22].

Additionally, bone flaps are the preferred technique in bone defects described as large [7], but how big the defect should be to consider a bone flap is a matter of great debate. It was traditionally considered from 6 cm onward for long bones, mainly because for smaller defects, many other, simpler and less morbid techniques exist as well (and will often suffice) [23, 24]. However, there is no evidence in the literature to support this (or any other) cutoff point [25]. The ability of bone flaps to improve local blood supply to infected and scarred areas in FRI sites has led many teams to challenge the size criterion [21, 26]. It is overall accepted that, in general, the larger the defect, the stronger the indication for a bone flap (some teams refer to a defect over 12 cm as an absolute indication [27]), but the opposite is not true: the smaller the defect, the more important other factors (e.g., previous failed attempts) are to take this decision.

Bone flaps are also especially suitable for critical bone defects in the upper limb, particularly in the forearm. This is because they preserve joint motion better than the rest of available techniques to manage bone defects, and due to the issues associated with external fixation in this location (difficult implantation, risk of nearby tendons' attritional rupture) [21].

Consider that patients must be fit enough for a lengthy surgical procedure, so very comorbid hosts (R4–5) are seldom candidates for bone flaps. In addition, deformity correction with bone flaps is challenging, so techniques such as bone transport are often more suitable in patients with malalignments.

What Are the Most Commonly Used Bone Flaps for FRI?

Many bone flaps have been described, such as the fibula, iliac crest, ribs, scapula, medial femoral condyle (MFC), distal radius, metacarpal, and carpal bones. Among them, the fibula flap is the most employed [8].

Fibula Flap

The fibula flap is the workhorse for bone reconstruction in FRI, mostly due to its structure and shape. The fibula flap is well-suited for long bones' reconstruction because it is long and tubular (its width and harvestable length resemble particularly well those of the forearm bones) and it provides a long, robust corticocancellous segment [11, 20]. Small segments must be preserved for proximal and distal tibiofibular joint stability (minimum 4 cm proximally and 6 cm from the distal fibula in adults), leaving a segment of over 25 cm (or even more in tall individuals) that can be safely harvested.

The fibula flap can be pedicled (by medializing it into the ipsilateral tibia, for segmental defects of the shaft) or free. It has dual vascularity, with endosteal and periosteal blood supply, which allows for corticotomies that then enable several insetting configurations [9, 10, 21]:

- A simple segment, such as for a long tibial defect.
- Double-barrel, to increase stability by duplicating cross-sectional area. It is the preferred configuration in the femur, where possible.
- In the humerus, tibia, and femur, the fibula flap can be encased into the medullary cavity

and/or embedded into a proximal and/or distal step-cut osteotomy, to increase stability of the construct and reduce the amount of hardware needed [9, 28]. These osteotomies are especially useful in the humerus to help deal with torsion forces but are technically demanding, as they must be done very precisely to obtain adequate bone contact and avoid secondary malrotations.

- Onlayed onto another bone, with or without vertical osteotomies.
- A vertical osteotomy can be performed along the fibula flap for simultaneous reconstruction of the radius and ulna [29].
- Multi-segment, when nonlinear shapes are needed (this scenario is rare in the setting of FRI).

The main arterial supply is endosteal, provided by branches from the peroneal artery (diameter of 1.5–2.5 mm) and its vena comitans, in a pedicle 2–6 cm long [9, 19]. This length can be extended by meticulously dissecting the periosteum on which the pedicle runs (beware, it is very easy to damage the pedicle with this maneuver). The pedicle gives branches to other tissues too, allowing inclusion of a skin paddle of up to about 10 × 20 cm and/or a muscle segment (flexor hallucis longus, soleus), if needed. It should be taken into account that when a skin paddle is harvested, primary closure is rarely possible and skin grafting is usually needed.

Donor-site morbidity, though not rare, is usually minor. A systematic review of 2534 free fibula flap procedures reported mostly wound healing complications in the early postoperative period (delayed wound healing, 17.4%) and functional complications at a later stage (limited ankle range of motion, 11.5%; temporary sensory deficit, 6.9%; ankle pain, 6.5%; claw toe, 6.1%; ankle instability, 5.8%), with a mean American Orthopedic Foot and Ankle Society score of 85.5% [30]. After healing of the free fibula flap, most patients are able to walk without gait aids [6]. In a study evaluating patients in which a free fibula flap had been performed to reconstruct a bone defect in the upper limb, all those who had suffered donor-site complications reported that the benefits of the fibula flap compensated their donor site morbidity [31].

Iliac Crest Flap

The iliac crest flap was first described in 1979 as an osteocutaneous flap [32, 33]. It provides a segment of 4–8 × 2–5 cm of corticocancellous bone (harvest of up to 15 cm has been described), uni- or bicortical, of predominantly cancellous composition. Its arterial supply, based on the deep circumflex iliac vessels, allows for composite harvest with a skin paddle of up to 10 × 20 cm (though direct closure is very unlikely if the paddle is over 8 cm wide) and/or an obliquus externus abdominis muscle strip if needed. The primary benefit of this flap is the large caliber of its pedicle (average 2.5 mm). Its curvature has been used advantageously to reconstruct the distal humerus, though only a few case reports exist, and long-term functional outcomes have not been reported on for this indication [28].

Its current use in FRI is scarce mostly due to its shape, as its curved anatomy restricts its utility in long bone reconstruction and usually implies the need of a corticotomy to allow insetting. Other disadvantages of this flap include its bulkiness (especially inconvenient in the upper limb), a demanding surgical technique, and the potential donor-site morbidity, which includes pain (26%), numbness (damage to lateral femoral cutaneous and ilioinguinal, >40%), gait disturbance (20%), limited walking or stair climbing (6%), herniation (3%), and contour deformity of the hip (patients struggle to wear belts) [34]. Small flaps have low morbidity, but donor morbidity increases rapidly as flap size increases. Due to these drawbacks, the iliac crest flap is mostly reserved for cases where the fibula flap is unavailable.

Medial Femoral Condyle Flap

The use of the MFC flap has grown since its description in 1991 [35, 36]. The pedicle provides a rich vascularity with a mean of 30 corticoperiosteal perforators before entering the cortex [36]. It is usually dependent on the descending geniculate artery (1.5 mm diameter), which provides a pedicle length of about 8–10 cm, but not infrequently stems from the superior medial genicular artery, which provides a much shorter (3–4 cm) and harder-to-dissect pedicle.

The MFC flap is most often harvested as a corticoperiosteal flap, but can also be a purely periosteal, a corticocancellous, or an osteoarticular flap by incorporating part of the medial femoral trochlea. Its main advantages are its thinness (minimal bulk) and adaptability, which allow it to be shaped to fit small and irregular bone defects, coupled with low donor-site morbidity. It is usually used for defects up to 5 cm (in which a fibula or iliac crest flap might feel excessive), such as the bones of the hand (scaphoid, phalanges), the clavicle, or more rarely, the talus [6]. Though it is possible to harvest up to 24 cm^2 of bone (without differences in femoral stability in cadaver models), the risk of femur fracture increases significantly if more than 7 cm of cortex are harvested. If size is kept under 5 cm and the bone harvested from the *anterior* half of the femoral cortex (the posterior half being more important for axial stability), morbidity is minimal (<2% of cases, usually knee pain) [37, 38]. Osteonecrosis of the femoral condyle has been anecdotally described [39], but the centrifugal blood flow from the medullary cavity to the cortical bone should not be damaged during this procedure so some authors hold the MFC unaccountable [38].

The periosteal variant of the MFC flap has intrinsic bone-forming potential and is thin and very pliable, allowing it to be wrapped around infected nonunion sites with minimal or no bone defect [40]. It is especially appropriate for the distal part of the upper limb (radius, ulna, metacarpals, phalanges), where there are many tendons, so minimal bulk is needed [21].

Other, less Often Used Flaps

Other periosteal flaps include the one based on the peroneal artery, which has been applied mostly in children with infected nonunions because these patients usually have minimal bone defects and a thick periosteum that lends itself to dissection nicely (unlike the periosteum in adults, which is thin and very fragile) [41, 42].

The distal radius flap can be used either free as a composite radial forearm flap, or (the more common scenario) as a pedicled bone flap based on the fourth and fifth compartment arteries for small defects of adjacent bones (hand and wrist). It can provide up to 1.5 × 6 cm of bone (no more than 25% of its circumference should be harvested). As with the MFC flap, it is best kept smaller to reduce the risk of radius fractures that are difficult to treat. In fact, some surgeons advocate for prophylactic plating if a flap on the larger end of the spectrum (5 cm or more) is needed [43].

The rib flap is a rare option due to the curvature of the ribs, which almost always imposes the need for unicortical corticotomies for insetting, and its potential donor-site morbidity, which is infrequent but serious (pneumo- or hemothorax).

The pedicle is long, and multiple ribs can be harvested (ideally, nonconsecutive ribs to reduce donor morbidity). It can also incorporate a latissimus dorsi or serratus anterior segment.

Rib flaps are usually reserved for situations in which the fibula flap is unavailable and/or in the rare event of infected spinal fractures, where substitution of hardware by pedicled rib flaps can be a viable option.

The scapula flap is based on the superficial circumflex scapular artery. About 10 cm of bone can be harvested, typically from the lateral edge as it provides greater bone stock. A variant is the scapular tip bone flap, of about 5–6 cm in length (2–3 cm wide), based on the angular branch of the thoracodorsal artery, which can be pedicled for the humerus. In both cases, the main advantage is the large caliber, long, consistent pedicle, and the great variety of composite flaps it allows. For example, the scapula can be harvested with a big skin paddle (8 × 20 cm) or a segment of latissimus dorsi muscle (plus/minus its overlying skin).

Both the scapula and the scapula tip flaps are bulky, as the surrounding soft tissues cannot be dissected off aggressively to ensure good osseous vascularization. This bulkiness and their shape make them well-suited for reconstructing the upper maxilla but much less so for long bones, especially those in the upper limb, where bulkiness will make the insetting particularly challenging. Moreover, though harvest in decubitus supinus position is possible, many teams are unaccustomed to this approach and harvest it in decubitus pronus, which most often implies an intraoperative change of patient position for insetting, lengthening surgical time. It is also worth noting that the harvest of these flaps requires detachment of the teres major muscle from the harvested bone (as well as teres minor muscle in large flaps), which is then reattached to the remaining scapula. Though long-term shoulder dysfunctions are rare, the ensuing postoperative shoulder rehabilitation is long and painful for patients, and persistent shoulder pain has been reported.

Choice of Flap

Reported union rates and time to union for the different flaps are similar and high (though evidence on flaps other than the fibula or iliac crest is mostly composed of small series of case reports) [44–47]. Thus, the choice of flap will depend on:

- The size and shape of the defect. For instance, small defects may be amenable to reconstruction with an MFC or distal radius flap, whereas a fibula flap will be needed for large defects.
- Structural needs of the recipient bone (e.g., to reconstruct weight-bearing bones, the fibula flap is preferred as it provides the highest amount of cortical bone).
- Other needs of the reconstruction, such as concomitant management of dead space (is a segment of muscle needed?) and/or the soft tissue envelope (the skin paddle must be large enough to cover the soft tissue defect, if one is present).
- Patient preferences or concerns about donor-site morbidity (e.g., the contour deformity after iliac crest flap harvest is a frequent complaint, especially in relation to wearing belts).
- The surgeons' skills and experience.

A Word on Preoperative Planning

As pointed out in previous chapters, thorough preoperative planning is crucial for bone reconstruction, particularly in cases of FRI [6]. Patient comorbidities, such as malnutrition, age, diabetes, and factors influencing wound healing or flap survival, must be optimized [5, 48]. In particular, smoking substantially affects flap viability and both bone and wound healing, so smokers must quit before reconstruction is initiated [49, 50]. Diabetes and malnutrition can impact surgical outcomes and increase the risk of postoperative complications, so nutritional (including both malnutrition and obesity) and glycemic optimization before surgery is also a must [51–53]. The patients' psychological state also plays a significant role, as reconstructive surgery requires a motivated and cooperative patient [54].

Consider also that these patients have often undergone severe injuries and multiple surgeries, so the presence or viability of the local arteries may be altered. At the very least, peripheral pulses (anterior and posterior tibial or radial and ulnar) should be palpated, and if altered, imaging studies such as angiography or ultrasound carried out [55]. If computed tomography (CT) imaging is available, it is generally wise to order an angio-CT to evaluate the state of potential recipient vessels, since CT imaging will be obtained from most patients anyway to evaluate bone healing and the presence of fistulae or sequestra, and because it will avoid intraoperative surprises.

What Are the Possible Complications of Bone Flaps?

In a meta-analysis comparing outcomes after (non-vascularized) bone grafts, Masquelet's induced membrane technique, bone transport, and bone flaps, *bone flaps* resulted in the lowest complication rate and the lowest amount of surgical revisions by far [11]. This may seem paradoxical, as bone flaps are the most demanding technique surgically out of those described, but is a direct and logical consequence of the intrinsic vascularization of flaps, which aids every aspect of healing (infection eradication, bone union, wound healing, etc.).

Recurrence of infection (<10%) and non-union (< 8%), common to all FRI surgeries, are lower after treatment with bone flaps than after treatment with (non-vascularized) bone grafts, Masquelet's induced membrane technique or bone transport [11, 44, 58, 59].

Stress fractures of bone flaps are not uncommon, especially of the fibula flap, as it is the preferred flap when a weight-bearing bone is involved. Wide ranges (0–25%) have been reported for this complication [1, 10, 11], probably as a result of differences in [21]:

- Bone fixation (minimal osteosynthesis confers a lower risk of infection recurrence, but a higher risk of stress fracture).
- Weight-bearing protocols (some teams allow earlier weight-bearing than others).
- The recipient bone's strain (the stress fracture risk is higher when the recipient bone sustains higher forces). Accordingly, stress fractures occur most often when the recipient is in the lower limb, though they can also occur in the upper extremities. The risk of stress fracture is maximal when the fibula flap is used to reconstruct a defect in the contralateral lower limb, because both patient's legs have been operated on, so the patient will tend to put some weight onto the recipient limb earlier than patients in which the recipient is in the same lower limb as the donor.

Bone flap stress fractures are more likely to happen in the first year after surgery, when not enough time has elapsed for the bone undergo hypertrophy [15, 56, 57]. Though these fractures promote callus formation and accelerate bone hypertrophy, it is important to limit weight-bearing until there is evidence of flap union and hypertrophy. In addition, it is crucial to select an adequate method of internal or external bone fixation to prevent the displacement and instability of fractures caused by stress (Fig. 6.1).

Donor-site morbidities have been previously described for each of the flaps discussed in this chapter.

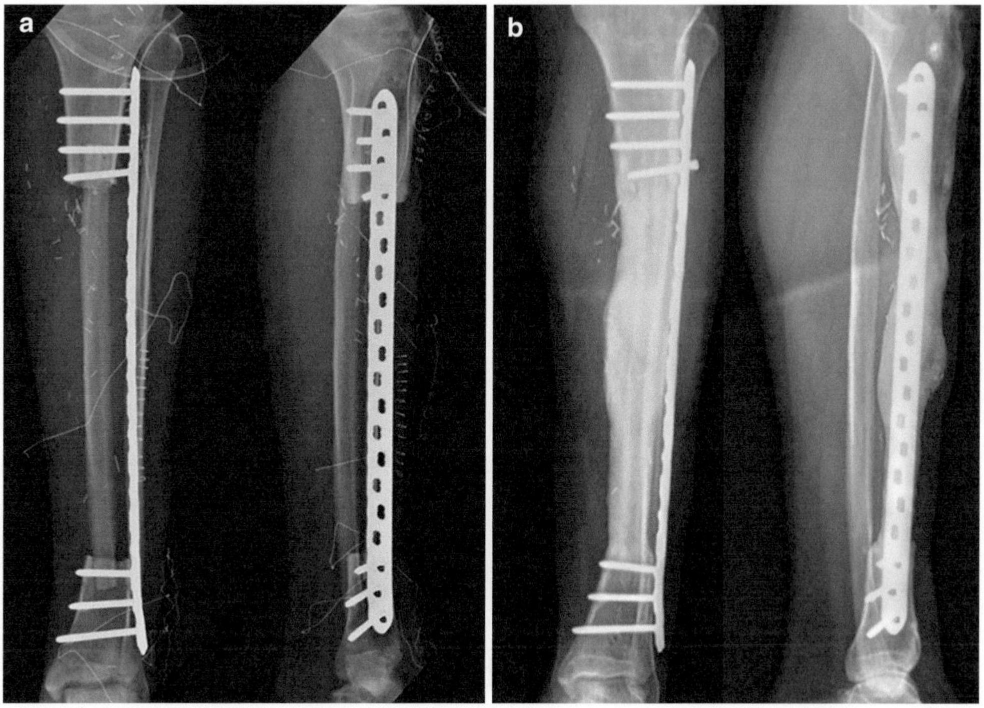

Fig. 6.1 Case 6.1, (**a**) Immediate postoperative X-rays after contralateral free fibula flap harvest to reconstruct a critical-size bone defect of the tibia. (**b**) X-rays after 4 years postoperatively show significant hypertrophy of the fibula flap

Finally, general complications of flap surgery, including bleeding/hematoma or wound healing problems, can arise. The most important of these complications is microanastomotic thrombosis, early revisions not being uncommon (5–10%), but flap loss being rare (<5% in experienced hands) [10, 60].

Clinical Cases

Case 6.1

A 33-year-old male patient, right-handed, nonsmoker and a factory worker, suffered a left forearm fracture as a result of high-energy trauma. He underwent surgery with a locked plate at another institution, despite which the patient continued with pain and functional limitations postoperatively for months. Subsequently, ulnar nonunion was confirmed. Five years after the initial surgery, the patient underwent surgery with aggressive resection of the devascularized tissue, resulting in a bone defect, so a cement spacer and pin were implanted, and the patient was referred to our center for further treatment.

We observed wound dehiscence and purulent discharge in the initial clinical evaluation (Fig. 6.2) and obtained X-rays (Fig. 6.3). In the first surgery at our institution, we collected samples for culture and pathology, replaced the cement spacer and resected the devitalized tissue until the bleeding bone was reached, resulting in an ulnar shaft defect of 6.5 cm (Fig. 6.4). Oxacillin/erythromycin-resistant *Staphylococcus (S.) epidermidis* and methicillin-resistant *S. aureus* (MRSA) grew in all culture samples, so treatment with levofloxacin and rifampicin was started. One week later, a second, more aggressive surgical debridement was performed, resulting in a bone defect of 8.3 cm and obtaining similar results from the microbial cultures. The patient had a good postoperative evolution, with no signs or symptoms of infection recurrence and normalization of laboratory parameters. After 10 weeks of antibiotic therapy, the bone defect was reconstructed with a free fibula flap from the contralateral leg, fixed using a 12-hole locking compression plate (LCP) as a bridge plate (Fig. 6.5), with a skin paddle for flap monitorization. An end-to-side anastomosis to the radial

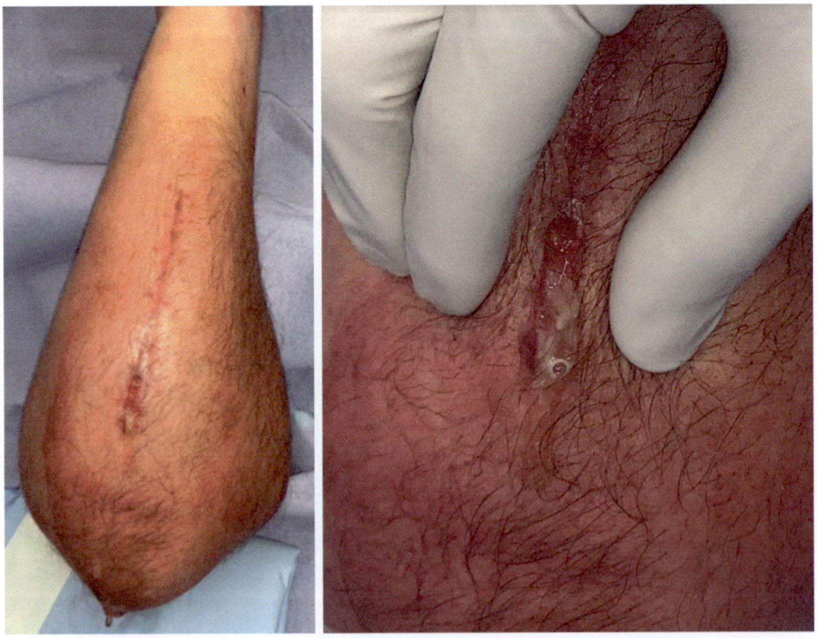

Fig. 6.2 Case 6.1, initial clinical images showed wound dehiscence, purulent discharge, and an exposed pin

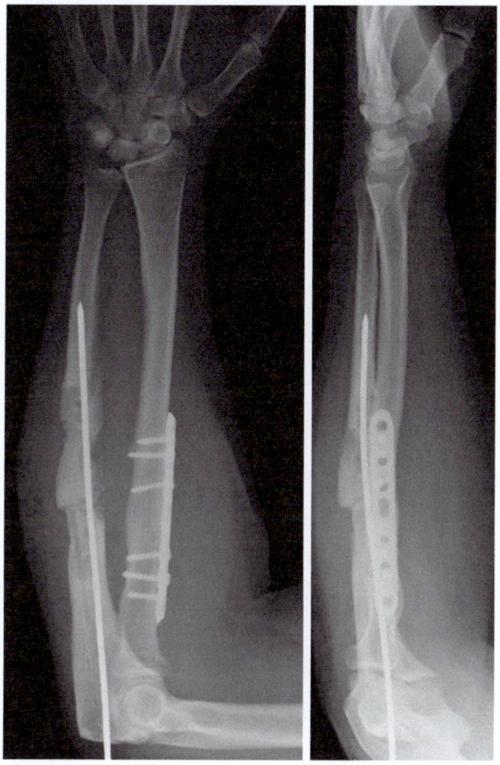

Fig. 6.3 Case 6.1, anteroposterior and lateral X-rays show the cement spacer in the ulnar bone defect, stabilized with a pin. A plate on the radius was used to treat the now-healed fracture

artery and two end-to-end anastomoses to the satellite vein of the ulnar-interosseous trunk and to the median vein of the elbow (superficial system) were performed, all with 8-0 Nylon. Postoperative recovery was uneventful, without pain and with good vitality of the skin paddle, and progressive integration of the fibula flap was observed in sequential X-rays until union was achieved at 12 weeks postoperatively (Fig. 6.6).

One year postoperatively, the patient reported 0 pain on the visual analog scale and during activity. He had an elbow range of motion of 130–20° for flexion and extension and of 70° and 40° for pronosupination (contralateral values: 80° and 80°, respectively). He is leading a normal life with a QuickDASH score of 0 (Fig. 6.7).

Case 6.2

A 69-year-old male farmer with no prior medical history suffered a left tibial plafond and distal fibula fracture due to crushing by a horse. The patient initially underwent open reduction and internal fixation (Fig. 6.8). In the early postoperative period, wound dehiscence and purulent discharge were observed. Antibiotics were prescribed for 3 months after surgery. Due to persistent poor healing, surgical irrigation and debridement were performed. An infected nonunion was confirmed, implants were removed, an external fixator was placed, and the patient was referred to a more complex hospital. At that second facility, the external fixator was removed, and the devitalized bone and soft tissue were resected. Samples were sent for culture, and an antibiotic-loaded cement spacer was placed. In the cultures, *Clostridium* and *Pseudomona* grew. After several months of antibiotic therapy and multiple surgical procedures for irrigation, debridement, and cement spacer exchanges with no progress, the patient was referred to our institution 1 year after the first surgery.

On admission, the patient presented with a swollen foot and ankle and many fistulas on the front, middle and lateral ankle. On the X-ray, the cement spacer on the front of the tibia and articular osteolysis of the talus were observed

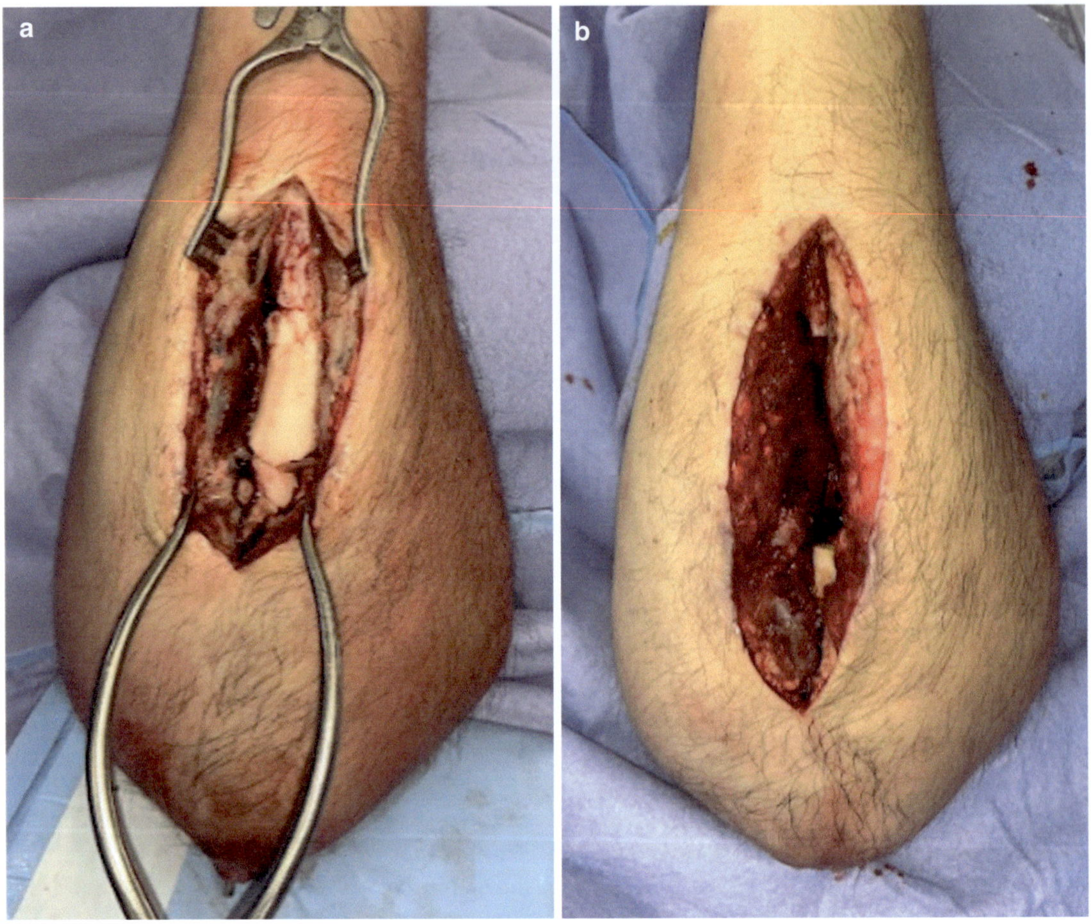

Fig. 6.4 Case 6.1, (**a**) Cement spacer and surrounding devitalized soft tissue. (**b**) Segmental bone defect of 6.5 cm after debridement

(Fig. 6.9). We performed a new surgical procedure for sample collection, debridement, and spacer replacement. The samples tested positive for methicillin-sensitive *S. aureus*. Laboratory parameters and clinical conditions were normalized after 45 days of antibiotic treatment. After two antibiotic-free weeks, reconstructive surgery was performed. An ankle arthrodesis was executed using a hindfoot arthrodesis nail complemented by a free osteocutaneous fibula flap from the opposite leg, which was interposed between the tibia and the talus (Fig. 6.10). End-to-side anastomosis to the anterior tibial artery and end-to-end anastomosis to one anterior tibial vein were performed with Nylon 9-0. The postoperative recovery was good, and bone union was achieved after 8 postoperative weeks. One year after surgery, the patient reported no pain while walking or standing and there were no signs or symptoms of infection recurrence (Fig. 6.11).

Case 6.3

A 19-year-old male patient, right-handed, veterinary student, nonsmoker and without comorbidities, consulted our institution for a nonunited fracture of the right radius. He had suffered a sports injury fracturing both his radius and ulna 2 years prior, and undergone surgery on two occasions at another institution with a torpid evolution. On physical examination, he presented deformity of the forearm, with a wrist range of motion compared to the healthy contralateral limb of 24°/72° for flexion, extension 62°/98°, ulnar deviation 4°/48°, radial deviation 28°/32°, pronation 92°/92°, supination 14°/88°, and pre-

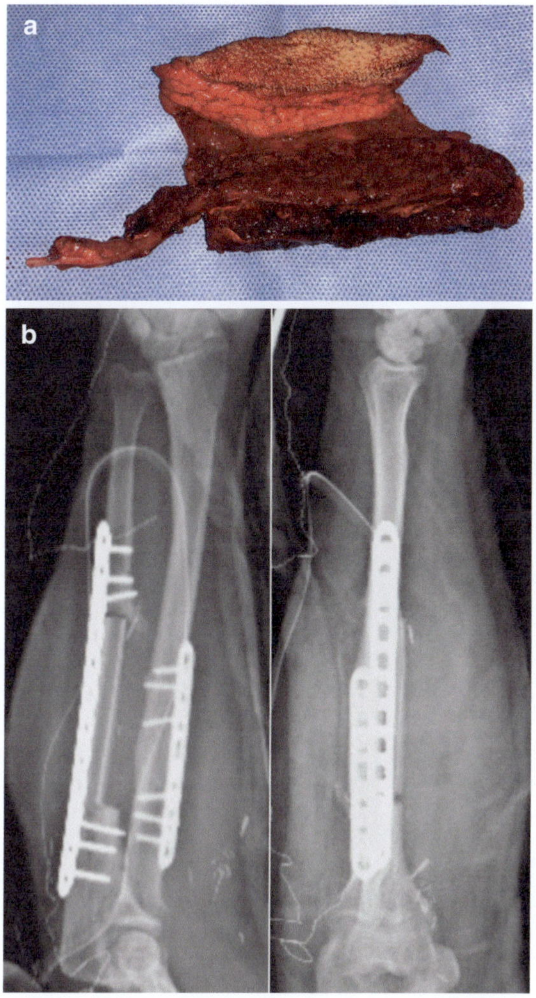

Fig. 6.5 Case 6.1, (**a**) free osteocutaneous fibula flap harvested to reconstruct the 8.3 cm ulnar bone defect. (**b**) Postoperative X-rays with the fibula flap fixed using a 12-hole locking compression bridge plate

served elbow range of motion (flexion 150°/150°, extension −4°/−4°). In the initial X-rays, there was evidence of nonunion of the radius together with radial shortening of 12 mm, volar angulation in the sagittal plane of 23° and radial angulation in the coronal plane of 20°, dislocation of the distal radioulnar joint, and persistence of osteosynthesis material in the ulna (Fig. 6.12). We took the patient into the operating room to obtain samples for culture and pathology, debride the nonunion and all other non-vital tissue, and correct the angular defects. This produced a 6 cm bone defect, into which we placed an antibiotic-loaded cement spacer together with an intramedullary pin to maintain radial alignment (Fig. 6.13a, b). The culture samples recovered *Bacillus* species and methicillin-sensitive *S. aureus*, so the patient underwent 3 months of antibiotic treatment with vancomycin and rifampicin until clinical and laboratory parameters were normalized.

We decided to reconstruct the radius using the induced membrane technique since an antibiotic-loaded cement spacer had already been placed. The cement spacer was removed, the radial shaft defect filled with a bone graft, and fixation using a 3.5 mm LCP bridge plate was performed. The lower radioulnar joint dislocation persisted after this maneuver, so a 7 mm ulnar shortening osteotomy was performed and fixed with a locking plate (Fig. 6.13c, d). The patient recovered well, without pain or signs of infection. However, 4 months after the surgery, there were signs of consolidation only at the ulna (Fig. 6.14a, b). As clinical recovery had been favorable (no pain, 95% mobility compared to the contralateral limb, no signs of infection) and there were no signs of implant loosening, a watchful waiting approach was decided on. At 16 months postoperatively his X-rays were compatible with nonunion of the bone graft, so we took him to the operating room for debridement and a medial condyle flap (Fig. 6.14c, d). The nonunion was confirmed, after the debridement of which a 2 cm bone defect was observed (Fig. 6.15a). We decided to use a medial condyle flap because of the size of the defect, multiple previous surgeries, and a history of infection. We harvested a 5 × 2 cm osteoperiosteal medial condyle flap (Fig. 6.15b, c) and fixed it into the radial defect under pressure (Fig. 6.15d). End-to-side anastomosis to the radial artery and end-to-end anastomosis to one radial vein were performed, both with Nylon 10-0.

Four months after the surgery, bone union was observed on the CT scan. Two years after the last surgery, the patient was pain-free, with wrist mobility (compared to contralateral) of flexion 55°/60°, extension 55°/90°, radial deviation 10°/20°, ulnar deviation 40°/50°, pronation 70°/90°, supination 90°/90°, a DASH score of 9, and X-rays showing full osseous consolidation (Fig. 6.16).

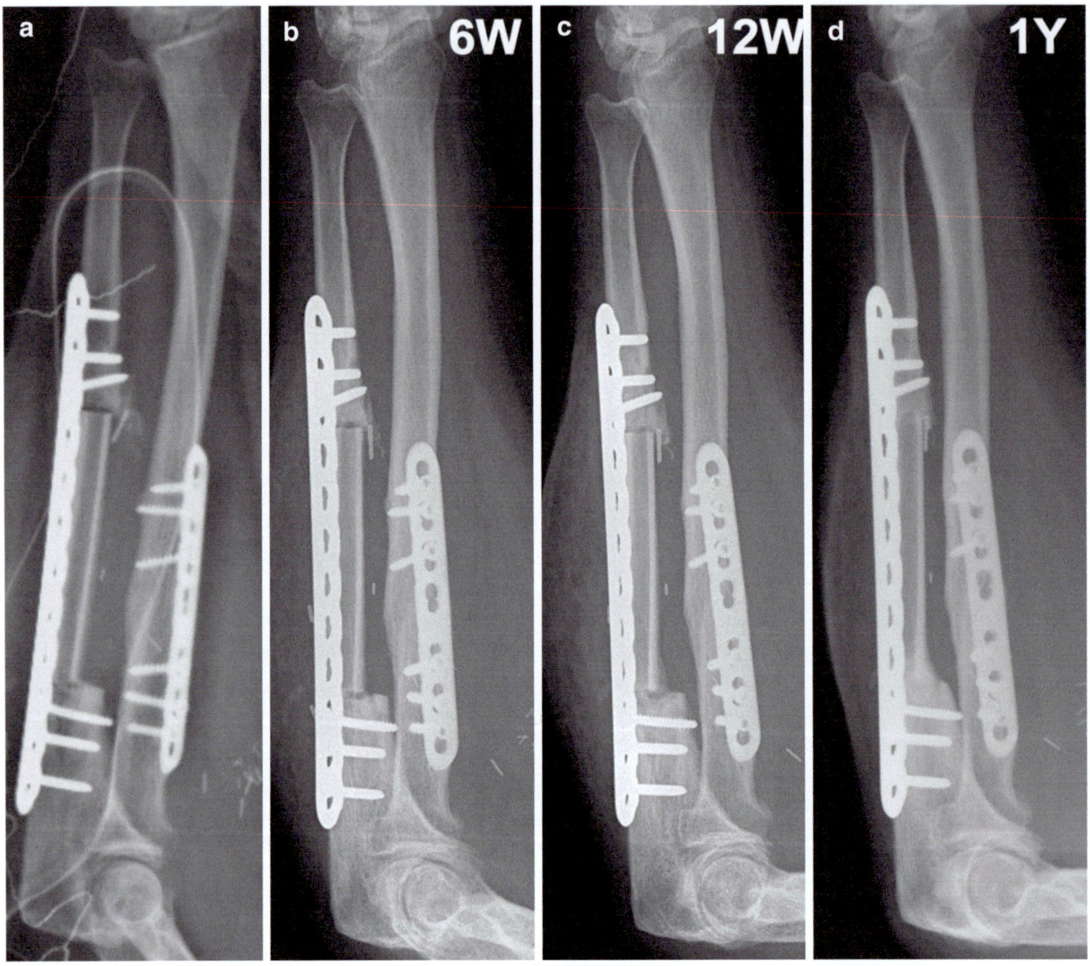

Fig. 6.6 Case 6.1, postoperative X-rays show consolidation progress from the initial postoperative period to 6 weeks, 12 weeks, and 1 year postoperatively

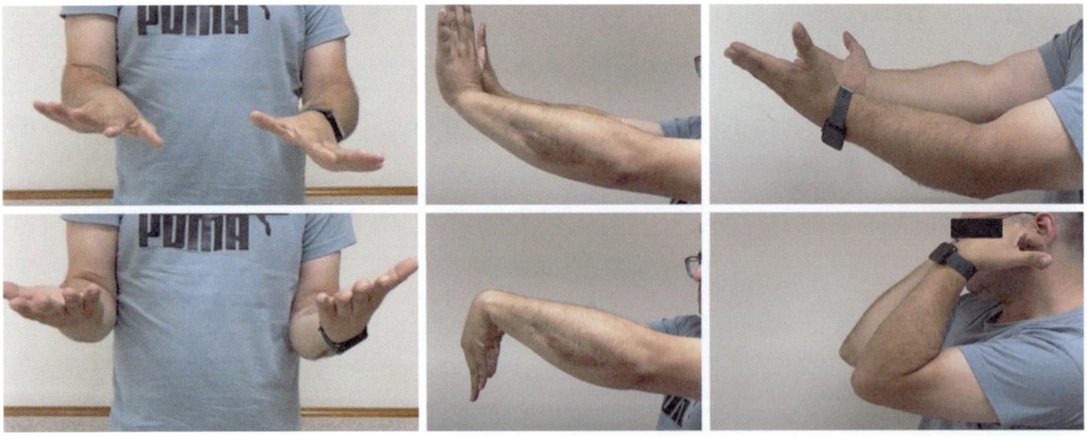

Fig. 6.7 Case 6.1, clinical assessment 1 year postoperatively showed excellent range of motion and a QuickDASH score of 0

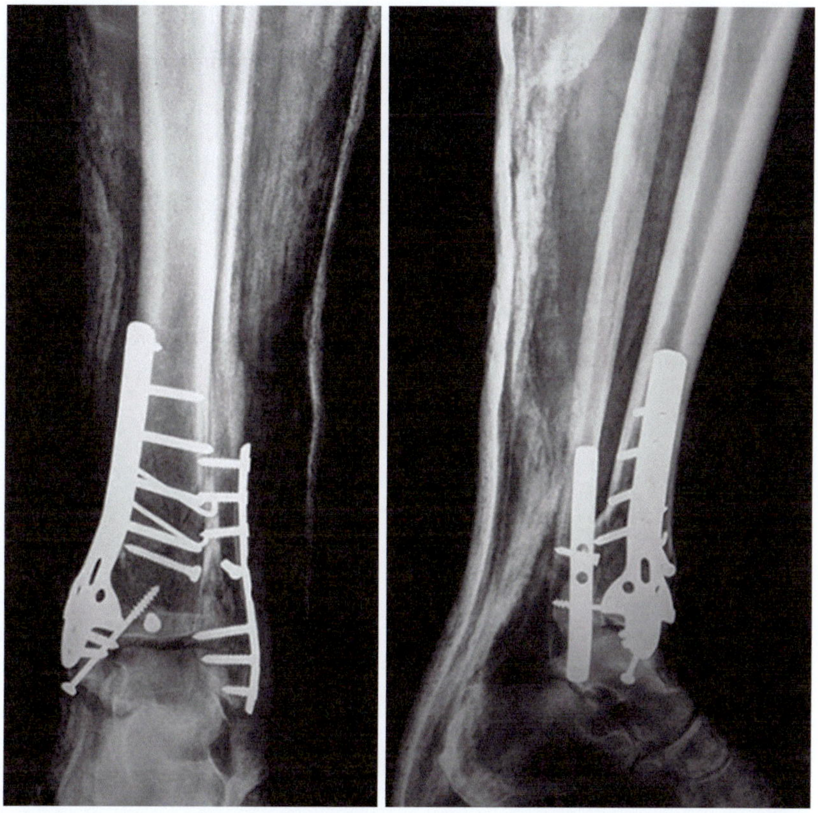

Fig. 6.8 Case 6.2, initial postoperative X-rays following open reduction and internal fixation of the tibia and fibula fracture

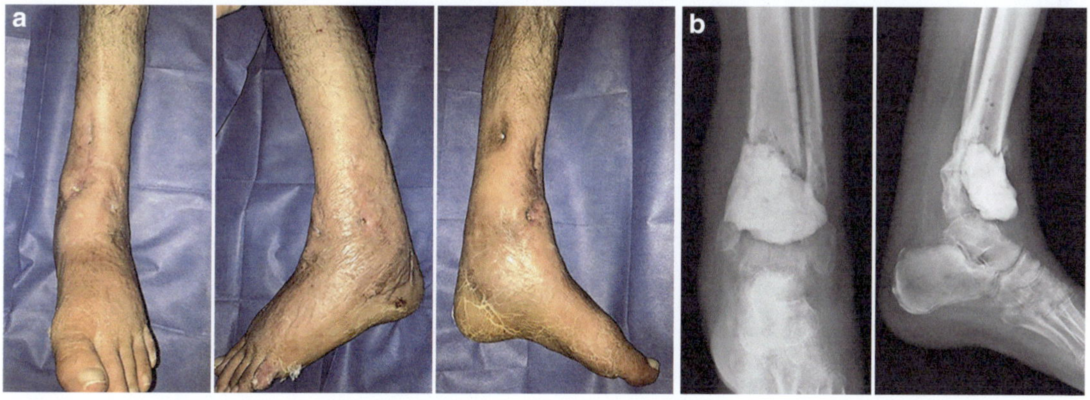

Fig. 6.9 Case 6.2, (**a**) The patient presented with ankle edema and multiple fistulas. (**b**) Anteroposterior and lateral radiographs of the ankle. The cement spacer was placed on the anterior aspect of the tibia. The articular surface of the talus shows radiolucencies

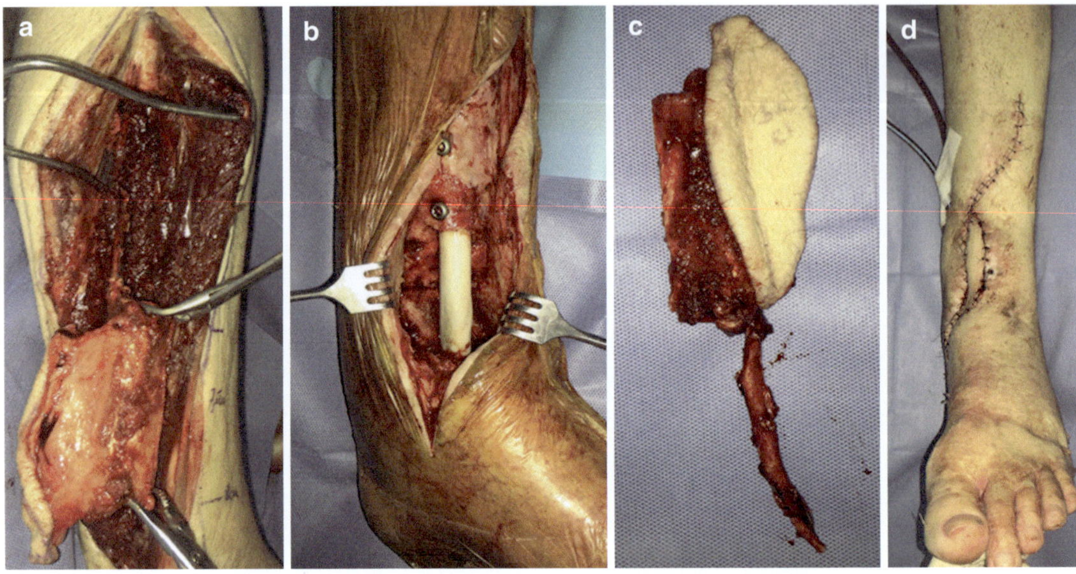

Fig. 6.10 Case 6.2, (**a**) Contralateral fibula flap harvest. (**b**) Ankle arthrodesis with a cemented nail. (**c**) The osteocutaneous fibula flap ready for transfer. (**d**) After wound closure, the skin paddle is left on the anterior aspect of the ankle to monitor the flap postoperatively

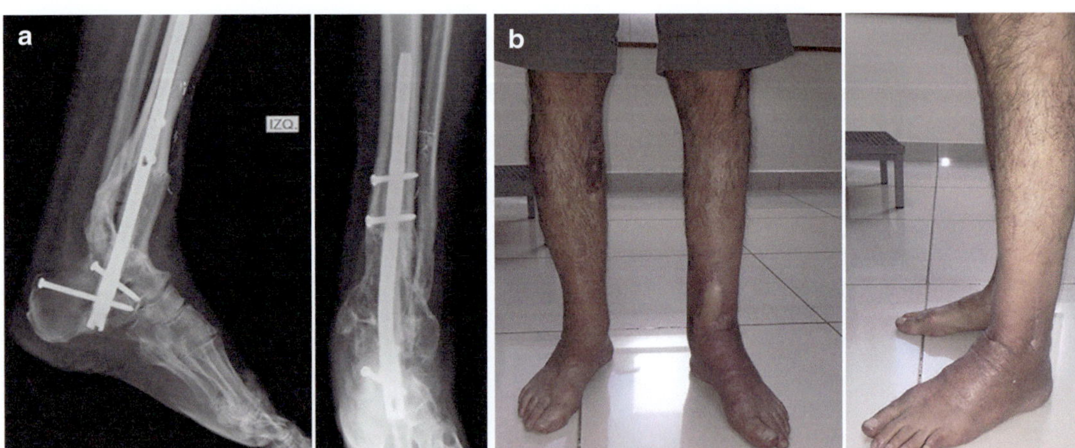

Fig. 6.11 Case 6.2, (**a**) One-year postoperative X-rays showing bone union. (**b**) Clinical result after 1 postoperative year. The patient was free of pain during walking or standing

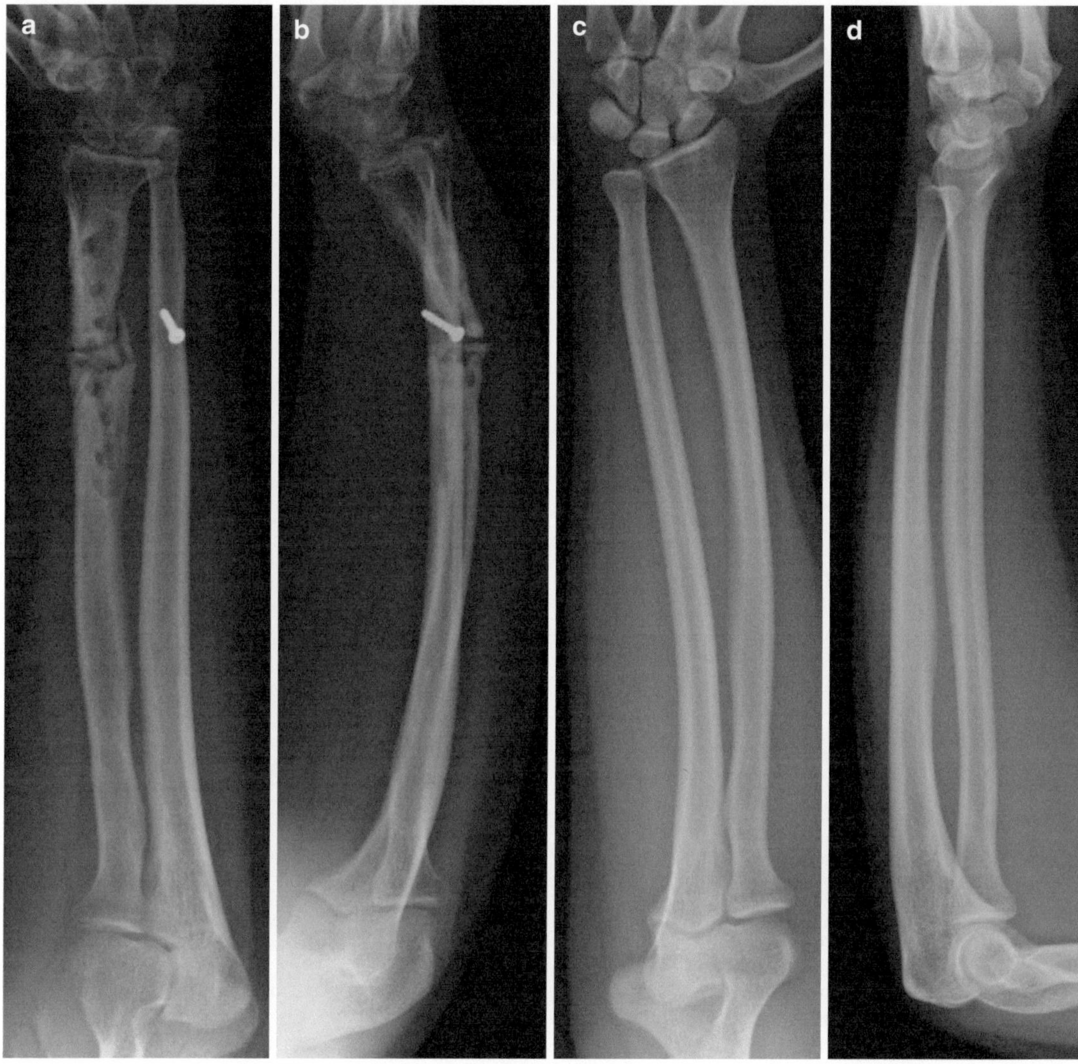

Fig. 6.12 Case 6.3, (**a**, **b**) Anteroposterior and lateral X-rays show nonunion at the distal third of the radial shaft. There was a radial shortening of 12 mm, increased volar angulation of 23°, deviation in the coronal plane of 20°, and dislocation of the distal radioulnar joint. (**c**, **d**) X-rays of the healthy opposite upper limb were used as a reference for the patient's normal anatomy

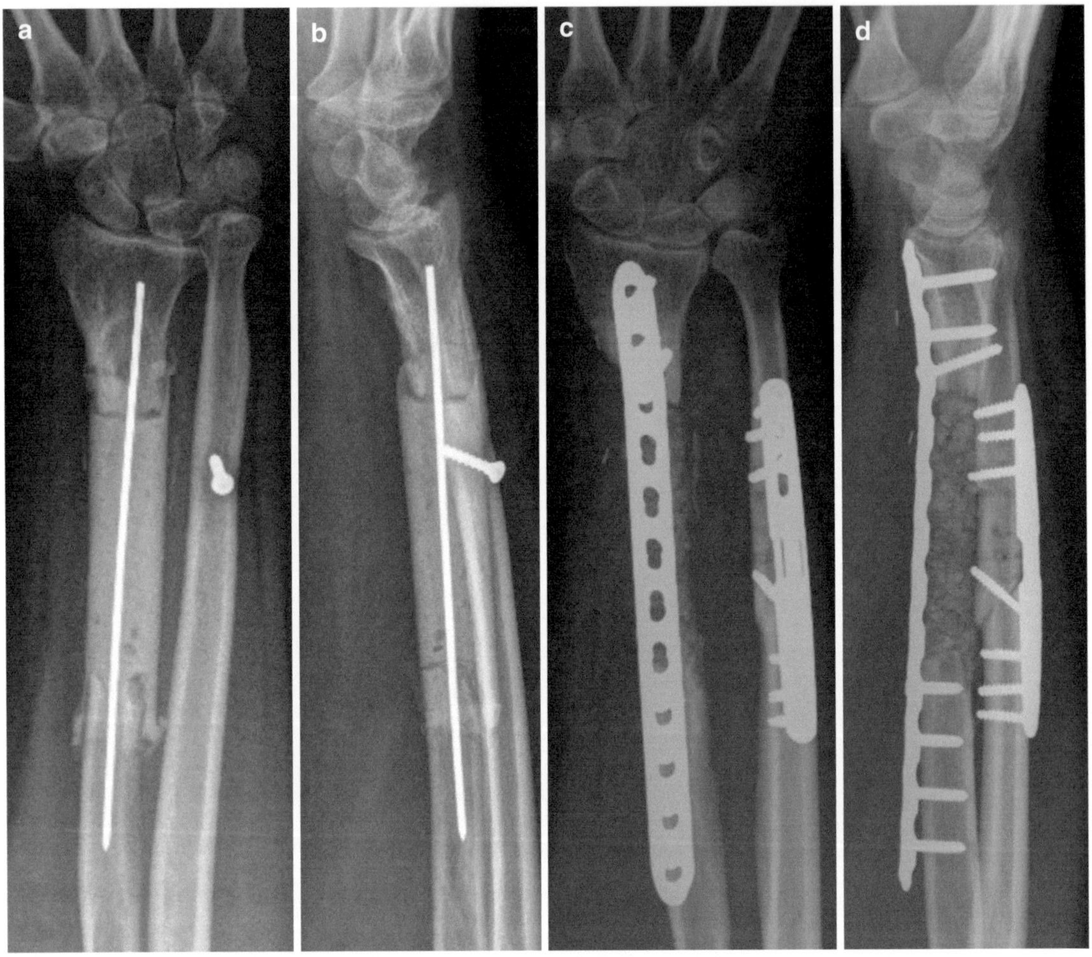

Fig. 6.13 Case 6.3, (**a**, **b**) Postoperative X-rays after surgical debridement and placement of an antibiotic-loaded cement spacer in the 6 cm bone defect of the radius. The spacer was fixed with an intramedullary pin to maintain radial alignment. (**c**, **d**) After antibiotic treatment, the second stage of the induced membrane technique was performed, and the radius was fixed with a 3.5 mm locking compression bridge plate. Due to persistent dislocation of the distal radioulnar joint, a 7 mm ulnar shortening was performed and plated

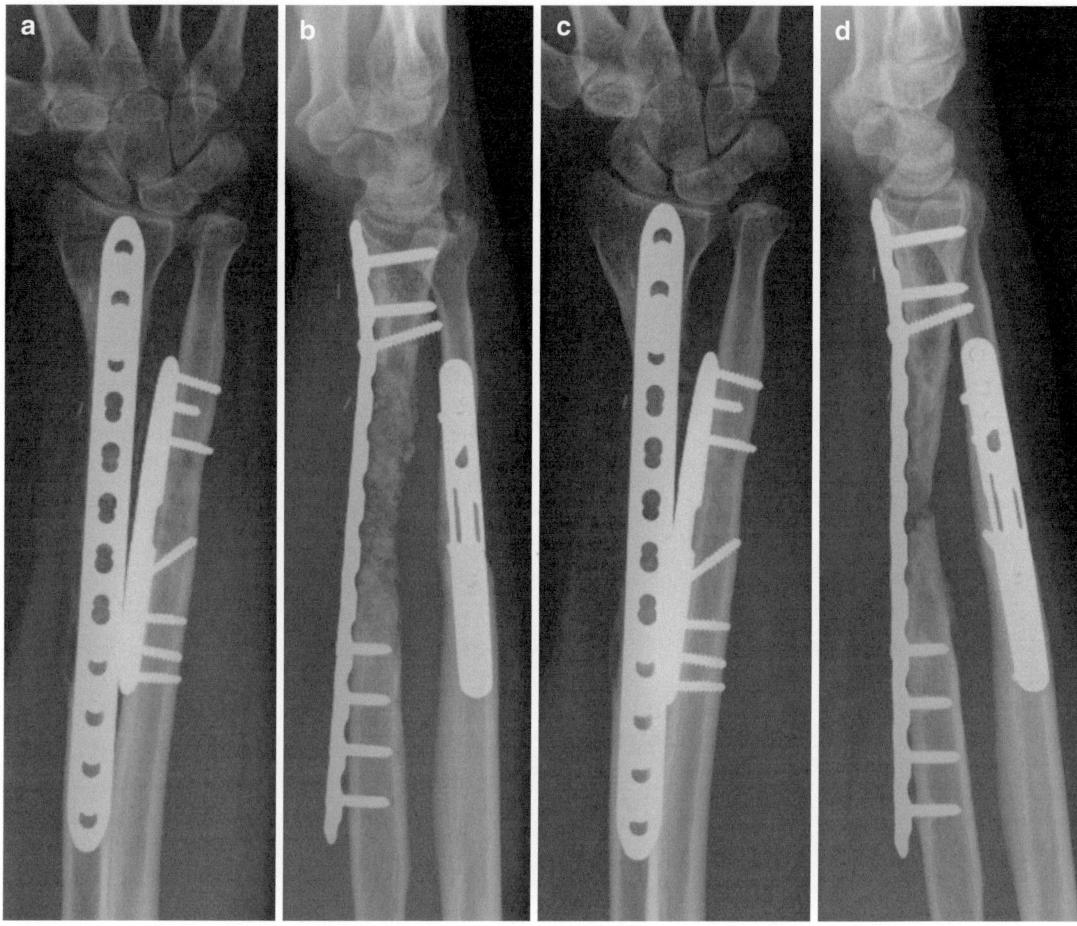

Fig. 6.14 Case 6.3, (**a**, **b**) Four months after the last surgery, X-rays show signs of bone union at the ulna but delayed healing at the radius. (**c, d**) At 16 months postoperatively, the X-ray shows a nonunion of the radius with resorption of the bone graft

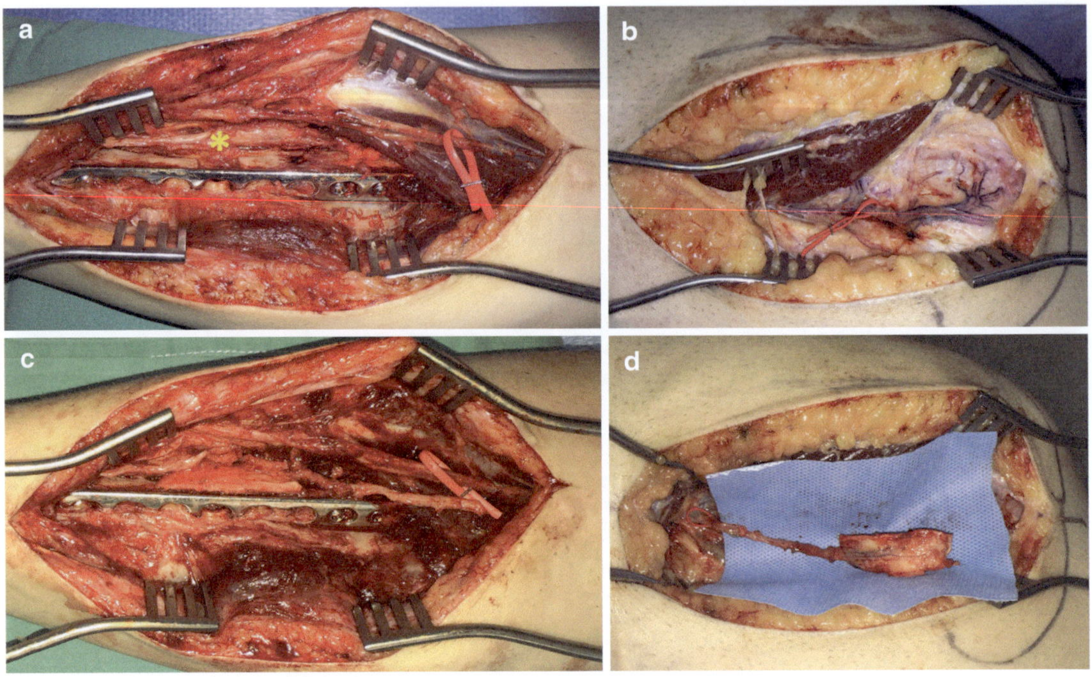

Fig. 6.15 Case 6.3, (**a**) After debridement of the non-union site, a 2 cm bone defect (yellow asterisk) ensued. (**b**) Medial femoral condyle flap harvest. Through a medial approach, dissection was performed until the medial femoral condyle was reached. The descending geniculate artery was repaired using a vessel loop. The division of the artery, located beyond the vessel loop, gives rise to the articular branch, which supplies blood to the flap. (**c**) Once the flap was placed into the defect, it was press-fixed. (**d**) The extent of pedicle dissection of this flap depends on the length necessary for adequate placement at the recipient site (up to 10 cm)

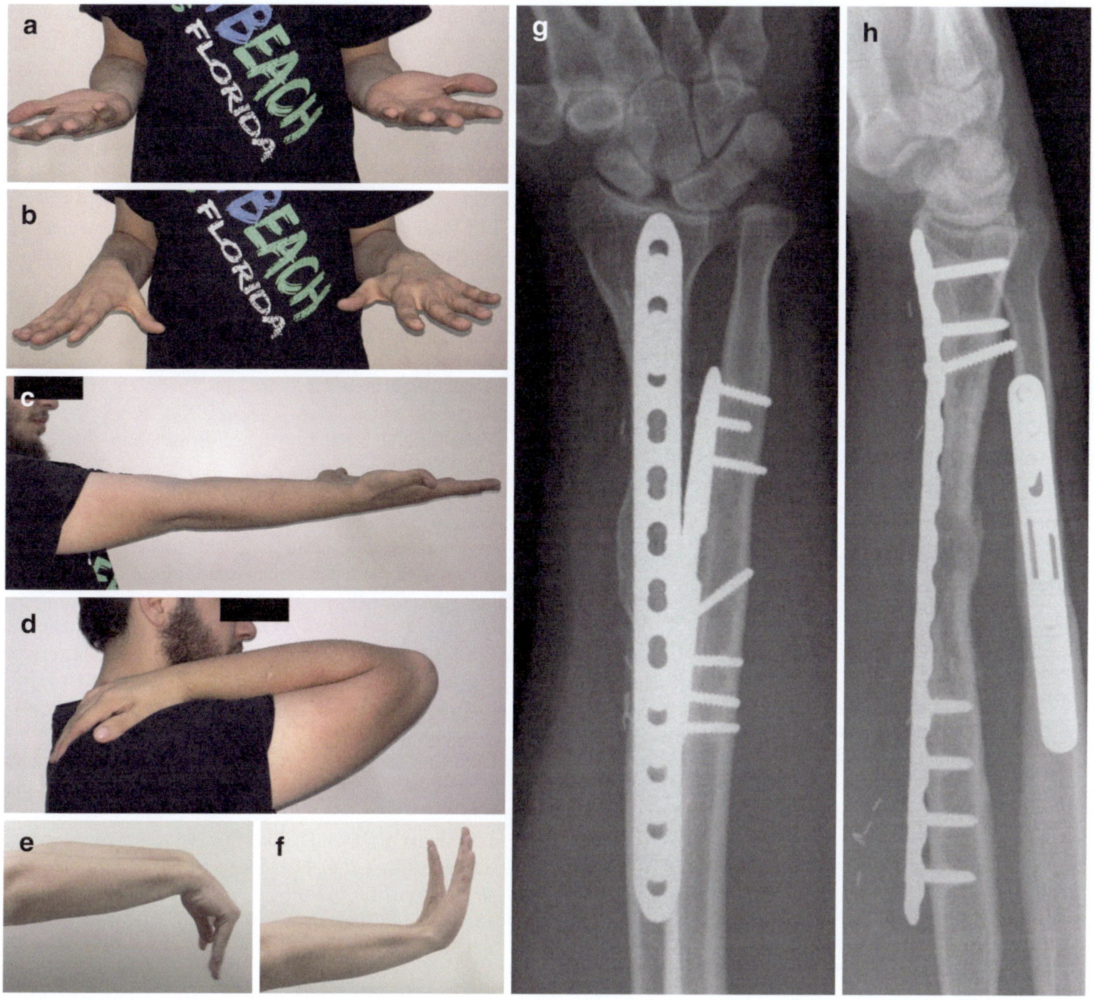

Fig. 6.16 Case 6.3. (**a–f**) Clinical images at 2 years of follow-up showing adequate range of motion. (**g**, **h**) Anteroposterior and lateral X-rays showing bone union with complete integration of the medial femoral condyle flap

Conclusions

Bone flaps allow reconstructive treatment even in the most complex scenarios. This is mostly due to their intrinsic blood supply, which allows flap survival regardless of the local conditions, and is responsible for bone flaps' improved bone healing and resistance to infection, as well as retention of their biomechanical properties (hypertrophy, minimal resorption). The result is that bone flaps have the lowest complication rate and lowest number of surgical revisions when compared to the rest of the techniques to treat infected critical bone defects.

The main disadvantages of bone flaps are the associated lengthy protected weight-bearing in lower limb FRIs, donor-site morbidity, longer surgical times (the patient must be fit enough to undergo this safely), and a higher technical demand.

The patients with FRI most benefited from bone flap surgery are those with poor vascularity of the FRI site (e.g., multiple previous unsuccessful attempts with other techniques), I4-type soft tissues of the FRI classification, and/or large segmental bone defects.

Large defects are usually reconstructed with a fibula flap, the workhorse for bone reconstruction in FRI. Donor-site morbidity is not rare but generally minor. To avoid stress fractures, limiting weight-bearing and adequate bone fixation are essential.

Small defects (< 5 cm) can be reconstructed with a MFC or distal radius flap. Donor-site morbidity is low if the size of these flaps is kept under 5 cm.

The iliac crest, scapula, and rib flaps are usually reserved for situations in which the fibula (or MFC and distal radius) flap is unavailable.

References

1. Kadhim M, Holmes L Jr, Gesheff MG, Conway JD. Treatment options for nonunion with segmental bone defects: systematic review and quantitative evidence synthesis. J Orthop Trauma. 2017;31:111–9.
2. Nauth A, Schemitsch E, Norris B, Nollin Z, Watson JT. Critical-size bone defects: is there a consensus for diagnosis and treatment? J Orthop Trauma. 2018;32(Suppl 1):S7–11.
3. He S-Y, Yu B, Jiang N. Current concepts of fracture-related infection. Int J Clin Pract. 2023;2023:4839701.
4. Rupp M, Walter N, Bärtl S, Heyd R, Hitzenbichler F, Alt V. Fracture-related infection-epidemiology, etiology, diagnosis, prevention, and treatment. Dtsch Arztebl Int. 2024;121:17–24.
5. Marais LC, Zalavras CG, Moriarty FT, Kühl R, Metsemakers W-J, Morgenstern M. The surgical management of fracture-related infection. Surgical strategy selection and the need for early surgical intervention. J Orthop. 2024;50:36–41.
6. Bishop AT, Shin AY. Vascularized bone grafting. In: Green's operative hand surgery. Elsevier; 2011. p. 1775–805.
7. Archual AJ, Bishop AT, Shin AY. Vascularized bone grafts in orthopaedic surgery: a review of options and indications. J Am Acad Orthop Surg. 2022;30:60.
8. Korompilias AV, Soucacos PN. Vascularized bone grafts in trauma and reconstructive microsurgery, part 1. Microsurgery. 2009;29:337–41.
9. Shin EH, Shin AY. Vascularized bone grafts in orthopaedic surgery. JBJS Rev. 2017;5:e1.
10. Tu Y-K, Yen C-Y. Role of vascularized bone grafts in lower extremity osteomyelitis. Orthop Clin North Am. 2007;38(37–49):vi.
11. Bezstarosti H, Metsemakers WJ, van Lieshout EMM, Voskamp LW, Kortram K, McNally MA, et al. Management of critical-sized bone defects in the treatment of fracture-related infection: a systematic review and pooled analysis. Arch Orthop Trauma Surg. 2021;141:1215–30.
12. Willems WF, Alberton GM, Bishop AT, Kremer T. Vascularized bone grafting in a canine carpal avascular necrosis model. Clin Orthop Relat Res. 2011;469:2831.
13. Soucacos PN, Kokkalis ZT, Piagkou M, Johnson EO. Vascularized bone grafts for the management of skeletal defects in orthopaedic trauma and reconstructive surgery. Injury. 2013;44(Suppl 1):S70–5.
14. de Boer HH, Wood MB, Hermans J. Reconstruction of large skeletal defects by vascularized fibula transfer. Factors that influenced the outcome of union in 62 cases. Int Orthop. 1990;14:121–8.
15. Han CS, Wood MB, Bishop AT, Cooney WP 3rd. Vascularized bone transfer. J Bone Joint Surg Am. 1992;74:1441–9.
16. Feltri P, Solaro L, Errani C, Schiavon G, Candrian C, Filardo G. Vascularized fibular grafts for the treatment of long bone defects: pros and cons. A systematic review and meta-analysis. Arch Orthop Trauma Surg. 2023;143:29–48.
17. Boretto JG, Holc F, Gallucci GL, Donndorff A, Rellán I, De Carli P. Fibula flap in upper extremity segmental/critical size bone defects fixed with locking plates. Single-institution observational cohort. Injury. 2023;54(Suppl 6):110737.
18. Copete González I, Vanaclocha N, Sánchez-García A, Thione A, Pérez-García A. Free vacularized fibula flap for septic bone defects of the lower limb. Int J Low Extrem Wounds. 2023;22:748–52.
19. Salgado CJ, Chim H, Moran SL, Wei FC, Mardini S. In: Wei FC, Mardini S, editors. Flaps and reconstructive surgery. Amsterdam: Elsevier Health Sciences; 2016.
20. Schaeffer CV, Stranix JT. Tackling bone loss of the lower extremity: vascularized bone grafting. Plast Aesthet Res. 2022;9:27.
21. del Piñal F, Innocenti M. Evolving concepts in the management of the bone gap in the upper limb. Long and small defects. J Plast Reconstr Aesthet Surg. 2007;60:776–92.
22. Ren G-H, Li R, Hu Y, Chen Y, Chen C, Yu B. Treatment options for infected bone defects in the lower extremities: free vascularized fibular graft or Ilizarov bone transport? J Orthop Surg Res. 2020;15:439.
23. Bumbasirevic M, Stevanovic M, Bumbasirevic V, Lesic A, Atkinson HDE. Free vascularised fibular grafts in orthopaedics. Int Orthop. 2014;38:1277–82.
24. Singh S, Toci GR, Kapadia K, Colon A, Greenberg P, Iyer H, et al. Vascularized bone grafting versus the 2-stage Masquelet technique for upper-extremity bone reconstruction: a meta-analysis. J Hand Surg Am. 2023;48:984–92.
25. Allsopp BJ, Hunter-Smith DJ, Rozen WM. Vascularized versus nonvascularized bone grafts: what is the evidence? Clin Orthop Relat Res. 2016;474:1319–27.

26. Antonini A, Rossello C, Salomone C, Iacoviello P, Chiarlone F, Burastero G. Bone defect management with vascularized fibular grafts in the treatment of grade III-IV osteomyelitis. Handchir Mikrochir Plast Chir. 2019;51:444–52.
27. El-Gammal TA, Shiha AE, El-Deen MA, El-Sayed A, Kotb MM, Addosooki AI, et al. Management of traumatic tibial defects using free vascularized fibula or Ilizarov bone transport: a comparative study. Microsurgery. 2008;28:339–46.
28. Cavadas PC, Landin L, Thione A, Ibañez J, Nthumba P, Roger I. Reconstruction of massive bone losses of the elbow with vascularized bone transfers. Plast Reconstr Surg. 2010;126:964–72.
29. Santanelli F, Latini C, Leanza L, Scuderi N. Combined radius and ulna reconstruction with a free fibula transfer. Br J Plast Surg. 1996;49:178–82.
30. Ling XF, Peng X. What is the price to pay for a free fibula flap? A systematic review of donor-site morbidity following free fibula flap surgery. Plast Reconstr Surg. 2012;129:657–74.
31. Miles MR, Jacobson L, Hill JB, Higgins JP, Giladi AM, Pet MA. Patient-reported lower extremity outcomes following fibula or medial femoral condyle free flaps for upper extremity defects. Hand (NY). 2023;18:1005–11.
32. Taylor GI, Townsend P, Corlett R. Superiority of the deep circumflex iliac vessels as the supply for free groin flaps. Clinical work. Plast Reconstr Surg. 1979;64:745–59.
33. Sanders R, Mayou BJ. A new vascularized bone graft transferred by microvascular anastomosis as a free flap. Br J Surg. 1979;66:787–8.
34. Gu Y, Ma H, Shujaat S, Orhan K, Coucke W, Amoli MS, et al. Donor- and recipient-site morbidity of vascularized fibular and iliac flaps for mandibular reconstruction: a systematic review and meta-analysis. J Plast Reconstr Aesthet Surg. 2021;74:1470–9.
35. Sakai K, Doi K, Kawai S. Free vascularized thin corticoperiosteal graft. Plast Reconstr Surg. 1991;87:290–8.
36. Scampa M, Mégevand V, Martineau J, Schaefer DJ, Kalbermatten DF, Oranges CM. Medial femoral condyle free flap: a systematic review and proportional meta-analysis of applications and surgical outcomes. Plast Reconstr Surg Glob Open. 2024;12:e5708.
37. Giladi AM, Rinkinen JR, Higgins JP, Iorio ML. Donor-site morbidity of vascularized bone flaps from the distal femur: a systematic review. Plast Reconstr Surg. 2018;142:363e–72e.
38. Guzzini M, Arioli L, Rugiero C, Rossini M, Argento G, Ferretti A. Donorsite defect of medial femoral condyle corticoperiostal flap in the treatment of lower limb infected nonunions. Handchir Mikrochir Plast Chir. 2021;53:376–82.
39. Boretto JG, Altube G, Gallucci GL, Narvaez HR, De Carli P. Femoral osteonecrosis after medial femoral condyle bone graft harvest. Plast Reconstr Surg Glob Open. 2018;6:e1792.
40. Jones DB Jr, Rhee PC, Bishop AT, Shin AY. Free vascularized medial femoral condyle autograft for challenging upper extremity nonunions. Hand Clin. 2012;28:493–501.
41. Soldado F, Knörr J, Haddad S, Corona PS, Barrera-Ochoa S, Collado D, et al. Vascularized tibial periosteal graft in complex cases of bone nonunion in children. Microsurgery. 2015;35:239–43.
42. Soldado F, Fontecha CG, Barber I, Velez R, Llusa M, Collado D, et al. Vascularized fibular periosteal graft: a new technique to enhance bone union in children. J Pediatr Orthop. 2012;32:308–13.
43. Taghinia AH, Upton J. In: Wei FC, Mardini S, editors. Flaps and reconstructive surgery. Elsevier Health Sciences; 2016.
44. Caterson EJ, Singh M, Turko A, Weaver MJ, Talbot S. The medial femoral condyle free osteocutaneous flap for osteomyelitis in pilon fractures. Injury. 2015;46:414–8.
45. Choudry UH, Bakri K, Moran SL, Karacor Z, Shin AY. The vascularized medial femoral condyle periosteal bone flap for the treatment of recalcitrant bony nonunions. Ann Plast Surg. 2008;60:174–80.
46. Bakri K, Shin AY, Moran SL. The vascularized medial femoral corticoperiosteal flap for reconstruction of bony defects within the upper and lower extremities. Semin Plast Surg. 2008;22:228–33.
47. Willemot L, Stewart D, Lawson R. Reconstruction of an infected midshaft radius and ulna nonunion using a free vascularized fibula and medial femoral condyle flap. Microsurgery. 2021;41:666–70.
48. Vincent A, Sawhney R, Ducic Y. Perioperative care of free flap patients. Semin Plast Surg. 2019;33:5–12.
49. Hwang K, Son JS, Ryu WK. Smoking and flap survival. Plast Surg (Oakv). 2018;26:280–5.
50. McNally M, Corrigan R, Sliepen J, Dudareva M, Rentenaar R, IJpma F, et al. What factors affect outcome in the treatment of fracture-related infection? Antibiotics (Basel). 2022;11:946.
51. Chen A, Garvey SR, Saxena N, Bustos VP, Jia E, Morgenstern M, et al. Is diabetes a contraindication to lower extremity flap reconstruction? An analysis of threatened lower extremities in the NSQIP database (2010-2020). Arch Plast Surg. 2024;51:234–50.
52. Goltsman D, Morrison KA, Ascherman JA. Defining the association between diabetes and plastic surgery outcomes: an analysis of nearly 40,000 patients. Plast Reconstr Surg Glob Open. 2017;5:e1461.
53. Crippen MM, Brady JS, Mozeika AM, Eloy JA, Baredes S, Park RCW. Impact of body mass index on operative outcomes in head and neck free flap surgery. Otolaryngol Head Neck Surg. 2018;159:817–23.
54. Krijgh DD, Teunis T, List EB, Mureau MAM, Luijsterburg AJM, Maarse W, et al. Mental health is strongly associated with capability after lower extremity injury treated with free flap limb salvage or amputation. Eur J Trauma Emerg Surg [Internet]. 2024; https://doi.org/10.1007/s00068-024-02459-1.

55. Weyh AM, Fernandes RP. Narrative review: fibula free flap, indications, tips, and pitfalls. Front Oral Maxillofac Med. 2021;3:4–4.
56. Minami A, Kaneda K, Itoga H, Usui M. Free vascularized fibular grafts. J Reconstr Microsurg. 1989;5:37–43.
57. Taylor GI. The current status of free vascularized bone grafts. Clin Plast Surg. 1983;10:185–209.
58. González C, Vanaclocha I, Sánchez-García N, Thione A, Pérez-García A. Free vacularized fibula flap for septic bone defects of the lower limb. Int J Low Extrem Wounds. 2023;22:748–52.
59. Lin C-H, Wei F-C, Chen H-C, Chuang DCC. Outcome comparison in traumatic lower-extremity reconstruction by using various composite vascularized bone transplantation. Plast Reconstr Surg. 1999;104:984–92.
60. Cavadas PC, Landín L, Ibáñez J, Nthumba P. Reconstruction of major traumatic segmental bone defects of the tibia with vascularized bone transfers. Plast Reconstr Surg. 2010;125:215–23.

Limb Salvage in Fracture-Related Infection of Unsalvageable Joints (F5)

7

Nieves Vanaclocha and Cristina Ojeda-Thies

Introduction

The multidisciplinary approach and advancements in surgical techniques continue to improve the success rates in treating fracture-related infection (FRI). However, sometimes, bone reconstruction is considered impossible or unadvisable (F5). This group includes cases in which the affected joint is unsalvageable, healing of the fracture is deemed unachievable (e.g., due to extensive bone involvement, poor vascularity, or lack of suitable bone reconstruction options), or the risk-benefit ratio and functional expectations advise against limb salvage [1, 2].

In this chapter, we will focus on the surgical options for limb salvage in cases in which the affected joint is unsalvageable. A joint may be considered unsalvageable after an FRI due to extensive cartilage damage and/or loss of the structures responsible for joint stability or mobility with no possibility of reconstruction (so even if bone continuity is reestablished, the joint will be unstable or unable to move). In such scenarios, the options for limb salvage include endoprosthetic joint replacement, excision arthroplasty, and arthrodesis.

The available literature to guide decision-making in these cases is scarce and heterogeneous. It suggests that all three of the abovementioned procedures are aggressive and have high complication and revision rates [3, 4]. A significant amount of patients finally undergo an amputation (mostly, due to recurring infection) [3–5]. Therefore, it is wise to plan and execute these limb salvage techniques in a way that avoids risking the best level of amputation (e.g., in a patient with a distal femoral FRI, not compromising the proximal femur to avoid potential involvement of the hip). In addition, the advisability of long-term antimicrobial suppressive therapy in these patients should be pondered, considering the specific microorganism strain (antibiotic resistance), patient condition, and their life expectancy [6]. For example, comorbidities such as end-stage renal disease or heart failure are particularly deleterious and associated to poor surgical outcomes, as well as many revisions, so these patients tend to benefit more from antibiotic suppression [1, 6]. Refer to Chap. 10 for more information on suppressive therapies, and to Chap. 8 for considerations in deciding whether to salvage the limb or to amputate.

Note that as in the rest of FRI patients, the principles reviewed in Chaps. 3 and 10, including

N. Vanaclocha (✉)
Orthoplastics Unit and Department of Plastic and Reconstructive Surgery, University and Polytechnic Hospital La Fe, Valencia, Spain

C. Ojeda-Thies
Bone Infection Unit, Department of Traumatology and Orthopedic Surgery, 12 de Octubre University Hospital, Madrid, Spain

Department of Surgery, School of Medicine, Complutense University, Madrid, Spain

N. Vanaclocha (ed.), *Treatment of Fracture-Related Infection*,
https://doi.org/10.1007/978-3-031-92452-1_7

preoperative patient optimization, are fundamental for success. The reader is referred to the abovementioned chapters for complementary reading.

Endoprosthetic Joint Replacement

Protocols for endoprosthetic joint replacement for cases of FRI are usually borrowed from two-stage reconstruction of periprosthetic joint infection (PJI) [4, 7].

In the first stage, the infection is debrided, tissue samples are obtained, the old hardware is removed, and the joint surfaces are prepared. An antibiotic-loaded spacer is implanted to fill the dead space, maintain the ligamentous and muscular tension across the joint, and release high-dose antibiotics locally. Spacers can immobilize the joint (a so-called static spacer) or allow for a range of motion (articulating spacer), there being no consensus on which is superior. On one hand, it has been postulated that static spacers could improve infection control by immobilizing the soft tissues. Further advantages are that they are easier to fashion and less expensive compared to articulating spacers. On the other hand, articulating spacers allow joint mobilization, easier exposure in the reimplantation stage and a better final range of motion [8]. Some randomized trials comparing articulating and static spacers in hip and knee PJI have shown better knee mobility and shorter length of stay for articulating spacers [9, 10], but other studies have found similar functional scores and similar rates of wound-related and spacer-related complication rates with both types of spacers. The type of pathogen does not appear to affect outcomes for static versus dynamic spacers, either [11].

After this first surgical stage, the patient's clinical status and inflammatory biomarkers are monitored. The ideal timing for the second stage is a matter of debate, but there is agreement that at least, all wounds must have healed and inflammatory biomarkers must have clearly improved in order to consider removal of the spacer and implantation of an endoprosthesis [6, 7, 12]. Note that biomarker levels within the normal range do not rule out persistent infection, and cultures of synovial fluid lack sensitivity. Some authors have proposed risk scores combining several markers to identify patients at risk for infection recurrence in PJI and calculate the (theoretical) optimal timing to perform the second stage [13], but validation is pending. Additionally, recent studies have placed into question the need for a two-week "antibiotic holiday" prior to proceeding with reimplantation [14, 15].

In the second stage, the spacer is removed and a joint endoprosthesis is implanted. Local antimicrobials are widely used, based on evidence favoring their use in other FRI cases (F1–4) and impregnating bone cement in aseptic revision joint arthroplasties, which are associated with significantly higher infection rates compared to primary procedures [16]. Cementing in reimplantation after PJI is routine for the knee joint but varies considerably between surgeons when the hip is affected. Some authors have used non-cemented implants coated in antibiotic-loaded calcium sulfate or hydrogels, with satisfactory outcomes [17, 18].

Often, surgeons must resort to constrained designs, augments, and tumor megaprostheses due to the extensive bone and soft tissue loss derived from the fracture and/or the subsequent infection [4, 6, 19, 20]. Many of these designs use stems to anchor the implant, potentially jeopardizing future bone preservation if another revision is needed. Considering the high reported revision rates, to preserve as much unaltered bone as possible, the use of stemless megaprostheses based on compressive osteointegration has been proposed [18, 21]. These prostheses allow eventual further shortenings while preserving the joint on the opposite end of the bone (e.g., the hip in cases of distal femoral replacement). Promising medium-term results have been reported [18, 21, 22], but experience is limited and to date, this is an off-label indication. More studies are needed to determine the safety and usefulness of this kind of prosthesis in FRI patients.

Which FRI Patients Benefit the Most from Endoprosthetic Joint Replacement?

Endoprosthetic joint replacement preserves joint function and allows earlier mobilization than if an arthrodesis, resection arthroplasty, or amputation are performed, with the added benefits of early mobilization and weight-bearing [7]. However, the trade-off is a high risk of infection recurrence, so endoprosthetic reconstruction in FRI has thus far been exceptional [23, 24]. Published experience is scarce, heterogeneous, and comprised by case series of patients with diverse reasons for replacement, mostly aseptic, with some secondary to septic arthritis or other causes of osteomyelitis (thus, FRI patients make only a small proportion of these case series) [4, 6, 25, 26]. Extrapolation from these studies to the FRI population should be done cautiously, as outcomes in FRI can differ significantly from that of cohorts with aseptic pathologies (which have higher success rates), lower average functional demands (lower wear-related failure rate, e.g., PJI), older age (worse conditions for osseointegration), or with shorter life spans (where prosthesis longevity is less of a concern, e.g., oncologic patients) [7, 19, 20].

The limited available literature suggests that endoprosthetic joint replacement in infectious contexts is able to achieve marked short-term functional improvement, but is associated to a high complication and revision rate, with limited endoprosthesis survivorship [4, 27, 28]. About a third of patients experience one or more major orthopedic complications [25, 29]. The most common cause for revision is infection recurrence (about 20%), followed by aseptic loosening (10–20% after 10 years) and dislocation (particularly in cases of hip arthroplasty) [4, 5, 20, 25]. Reported endoprosthesis revision-free survivorship in cases of distal femoral replacement, which are the most frequent, is between 70% and 80% at 5 years [25, 28–30]. Survivorship until first reoperation for any cause is around 50–60% at 5 years [28, 30]. It is important to consider that the study participants of the referenced publications were on average over 65 years old, which is considerably older than the FRI population. Endoprosthesis survivorship rates are likely to be *lower* in the younger FRI patients, as their greater functional demand will lead to increased rates of mechanical failure of the endoprosthesis [4, 28]. Accordingly, younger patient age has been associated to higher risk of megaprosthesis reoperation and revision (for any cause and due to aseptic loosening) [28]. Patients and surgeons should also be aware that the rate of secondary amputation is just over 5%, mostly due to infection recurrence.

In evaluating an FRI patient for a potential endoprosthetic joint replacement, muscular sufficiency and ligamentous stability must be assessed as they are important for the endoprosthetic joint to function (e.g., the knee extensor mechanism). Patients in whom these structures have been lost or damaged enough that they would require a complex reconstruction are poor candidates for endoprosthetic joint replacement, and likely better served with another form of treatment (e.g., arthrodesis) [20]. Consider also that the outcomes of arthrodesis in some joints (e.g., ankle or wrist) are similar or even superior to endoprosthesis, particularly for high-demand patients. These patients are also likely to benefit more from arthrodesis. Patients should be aware that joint replacement will only partially correct limb-length discrepancy. Finally, revision arthroplasties are usually bulky, and soft tissue coverage can be challenging, even requiring additional techniques for soft tissue coverage (e.g., flap) for the joint replacement to be successful.

The abovementioned considerations, risks, and trade-offs should be weighed against the potential functional benefits in the context of the patient's baseline functionality, and thoroughly discussed with the patient when considering endoprosthetic joint replacement in FRI [4, 20]. The FRI patients most likely to benefit from endoprosthetic joint replacement are F5 R1–3 I1–4 patients in the FRI classification [1] who are expected to have an active lifestyle after arthroplasty, in whom the structures needed for optimal prosthetic joint function are preserved (e.g., functional knee extensor mechanism) and in whom the estimated risk of postoperative recurrence is low (good infection control).

The development of special coatings and surface modifications to prevent bacterial adherence could change susceptibility of hardware to harnessing biofilm and expand the indications of endoprosthetic joint replacement in FRIs [31, 32]. The most researched coatings are silver, iodine, and gentamicin poly(D,L-lactide) [31, 33, 34]. Other coatings, studied mostly preclinically, include polyethylene oxide, bioactive copper, nanostructured surface finishing (nanotubes containing antimicrobials such as antibiotics or fluorine), and antimicrobial peptides, among others [31].

Early clinical experience with silver, iodine, and gentamicin poly(D,L-lactide) has been published in a few mixed cohorts made up mostly of oncologic cases, with a few FRI cases. Some promising results have been observed, with good osseointegration and low infection recurrence rates at medium-term follow-up [31, 34, 35]. For example, iodine-coated prostheses seem to be associated with a low postoperative infection risk (<5% recurrence in mixed cohorts), and their use appears to be safe. Gentamicin poly(D,L-lactide)-coated nails have been used for tibial fractures, both as a primary treatment and in infected nonunions, with good clinical outcomes and no adverse effects. For silver-coated prostheses, evidence on their effectiveness for reducing infection risk is contradictory, with some studies finding considerable risk reduction and others finding no statistically significant difference. Survivorship appears to be no different than that reported with uncoated prostheses [33–35].

Concerns exist regarding the true benefit of these antimicrobial-coated endoprostheses compared to conventional arthroplasties, as there are no clinical comparative studies to date evaluating the respective rates of infection recurrence [33]. These antimicrobial-coated prostheses are significantly more expensive than regular endoprostheses, so it is critical to find out whether they provide any added value and, if so, how much. Furthermore, the spectrum of activity and the duration of the protection that these coatings purportedly provide are largely unknown, and while some coatings have antibacterial properties inherent to their chemical properties, those coated in antibiotics could favor the development of antibiotic resistance if the pathogens are exposed to subinhibitory antimicrobial concentrations for a prolonged amount of time. Another concern is biocompatibility, especially in the case of heavy metals. Hypersensitivity reactions appear to be uncommon based on the published studies, probably owing to the low allergenic profiles of the selected molecules, but not entirely rare. For example, local silver toxicity (argyria) is a well-known possibility with silver-coated implants, especially dermatological manifestations [31, 33]. It is also worth highlighting that the behavior of these prostheses in the human body over time is unknown (effects of the surface modifications on biomechanical stability, osseointegration, useful life of the implant, etc.).

Three-dimensional printing technology has been experimentally applied to bone defects of other etiologies (mostly oncologic), and could play a part in the treatment of FRIs in the future [36].

Resection Arthroplasty

Resection arthroplasty involves debridement and resection of joint surfaces without further bone reconstruction, leaving the defect to be filled with a scar. Most of the literature regarding resection arthroplasty refers to the hip, though the procedure can also be applied in other joints such as the shoulder, elbow, or joints of the hands and feet. As with the rest of FRI patients, several techniques can be used to fill the dead space to prevent seroma and infection recurrence. The use of antibiotic-loaded spacers has been shown to increase infection eradication in patients with septic arthritis [37]. Eventual conversion to total hip arthroplasty is low, and quality of life is reduced, with a great impact on physical function [38, 39]. The scar will be able to handle only small axial loads, but joint motion is partially preserved, as patients can employ compensatory mechanisms to generate joint movement. In the hip joint, filling the defect with muscular flaps of the internal and external rotators as well as the gluteus minor muscle can help cushion the proximal femur against the ilium. Nevertheless, revision rates are high, with one in four patients requiring reoperation for persistent infection [3, 40, 41].

Which FRI Patients Benefit the Most from Resection Arthroplasty?

This treatment modality is generally considered for F5 R3–4 I1–4 patients with very low functional demands in which endoprosthetic joint replacement is not advisable (e.g., poor infection control, unfit enough for a joint replacement) or has an extremely high risk of other complications such as periprosthetic fracture or dislocation, an arthrodesis would be more functionally limiting (e.g., the hip), but long-term suppressive antimicrobial therapy is inadvisable or not feasible (e.g., multiresistant microorganism).

Arthrodesis

Arthrodesis involves fusion of the joint involved. Advantages of this procedure in FRI include the stability it provides, which favors infection control, and that volume augmentation at the FRI site is minimal, favoring wound closure (tensionless direct closure is usually possible even in patients with a soft tissue defect).

Arthrodesis due to FRI is most commonly performed in the ankle and foot, though ample experience also exists with knee, wrist, and elbow fusions [42–44]. It can be done without graft, with different types of non-vascularized bone graft (allograft, autograft) or even with a bone flap, and can be stabilized with different types of fixation until achieving union (e.g., intramedullary nail, external fixator) [42, 45, 46]. Alternately, fusion endoprostheses can also be used in the ankle or knee [47, 48]. Arthrodesis can be performed in one stage, or, more often, in two (after a period with an antibiotic-impregnated spacer) [42, 43].

However, arthrodesis entails the loss of the joint's function and thus functional compromise. Moreover, the published experience for FRI is scarce and mainly limited to case series. Limb-length discrepancy cannot be corrected without bone transport, so some shortening can be expected, especially if <2 cm of limb shortening is needed for bone contact [49]. Note that a small shortening can be desirable, particularly in knee fusions, to aid with the swing phase during the gait cycle and avoid overloading of the contralateral hip and lower back muscles. It can also facilitate wound closure further.

Most of the published experience for arthrodesis as treatment for FRI stems from ankle or tibio-talocalcaneal fusions for infections following fractures of the ankle, pilon, talus, or calcaneus. Satisfactory fusion of the ankle joint and eradication of the infection can be achieved in 80–90% of patients. When successful, ankle arthrodesis improves pain and function and allows durable loading across the ankle joint, enabling performance of activities of daily living and even professional occupations. However, gait analysis studies show significant differences compared to normal controls regarding cadence and stride length [50, 51], and many patients have a degree of remaining disability. Moreover, complications and reoperations are common, and ankle fusions due to infection have inferior outcomes to those performed for aseptic indications [42, 45, 52–54]. Less has been published on knee arthrodesis, most of it in relation to PJI, with some authors observing improved functional outcomes, quality of life and survival in comparison with above-knee amputations, but others finding no differences or with results favoring amputation [47, 55, 56]. In any case, patients with a knee arthrodesis will commonly require technical aids for ambulation [57].

Overall, the rate of complications following arthrodesis seems to be around 30%, and the rate of infection recurrence between 10% and 20% (depending on the method of fusion) [42, 43, 45, 47]. Survivorship for implants left inside the body at 5 and 10 years is comparable to that of endoprosthetic joint replacement (between 70% and 80% at 5 years for implant revision), and rates of nonunion are variable but generally over 10% [42, 45]. Outcomes for union are similar for external and internal fixation techniques, but patients treated with external fixation seem to have higher odds of deep infection and amputation (severity of FRI is likely a confounding factor) [58]. Amputation rates due to complications (mostly, infection recurrence) remain over 5% [42, 43, 45, 47].

Which FRI Patients Benefit the Most from Arthrodesis?

Once again, when deciding on whether to opt for this treatment, the patient's baseline functionality must be considered. Unlike amputations, the patient's age does not seem to affect postoperative functionality after arthrodesis [47]. The F5 FRI patients most likely to benefit from arthrodesis are R1–3-type hosts with good infection control and adequate bone stock in whom endoprosthetic replacement is either not possible (e.g., due to inability to provide adequate prosthetic coverage) or not advisable (e.g., due to mechanical problems such as nonfunctional knee extensor apparatus, or extensive muscle atrophy because the patient no longer walks due to severe deconditioning), or the patient is unlikely to be able to wear an external prosthesis if an amputation were performed (see Chap. 8). For some joints, such as the knee, amputation in young patients with good orthotic care leads to better patient satisfaction than an arthrodesis, particularly if they are fitted with a microprocessor-controlled-knee joint [47]. Another indication would be if the patients' functional demands cannot be satisfactorily served with a resection arthroplasty or antibiotic suppression.

Limb Salvage in Unsalvageable Joints with FRI

Based on the limited available literature, endoprosthetic joint replacement, resection arthroplasty and arthrodesis in FRI:

- Are aggressive procedures, with a 50% revision rate at 5 years.
- Are associated with an approximately 20% risk of infection recurrence.
- Have secondary amputation rates of just over 5%.

Joint replacement and arthrodesis tend to be considered in the same types of patients: R1–3 patients who would be active after the surgery and have good infection control. Joint replacement is preferred if a better functional outcome is expected with it (e.g. a knee with a preserved extensor mechanism), otherwise, arthrodesis is wiser. Revision-free implant survivorship in both cases is about 70–80% at 5 years.

In patients who are poor candidates for joint replacement or arthrodesis and have very low functional demands, excision arthroplasty can be considered. Long-term antimicrobial suppressive therapy is the main alternative in such patients, as they tend to be in a poor physical condition.

Clinical Cases

Case 7.1

A 45-year-old female with a history of alcohol abuse disorder and longstanding mixed eating disorder suffered a comminuted intertrochanteric fracture after a fall from standing height (Fig. 7.1). It was fixed with a proximal femur nail antirotation (Fig. 7.2). She presented 9 weeks after surgery with a methicillin-sensitive *Staphylococcus aureus* infection of the trochanteric bursa involving the internal fixation (F2 R2 I1). After several unsuccessful debridements with retention of the implanted nail, the nail was exchanged in a single stage for a 150° sliding hip screw augmented with vancomycin- and gentamycin-impregnated calcium sulfate-phosphate (F3 R2 I1, Fig. 7.3). Rice body bursitis was observed. The patient suffered several dislocations of the affected hip despite an abduction orthosis (Fig. 7.4), and was eventually able to self-reduce. The hip instability did not improve despite revising the fixation with a fixed-angle blade plate (Fig. 7.5). *Klebsiella aerogenes* grew in cultures from the intraoperative samples, and

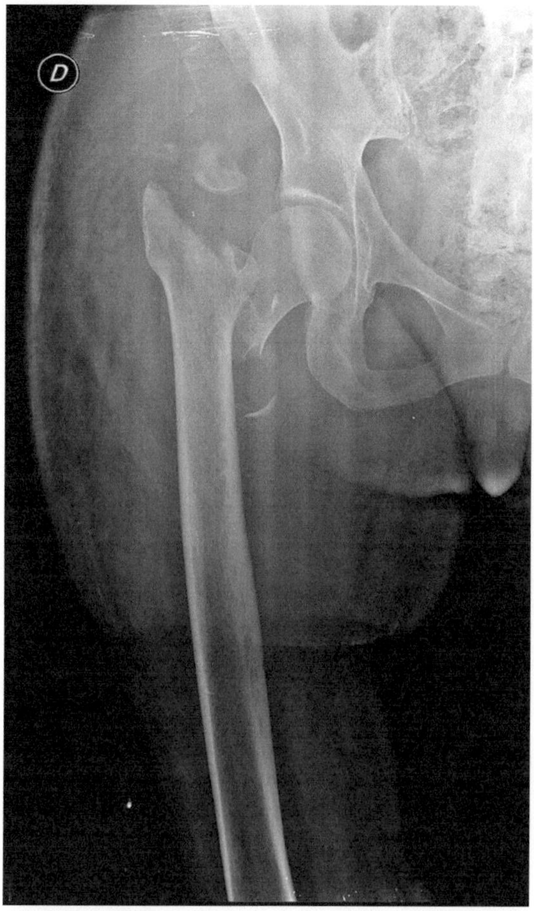

Fig. 7.1 Case 7.1, anteroposterior radiograph of the right hip showing an intertrochanteric fracture with avulsion of the tip of the greater trochanter

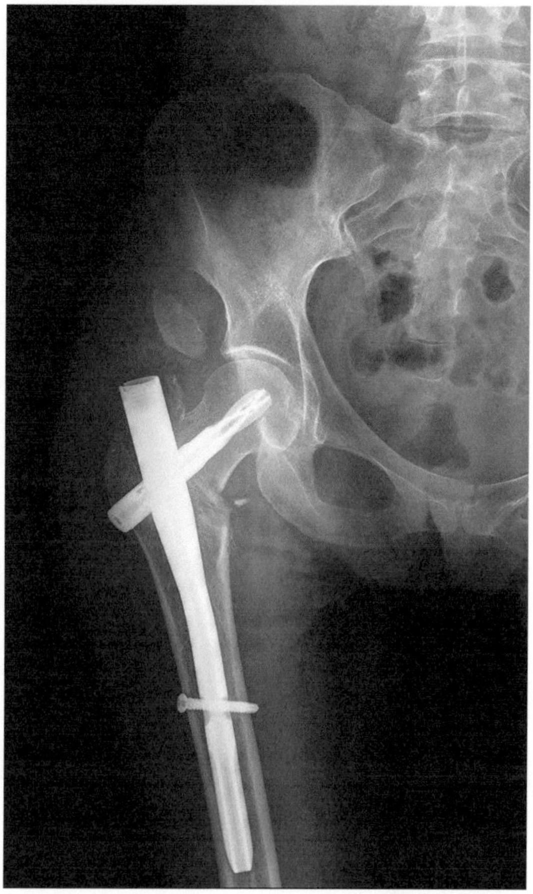

Fig. 7.2 Case 7.1, postoperative anteroposterior radiograph of the right hip after internal fixation of the intertrochanteric fracture with a cephalomedullary nail (PFNA, DePuy Synthes, Raynham, Massachusetts, United States of America)

the patient was treated with intravenous antibiotics.

Nine months after commencing treatment, the nonunion persisted and the patient continued suffering hip dislocations (F5 R2 I1, Fig. 7.6). During this period, she had also suffered fragility fractures of the left shoulder, right tibia, and left ankle. Girdlestone resection arthroplasty was performed 10 months after the initial fracture. The patient required two further debridements due to postoperative seroma at the resection site; in one of the surgeries, *Staphylococcus aureus* was again cultured in tissue samples, so she was treated with dalbavancin. Her recovery was satisfactory. However, she later developed a chronic polymicrobial infection of the right tibial nail (*Bacteroides fragilis, Streptococcus mitis*), which was treated with a single-stage exchange for an antibiotic-loaded cement-coated nail due to the refracture risk despite having a healed fracture.

Three years after the resection arthroplasty, the patient uses a walking frame indoors but requires a wheelchair for outdoor displacements. The 8 cm limb-length discrepancy was corrected with a shoe lift (Fig. 7.7). The hip shows no signs of infection and is pain-free. Elective conversion to a total hip arthroplasty has been rejected by several arthroplasty surgeons due to the high risk of complications.

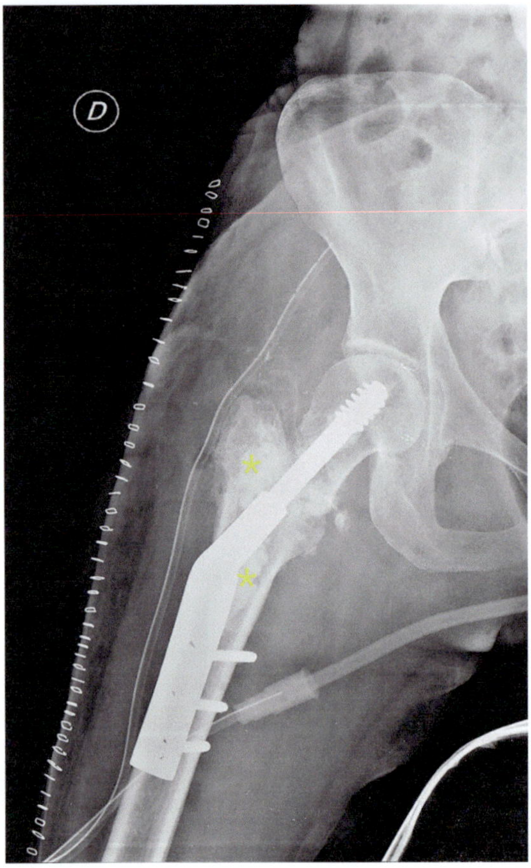

Fig. 7.3 Case 7.1, postoperative anteroposterior radiograph of the right hip after removal of the cephalomedullary nail and re-osteosynthesis with a sliding hip screw (DHS, DePuy Synthes, Raynham, Massachusetts, United States of America). Local antibiotic was placed in the trajectories of the blade and nail (asterisks) in the form of calcium sulfate-phosphate mixed with vancomycin and gentamycin (Cerament, Bonesupport, Lund, Sweden)

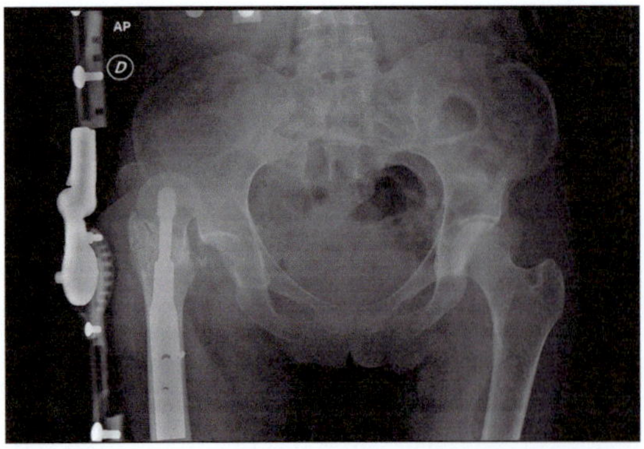

Fig. 7.4 Case 7.1, anteroposterior radiograph of the pelvis showing a right hip dislocation, despite wearing an anti-dislocation orthosis

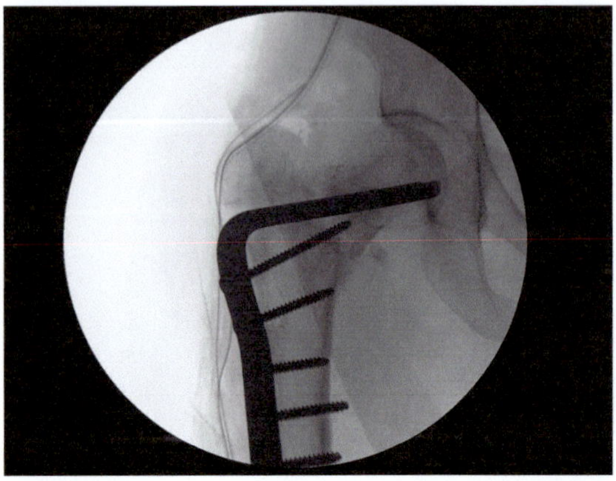

Fig. 7.5 Case 7.1, intraoperative fluoroscopy of the right hip during revision of the internal fixation with a blade plate

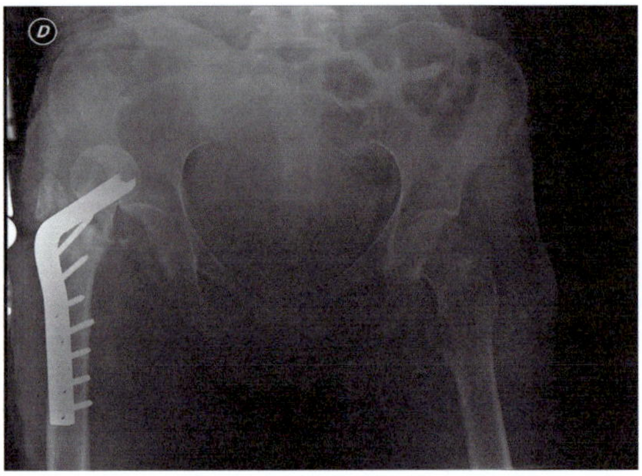

Fig. 7.6 Case 7.1, anteroposterior radiograph of the pelvis showing a right hip dislocation, despite wearing an anti-dislocation orthosis. Note the secondary displacement of the femoral neck in the coronal plane

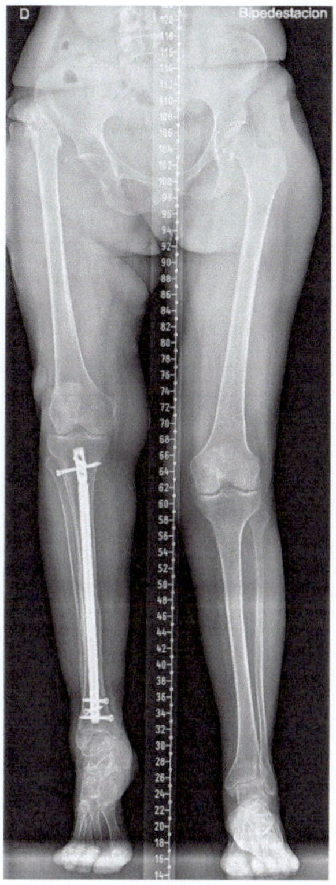

Fig. 7.7 Case 7.1, anteroposterior standing long leg radiograph 3 years after girdlestone resection arthroplasty. Elevation of the right hip toward the ilium can be observed, leading to a significant limb-length discrepancy

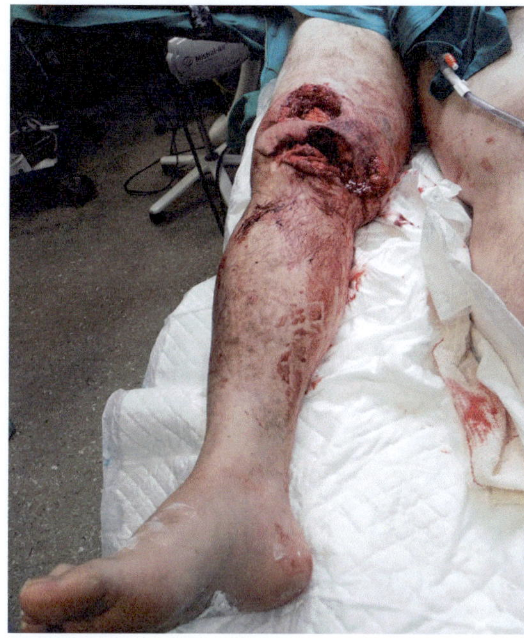

Fig. 7.8 Case 7.2, clinical photograph of the gunshot injury at first presentation at the hospital that initially treated the patient

Case 7.2

A 56-year-old male with a history of rheumatoid arthritis treated with leflunomide and hydroxychloroquine, as well as arterial hypertension, obesity and a right femoral fracture 20 years earlier treated with a slotted Fernández Domingo nail, suffered an accidental shotgun injury to the right knee with disruption of the extensor mechanism (Fig. 7.8). He was transferred to our hospital after initial debridement and provisional fixation with a K-wire (Fig. 7.9). Re-debridement with removal of the femoral nail (through the knee after trying several other methods, Fig. 7.10) was performed. A gentamicin-loaded bone cement spacer was implanted, and a provisional negative-pressure wound therapy device applied. The joint was stabilized with a bridging temporary external fixator (Fig. 7.11). Due to logistic problems, the soft tissue defect was covered almost 4 weeks after the fracture with a latissimus dorsi flap (Fig. 7.12), and the fracture treated with a knee arthrodesis prosthesis (Endo-Model, Waldemar Link, Hamburg, Germany; Fig. 7.13). *Paenibacillus larvae, Candida albicans,* and *Staphylococcus epidermidis* grew on cultures from intraoperative samples (F5 R3 I4). The latissimus dorsi flap suffered an arterial microthrombosis, unsalvageable despite revision, and a new attempt with the contralateral latissimus dorsi was also unsuccessful (the patient's autoimmune disorder was credited for these repeated microthromboses).

Above the knee amputation was initially considered, but in light of the patient having an intact, sensate foot, his age, and comorbidities, knee fusion was proposed to treat the soft tissue and bony defect (Fig. 7.14). The prosthesis was removed, the popliteal vascular bundle freed from the proximal and distal tethers at the tibia and femur, respectively, and acute shortening performed, closing the defect at the level of the knee. In the same stage, a percutaneous lengthening osteotomy was done at the proximal tibia

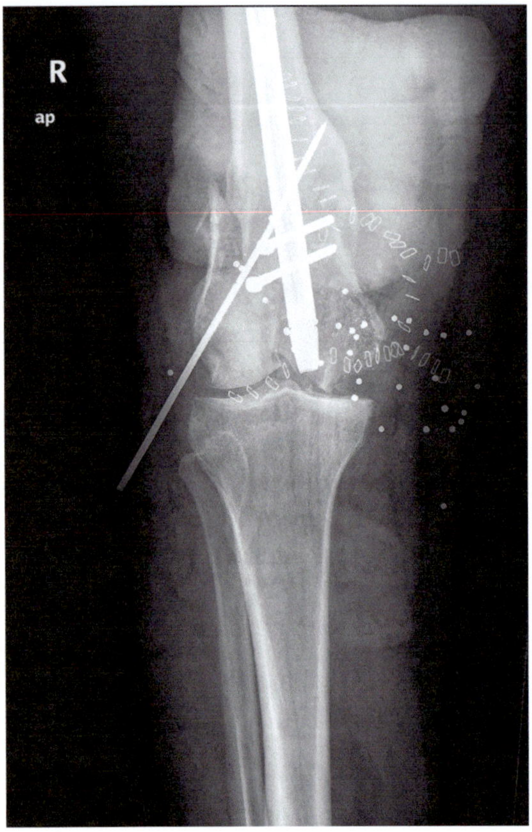

Fig. 7.9 Case 7.2, anteroposterior radiograph of the right knee upon transfer to our trauma center. The fracture had been fixed with a percutaneous K-wire and the joint immobilized with a plaster backslab. Note femoral nail from an injury 20 years prior

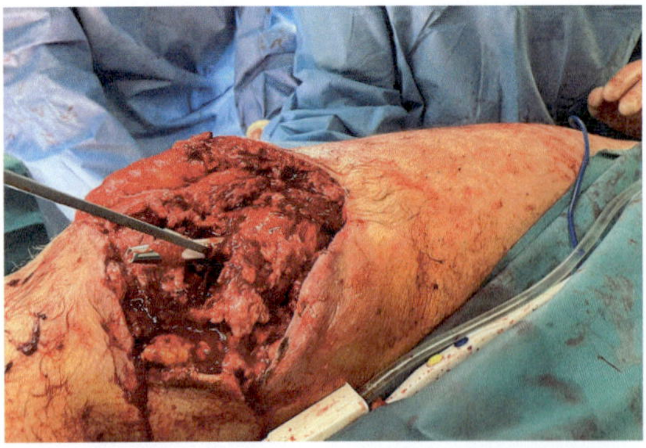

Fig. 7.10 Case 7.2, intraoperative photograph of the emergency debridement performed at the trauma center. There is a defect of the distal quadriceps muscle. The distal end of the slotted femoral Fernández Domingo nail (Surgival; Paterna, Valencia, Spain) is held with a Lambotte bone hook

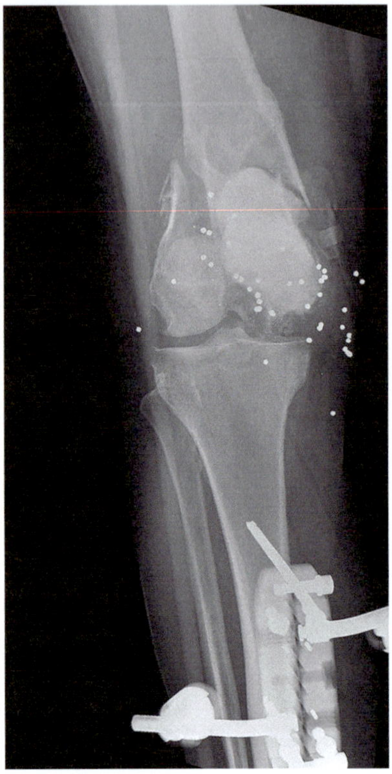

Fig. 7.11 Case 7.2, postoperative anteroposterior radiograph of the right knee after removal of the femoral nail, debridement, implantation of an antibiotic-loaded bone cement spacer in the bony defect and temporary fixation with a bridging external fixator

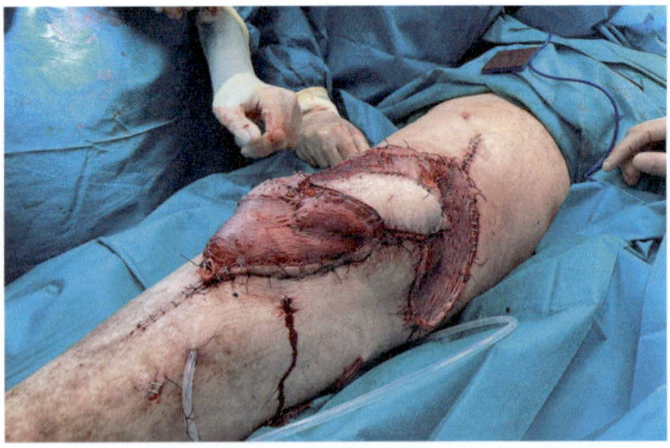

Fig. 7.12 Case 7.2, intraoperative photograph after closure of the defect with a latissimus dorsi free flap and split thickness skin graft

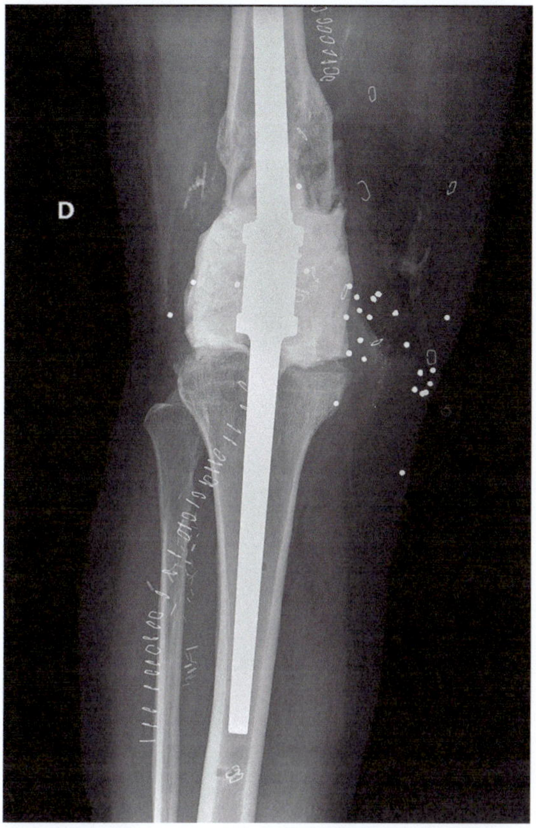

Fig. 7.13 Case 7.2, anteroposterior radiograph of the right knee after treatment with a knee arthrodesis prosthesis (Endo-Model, Waldemar Link, Hamburg, Germany)

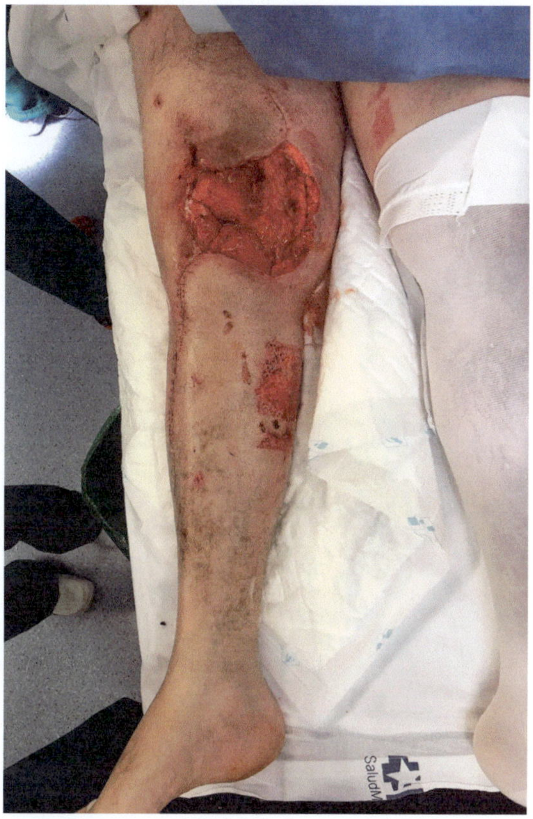

Fig. 7.14 Case 7.2, clinical photograph of the soft tissue defect of the right knee after two failed attempts at coverage with latissimus dorsi flaps. The defect is filled with friable granulation tissue and the prosthesis underneath is infected

(Figs. 7.15 and 7.16). The acute shortening allowed the defect to be closed with skin and muscles from the anterolateral tibial compartment. Compression was applied to the arthrodesis site, and a gradual lengthening of 8 cm performed at the proximal tibia (Figs. 7.17 and 7.18). A further ring system had to be applied to avoid equinovarus deformity of the foot and ankle due to the deformity (Fig. 7.19). The infection resolved uneventfully after the wounds had healed.

At 18 months postoperatively, the fixator was removed and substituted in the same stage with a minimally invasive percutaneous locking anterolateral plate crossing the fusion, covered in calcium sulfate loaded with vancomycin and gentamycin (Fig. 7.20). Three years after the hunting accident, the patient walks without technical aid on level ground and uses a hiking stick for irregular terrain. He remains infection-free and goes for long walks in the countryside, having taken up birdwatching instead of hunting (Fig. 7.21).

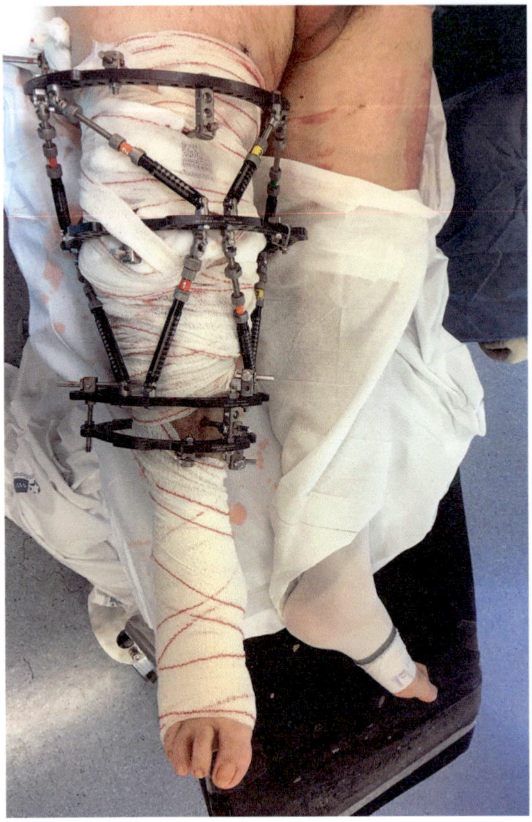

Fig. 7.15 Case 7.2, clinical photograph immediately after arthrodesis of the right knee and distraction osteogenesis with a circular hexapod fixator (Taylor Spatial Frame, Smith & Nephew, London, United Kingdom)

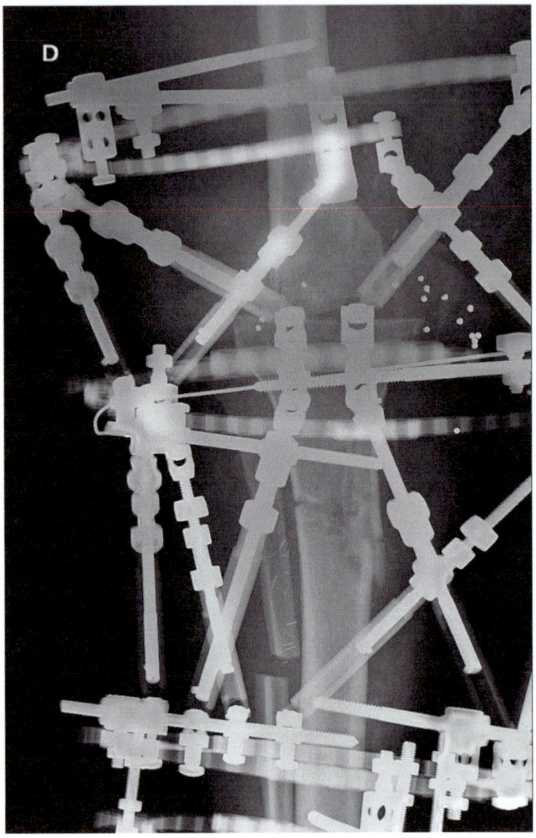

Fig. 7.16 Case 7.2, anteroposterior radiograph immediately after surgery for arthrodesis of the right knee and distraction osteogenesis with a circular hexapod fixator. (Taylor Spatial Frame, Smith & Nephew, London, United Kingdom)

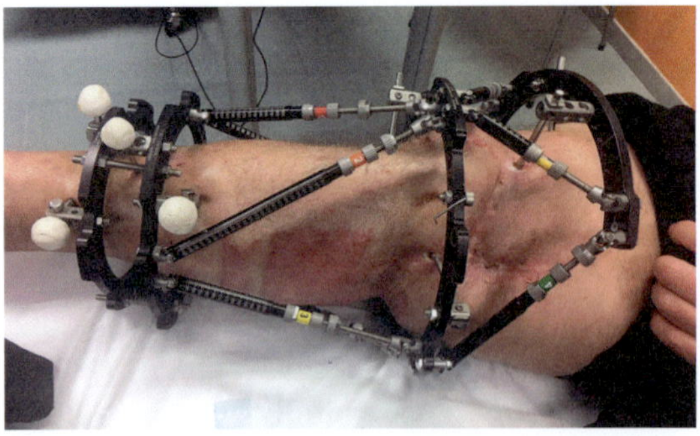

Fig. 7.17 Case 7.2, clinical photograph at 2 months postoperatively, after commencing lengthening. Note the scars around the knee, relative to the soft tissue defect shown in Fig. 7.14, and the distance between the two distal rings, at the distraction osteogenesis site, compared to Fig. 7.15

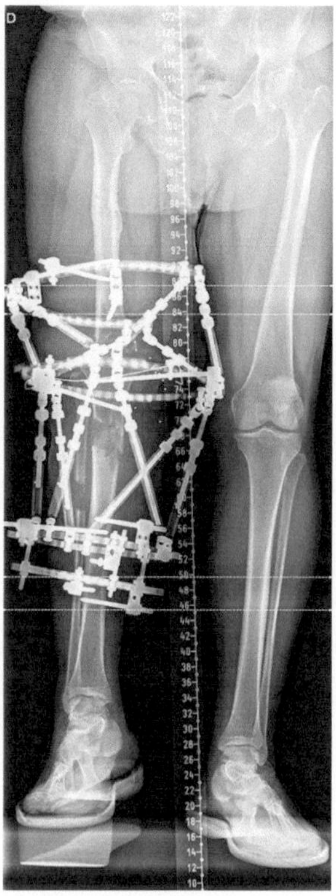

Fig. 7.18 Case 7.2, anteroposterior long-leg standing radiograph 2 months after hexapod fixator implantation, showing bony contact at the arthrodesis site, distraction osteogenesis of the proximal tibia and limb-length discrepancy. An equinus deformity was starting to develop

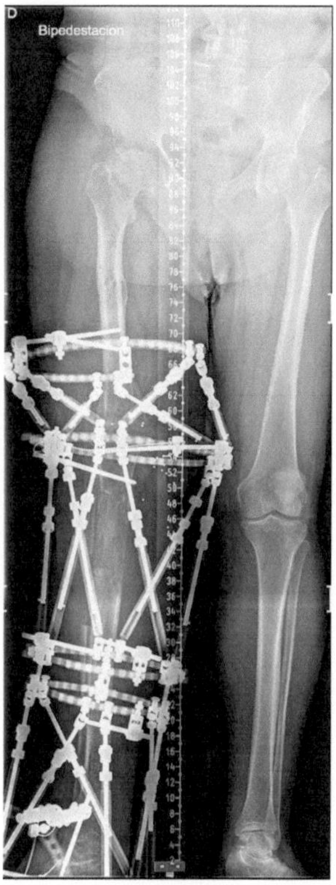

Fig. 7.19 Case 7.2, anteroposterior long-leg standing radiograph 12 months after hexapod fixator implantation, upon completion of osteogenesis distraction. Note the addition frame crossing the ankle joint to control the equinus deformity

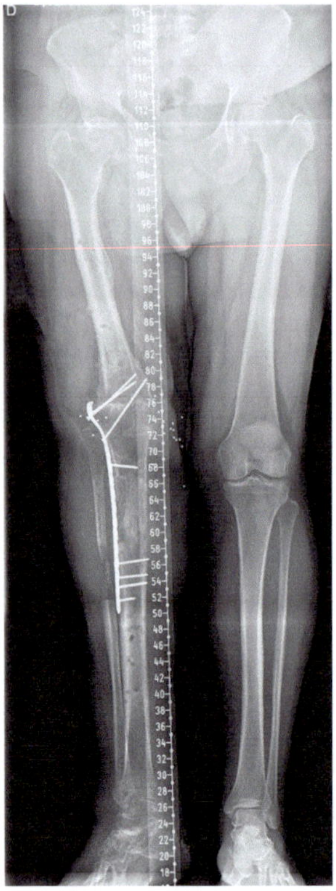

Fig. 7.20 Case 7.2, anteroposterior long-leg standing radiograph after removal of the circular fixator, and prophylactic fixation with a VA-LCP proximal tibia plate. (DePuy Synthes, Raynham, Massachusetts, United States of America)

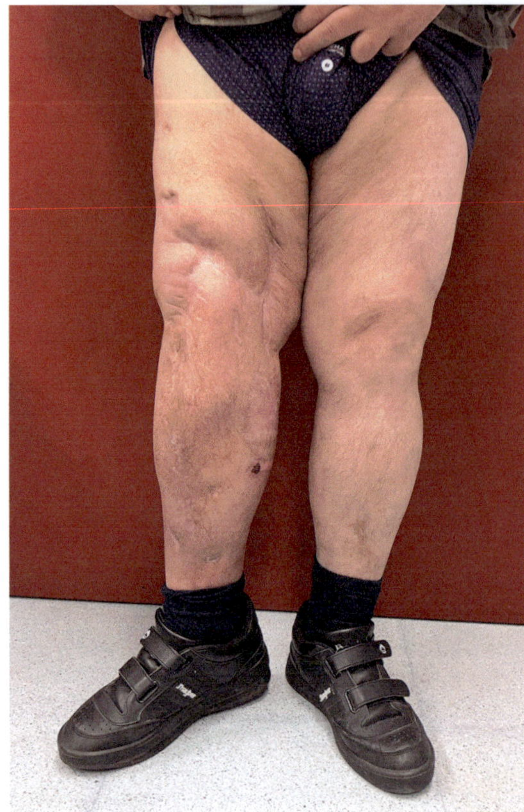

Fig. 7.21 Case 7.2, clinical appearance 3 years after the gunshot injury

Conclusions

When reconstruction of a joint affected by FRI is considered impossible or unadvisable (F5), the available surgical options for limb salvage are endoprosthetic joint replacement, excision arthroplasty, and arthrodesis. They are all aggressive procedures and associate high revision rates (around 50% at 5 years).

The available literature to guide decision-making in these cases is studies scant and heterogeneous. Often, it is based on PJI cases.

Endoprosthetic joint replacement provides considerable short-term improvement, at the cost of high rates of failure in the medium term (mostly, due to infection recurrence). The patients that will benefit from it the most are F5 R1–3 I1–4 with good infection control who are expected to have an active lifestyle after the procedure and in whom the structures needed for optimal prosthetic joint function are preserved.

Resection arthroplasty candidates are mostly F5 R3–4 I1–4 with an infected hip and very low functional demands.

Arthrodesis favors wound closure. It often includes a small shortening to collapse the bone defect. It has similar complications to endoprosthetic joint replacement (revision-less survivorship between 70% and 80% at 5 years). It is usually an alternative to endoprosthetic joint replacement when arthroplasty is not possible or unadvisable, in patients who are unlikely to wear an external prosthesis if amputation were performed.

References

1. Alt V, McNally M, Wouthuyzen-Bakker M, et al. The FRI classification – a new classification of fracture-related infections. Injury. 2024;55:111831. https://doi.org/10.1016/j.injury.2024.111831.
2. Morgenstern M, Clauss M, Sendi P, et al. Treatment of fracture-related infections. In: Textbook of polytrauma management: a multidisciplinary approach. 3rd ed. Berlin: Springer; 2022. p. 573–81.
3. Leitner L, Posch F, Amerstorfer F, et al. The dark side of arthroplasty: competing risk analysis of failed hip and knee arthroplasty with periprosthetic joint infection. J Arthroplast. 2020;35:2601–2606.e1. https://doi.org/10.1016/j.arth.2020.04.078.
4. Sambri A, Parisi SC, Zunarelli R, et al. Megaprosthesis in non-oncologic settings-a systematic review of the literature. J Clin Med. 2023;12:4151. https://doi.org/10.3390/jcm12124151.
5. Di Martino A, Pederiva D, Bordini B, et al. Proximal femoral replacement for non-neoplastic conditions: a systematic review on current outcomes. J Orthop Traumatol. 2022;23:18. https://doi.org/10.1186/s10195-022-00632-z.
6. Theil C, Schneider KN, Gosheger G, et al. Revision TKA with a distal femoral replacement is at high risk of reinfection after two-stage exchange for periprosthetic knee joint infection. Knee Surg Sports Traumatol Arthrosc. 2022;30:899–906. https://doi.org/10.1007/s00167-021-06474-2.
7. Vertesich K, Puchner SE, Staats K, et al. Distal femoral reconstruction following failed total knee arthroplasty is accompanied with risk for complication and reduced joint function. BMC Musculoskelet Disord. 2019;20:47. https://doi.org/10.1186/s12891-019-2432-4.
8. Voleti PB, Baldwin KD, Lee G-C. Use of static or articulating spacers for infection following total knee arthroplasty: a systematic literature review. J Bone Joint Surg Am. 2013;95:1594–9. https://doi.org/10.2106/JBJS.L.01461.
9. Nahhas CR, Chalmers PN, Parvizi J, et al. A randomized trial of static and articulating spacers for the treatment of infection following total knee arthroplasty. J Bone Joint Surg Am. 2020;102:778–87. https://doi.org/10.2106/JBJS.19.00915.
10. Nahhas CR, Chalmers PN, Parvizi J, et al. Randomized trial of static and articulating spacers for treatment of the infected Total hip arthroplasty. J Arthroplast. 2021;36:2171–7. https://doi.org/10.1016/j.arth.2021.01.031.
11. Grant C, Chang J, Poehlein E, et al. Static versus articulating spacer: does infectious pathogen type affect treatment success? Clin Orthop Relat Res. 2024;482:1850–5. https://doi.org/10.1097/CORR.0000000000003075.
12. Sousa R, Carvalho A, Soares D, Abreu MA. Interval between two-stage exchanges: what is optimal and how do you know? Arthroplasty. 2023;5:33. https://doi.org/10.1186/s42836-023-00185-4.
13. Ascione T, Balato G, Festa E, et al. Ideal timing of reimplantation in patients with periprosthetic knee infection undergoing 2-stage exchange: a diagnostic scoring system. J Bone Joint Surg Am. 2024;106:984–91. https://doi.org/10.2106/JBJS.23.00424.
14. Akgün D, Müller M, Perka C, Winkler T. High cure rate of periprosthetic hip joint infection with multidisciplinary team approach using standardized two-stage exchange. J Orthop Surg Res. 2019;14:78. https://doi.org/10.1186/s13018-019-1122-0.
15. Ascione T, Balato G, Mariconda M, et al. Continuous antibiotic therapy can reduce recurrence of prosthetic joint infection in patients undergoing 2-stage exchange. J Arthroplast. 2019;34:704–9. https://doi.org/10.1016/j.arth.2018.12.017.
16. Gandhi R, Backstein D, Zywiel MG. Antibiotic-laden bone cement in primary and revision hip and knee arthroplasty. J Am Acad Orthop Surg. 2018;26:727–34. https://doi.org/10.5435/JAAOS-D-17-00305.
17. McPherson EJ, Crawford BM, Kenny SG, et al. Point-of-care coating of revision femoral stems with antibiotic-loaded calcium Sulfate: reduction in infection after 2nd stage Reimplantation but not with aseptic revisions. Arthroplast Today. 2024;25:101302. https://doi.org/10.1016/j.artd.2023.101302.
18. Corona PS, Altayó M, Amat C, et al. Reconstruction of infected post-traumatic bone defects of the distal femur with the compress® implant. Preliminary results of a staged non-biological strategy. Injury. 2021;52:606–15. https://doi.org/10.1016/j.injury.2020.10.016.
19. Aebischer AS, Hau R, de Steiger RN, et al. Distal femoral replacement for Periprosthetic fractures after TKA: Australian Orthopaedic Association National Joint Replacement Registry review. J Arthroplast. 2022;37:1354–8. https://doi.org/10.1016/j.arth.2022.02.115.
20. Calori GM, Colombo M, Malagoli E, et al. Megaprosthesis in post-traumatic and periprosthetic large bone defects: issues to consider. Injury. 2014;45(Suppl 6):S105–10. https://doi.org/10.1016/j.injury.2014.10.032.
21. Li H, Zhang X, Li X, et al. The survival and complication profiles of the compress® Endoprosthesis: a systematic review and meta-analysis. J Bone Oncol. 2024;47:100623. https://doi.org/10.1016/j.jbo.2024.100623.

22. Parlee L, Kagan R, Doung Y-C, et al. Compressive osseointegration for endoprosthetic reconstruction. Orthop Rev (Pavia). 2020;12:8646. https://doi.org/10.4081/or.2020.8646.
23. Depypere M, Morgenstern M, Kuehl R, et al. Pathogenesis and management of fracture-related infection. Clin Microbiol Infect. 2020;26:572–8. https://doi.org/10.1016/j.cmi.2019.08.006.
24. Panteli M, Giannoudis PV. Chronic osteomyelitis: what the surgeon needs to know. EFORT Open Rev. 2016;1:128–35. https://doi.org/10.1302/2058-5241.1.000017.
25. Sobol KR, Fram BR, Strony JT, Brown SA. Survivorship, complications, and outcomes following distal femoral arthroplasty for non-neoplastic indications. Bone Jt Open. 2022;3:173–81. https://doi.org/10.1302/2633-1462.33.BJO-2021-0202.R1.
26. Mancino F, Di Matteo V, Mocini F, et al. Survivorship and clinical outcomes of proximal femoral replacement in non-neoplastic primary and revision total hip arthroplasty: a systematic review. BMC Musculoskelet Disord. 2021;22:933. https://doi.org/10.1186/s12891-021-04711-w.
27. Korim MT, Esler CNA, Reddy VRM, Ashford RU. A systematic review of endoprosthetic replacement for non-tumour indications around the knee joint. Knee. 2013;20:367–75. https://doi.org/10.1016/j.knee.2013.09.001.
28. Wyles CC, Tibbo ME, Yuan BJ, et al. Long-term results of total knee arthroplasty with contemporary distal femoral replacement. J Bone Joint Surg Am. 2020;102:45–51. https://doi.org/10.2106/JBJS.19.00489.
29. Angers-Goulet M, Pelet S, Belzile EL, Bédard M. Total knee arthroplasty with distal femoral replacement is associated with an important complication rate. A case series. Knee. 2019;26:1080–7. https://doi.org/10.1016/j.knee.2019.07.013.
30. Sukhonthamarn K, Strony JT, Patel UJ, et al. Distal femoral replacement and periprosthetic joint infection after non-oncological reconstruction: a retrospective analysis. J Arthroplast. 2021;36:3959–65. https://doi.org/10.1016/j.arth.2021.08.013.
31. Metsemakers W-J, Fragomen AT, Moriarty TF, et al. Evidence-based recommendations for local antimicrobial strategies and dead space management in fracture-related infection. J Orthop Trauma. 2020;34:18–29. https://doi.org/10.1097/BOT.0000000000001615.
32. Moriarty TF, Metsemakers W-J, Morgenstern M, et al. Fracture-related infection. Nat Rev Dis Primers. 2022;8:67. https://doi.org/10.1038/s41572-022-00396-0.
33. Alt V. Antimicrobial coated implants in trauma and orthopaedics-A clinical review and risk-benefit analysis. Injury. 2017;48:599–607. https://doi.org/10.1016/j.injury.2016.12.011.
34. Vicente M, Nomdedeu J, Lakhani K, Corona PS. Are silver-coated megaprostheses superior to uncoated megaprostheses in managing chronic end-stage periprosthetic hip and knee infection? Arch Orthop Trauma Surg. 2024;144:2197–205. https://doi.org/10.1007/s00402-024-05244-2.
35. Fiore M, Sambri A, Morante L, et al. Silver-coated distal femur megaprosthesis in chronic infections with severe bone loss: a multicentre case series. J Clin Med. 2023;12:6679. https://doi.org/10.3390/jcm12206679.
36. He S-Y, Yu B, Jiang N. Current concepts of fracture-related infection. Int J Clin Pract. 2023;2023:4839701. https://doi.org/10.1155/2023/4839701.
37. Shu HT, Ghanem D, Covarrubias O, et al. Poor outcomes of Girdlestone resection arthroplasty in injection drug users: a retrospective study. Antibiotics (Basel). 2024;13:782. https://doi.org/10.3390/antibiotics13080782.
38. Wixted CM, Polascik BA, Cochrane NH, et al. A multicenter prospective investigation on patient physical and mental health after Girdlestone resection arthroplasty. J Arthroplast. 2023;38:899–902. https://doi.org/10.1016/j.arth.2022.12.016.
39. Vincenten CM, Den Oudsten BL, Bos PK, et al. Quality of life and health status after Girdlestone resection arthroplasty in patients with an infected total hip prosthesis. J Bone Jt Infect. 2019;4:10–5. https://doi.org/10.7150/jbji.28390.
40. Corap Y, Brix M, Emmeluth C, Lindberg-Larsen M. Patient safety in distal femoral resection knee arthroplasty for non-tumor indications: a single-center consecutive cohort study of 45 patients. BMC Musculoskelet Disord. 2022;23:199. https://doi.org/10.1186/s12891-022-05100-7.
41. Brunet L, Fernández-Valencia JA, Torner P, et al. Is hip resection arthroplasty a successful definitive treatment? J Orthop. 2023;35:93–8. https://doi.org/10.1016/j.jor.2022.11.008.
42. Hulscher JB, te Velde EA, Schuurman AH, et al. Arthrodesis after osteosynthesis and infection of the ankle joint. Injury. 2001;32:145–52. https://doi.org/10.1016/s0020-1383(00)00156-x.
43. Mercurio M, Gasparini G, Cofano E, et al. Knee arthrodesis for periprosthetic knee infection: fusion rate, complications, and limb salvage-a systematic review. Healthcare (Basel). 2024;12:804. https://doi.org/10.3390/healthcare12070804.
44. McAuliffe JA, Burkhalter WE, Ouellette EA, Carneiro RS. Compression plate arthrodesis of the elbow. J Bone Joint Surg Br. 1992;74:300–4. https://doi.org/10.1302/0301-620X.74B2.1544974.
45. Kienast B, Kiene J, Gille J, et al. Posttraumatic severe infection of the ankle joint – long term results of the treatment with resection arthrodesis in 133 cases. Eur J Med Res. 2010;15:54–8. https://doi.org/10.1186/2047-783x-15-2-54.
46. Ring D, Jupiter JB, Toh S. Transarticular bony defects after trauma and sepsis: arthrodesis using vascularized fibular transfer. Plast Reconstr Surg. 1999;104:426–34. https://doi.org/10.1097/00006534-199908000-00016.
47. Hungerer S, Kiechle M, von Rüden C, et al. Knee arthrodesis versus above-the-knee amputation after septic failure of revision total knee arthroplasty: comparison of functional outcome and complication rates.

BMC Musculoskelet Disord. 2017;18:443. https://doi.org/10.1186/s12891-017-1806-8.
48. Caravelli S, Ambrosino G, Vocale E, et al. Custom-made implants in ankle bone loss: a retrospective assessment of reconstruction/arthrodesis in sequelae of septic Non-Union of the Tibial Pilon. Medicina (Kaunas). 2022;58:1641. https://doi.org/10.3390/medicina58111641.
49. Chalak A, Singh S, Ghodke A, et al. Ilizarov ankle arthrodesis: a simple salvage solution for failed and neglected ankle fractures. Indian J Orthop. 2022;56:1587–93. https://doi.org/10.1007/s43465-022-00669-6.
50. Brauns A, Lammens J. The challenge of the infected pilon tibial non-union: treatment with radical resection, bone transport and ankle arthrodesis. Acta Orthop Belg. 2020;86:335–41.
51. Singer S, Klejman S, Pinsker E, et al. Ankle arthroplasty and ankle arthrodesis: gait analysis compared with normal controls. J Bone Joint Surg Am. 2013;95:e191. (1–10. https://doi.org/10.2106/JBJS.L.00465.
52. Rosteius T, Lotzien S, Königshausen M, et al. Analysis of bone transport for ankle arthrodesis as a limb salvage procedure for the treatment of septic pilon fracture nonunion. Sci Rep. 2021;11:24472. https://doi.org/10.1038/s41598-021-04187-7.
53. Choi W, Park K-H, Oh C-W, et al. Treatment of critical-sized bone defects involving the ankle joints: staged Tibiotalocalcaneal arthrodesis with induced membrane technique and intramedullary nail. J Orthop Trauma. 2022;36:474–80. https://doi.org/10.1097/BOT.0000000000002363.
54. Meinert M, Colcuc C, Herrmann E, et al. Septic history limits the outcome of Tibiotalocalcaneal arthrodesis. J Clin Med. 2023;12:3422. https://doi.org/10.3390/jcm12103422.
55. Trouillez T, Faure PA, Martinot P, et al. Above-the-knee amputation versus knee arthrodesis for revision of infected total knee arthroplasty: recurrent infection rates and functional outcomes of 43 patients at a mean follow-up of 6.7 years. Orthop Traumatol Surg Res. 2021;107:102914. https://doi.org/10.1016/j.otsr.2021.102914.
56. Schnetz M, Maluki R, Ewald L, et al. Above-knee amputation shows higher complication and mortality rates in line with lower functional outcome compared to knee arthrodesis in severe periprosthetic joint infection. Bone Joint J. 2024;106-B:669–79. https://doi.org/10.1302/0301-620X.106B7.BJJ-2023-0978.R2.
57. Mayes WH, Severin AC, Mannen EM, et al. Management of periprosthetic joint infection and extensor mechanism disruption with modular knee fusion: clinical and biomechanical outcomes. Arthroplast Today. 2021;8:46–52. https://doi.org/10.1016/j.artd.2020.12.008.
58. Al-Naseem AO, Hayat J, Addar A, Marwan Y. External versus internal fixation techniques for ankle arthrodesis: a systematic review and meta-analysis. J Foot Ankle Surg. 2024;63:769–75. https://doi.org/10.1053/j.jfas.2024.05.010.

Amputation in Fracture-Related Infection

8

Nieves Vanaclocha, Alessandro Thione,
Alberto Pérez-García, and Cristina Ojeda-Thies

Introduction

Limb salvage has become a critical consideration in the treatment of patients with FRI, emphasizing the preservation of the limb over amputation [1]. In fact, amputation is quoted among the complications in FRI treatment, currently at just over 3% [2, 3]. Despite this, amputation is a therapeutic option, not necessarily a failure, because the goal is above all an infection-free functional limb, and this can be achieved with an amputation [4, 5]. Additionally, limb salvage is a long, debilitating journey, the benefits of which are generally reaped in the long term, so not every patient will obtain a high enough return on their investment for limb salvage to be in their best interest [5, 6]. In fact, amputation can provide a *better* functional outcome than a poorly salvaged limb [4, 7, 8]. Medium-term functional outcome (1–5 years) has been found to be no different between amputation and limb reconstruction for tibial or calcaneal FRIs, where the options for external prostheses are numerous and able to mitigate most of the impairment of a below-knee amputation [5, 9–11]. Furthermore, amputation usually allows early mobilization after a first-stage procedure, so recovery is usually achieved earlier than with limb salvage [6, 12].

However, amputation entails greater functional compromise the more proximal the level of amputation. For example, having to fasten on the external prosthesis in the dark if they wish to go to the bathroom during nighttime (to avoid waking up their partner) is a frequent complaint in middle-aged male patients, which make up a large proportion of FRI patients. The physical impairments derived from amputation are only partially mitigated by prostheses, in different degrees (see section *When is a satisfactory functional outcome after amputation considered likely?* below). For example, due to prosthesis design, control and suspension mechanisms, limb biomechanics are altered, and the kinetic transmission to the prosthesis is less efficient than to the native limb, increasing the energy expenditure required. Consequently, patients tend to reduce their residual limb's range of motion. Moreover, the functional

N. Vanaclocha (✉) · A. Thione
Orthoplastics Unit and Department of Plastic and Reconstructive Surgery, University and Polytechnic Hospital La Fe, Valencia, Spain

A. Pérez-García
Department of Surgery, Universitat de València, Valencia, Spain

Orthoplastics Unit and Department of Plastic and Reconstructive Surgery, University and Polytechnic Hospital La Fe, Valencia, Spain

C. Ojeda-Thies
Bone Infection Unit, Department of Traumatology and Orthopedic Surgery, 12 de Octubre University Hospital, Madrid, Spain

Department of Surgery, School of Medicine, Complutense University, Madrid, Spain

N. Vanaclocha (ed.), *Treatment of Fracture-Related Infection*,
https://doi.org/10.1007/978-3-031-92452-1_8

envelope (space in which the prosthesis can be used reliably, in relation to the patient's body) is more limited than for native limbs, and weight loading (e.g., lifting objects or walking with a pack) is limited by prosthetic tolerance and the patient-socket interface, with the socket potentially slipping away from the residual limb for objects heavier than a certain weight (this weight varies depending on the stability of the residual limb-socket interface) [13–15]. In addition, a painless stump with stable, nonredundant coverage may not be easy to obtain. Unplanned revision surgeries to treat infection or remodel the stump can be needed, and chronic neuropathic pain is common [16, 17]. Functional outcomes are similar between early and late posttraumatic amputations, but a late amputation may not alleviate mental health issues or pain sensitization that may arise while attempting to salvage the limb [17, 18].

The authors of this chapter were unable to find any literature reporting on the risk of infection recurrence after amputation in FRI patients. In patients undergoing above-knee amputation due to an infected knee arthroplasty, reported rates of infectious recurrence range between 10% and 35%, without statistically significant differences in the rates after amputation vs. after knee arthrodesis [9, 19]. A study on below-knee amputations due to traumatic injury reported a postoperative infection rate over 40% [17]. Though the populations differ in significant ways to the FRI population, in the absence of studies with FRI patients, these rates can give clinicians an idea of the infection rates that can be expected after an amputation due to FRI.

It is worth highlighting that mortality after amputation in the first postoperative 6 months in an FRI-only cohort was found to be 0% [4]. This differs from the mortality reported in patients amputated for other reasons (e.g., PJI, diabetes mellitus) who have a reduced life expectancy in comparison with FRI patients.

Amputation is likely to be in the patients' best interest when satisfactory functional outcome after limb salvage is *unlikely,* while a satisfactory functional outcome after amputation is *likely*.

When Is a Satisfactory Functional Outcome After Limb Salvage Considered Unlikely?

Two factors stand out regarding the overall postoperative functionality and quality of life of individuals who undergo limb salvage procedures: fracture union and limb sensation.

Fracture Union is a *requirement* for a satisfactory functional outcome, and a priority in FRI treatment due to its importance for both limb functionality and infection control [20–22]. The main strategy to enhance bony union in patients with FRI is preoperative optimization of the patient's health status (including nutrition and illnesses such as diabetes mellitus) and of the blood supply to the limb (e.g., smoking cessation), in addition to mechanical stability and availability of osteogenic potential, scaffolding, and growth factors to enable healing [2, 23, 24].

Several methods can stimulate bone formation postoperatively, such as low-intensity pulsed ultrasound, shockwave therapy, or pulsed electromagnetic fields. These mechanical stimulation techniques purportedly promote bone healing by enhancing cellular activity and blood flow. They have been reported to shorten external fixator time in small cohorts of patients undergoing distraction osteogenesis (though this is an off-label application) [25, 26]. However, complications including infections and fractures are not rare [23], and the available meta-analyses on the use of these techniques have reported inconsistent outcomes [25, 26]. Sufficiently powered controlled clinical trials are needed to clarify their benefits and potential risks.

Sensation of the plantar and palmar surfaces of the foot and hand, respectively, though not a requirement, is *crucial for a satisfactory functional outcome*. This is because continuous and dynamic sensory feedback is critical to fine-tune movements, generate adaptative responses to environmental changes (e.g., uneven terrain), and adjust pressure distribution dynamically [13–15]. Foot sensitivity (especially plantar sensitivity) is important to maintain balance and stability, coordinate movements during the gait cycle, and to protect the foot from lesions due to pressure and other stressors. Hand sensation is necessary to adjust pinch and grip pressures to properly grasp objects, it is indispensable for manual tasks. Consequently, few patients have a satisfactory functional outcome with an insensitive foot, and almost none with an insensitive hand. The opposite is also true—a limb with good sensory feedback is preferable to a prosthesis, because the currently available prosthetic options provide an inferior functional outcome to a well-reconstructed limb [13–15]. This is not only due to the abovementioned advantages of having continuous and dynamic sensory feedback, but also because natural and efficient mobility requires sensitive input, and the currently commercially available prostheses do not provide haptic feedback [13, 27]. Lack of plantar sensation results in worsened balance and stability, so prosthetic users have a higher risk of stumbling and falling than patients with two native limbs [14, 15]. In the hand, rehabilitated amputees must rely mostly on their vision to regulate grip force, which is challenging and prone to them making the grip too weak (the object slips and falls) or too strong (fragile objects can be crushed) [13]. With sensorized prostheses (thus far, experimental), the dominant limb of patients that have a native and a prosthesized limb is always the native one, even if it implies a handedness shift [28].

The limited available research suggests that protective sensation is the minimum required to obtain a satisfactory outcome in both the upper and lower limbs. Sensory disturbances in FRI patients usually result from nerve lesions secondary to the initial trauma, so, if a good nerve repair is possible and a minimum of protective sensation is expected, limb salvage (with nerve repair) is the preferred choice [1, 29]. Some patients recover protective sensation months or years after the injury, so nerve injury is not an absolute indication for amputation [30]. In the absence of protective sensation of the hand or foot, amputation will generally be a better option, but it is rarely necessary for it to be performed in an emergency setting. Patients do psychologically better if they have a chance to discuss the possibility or need of amputation with their surgeon and participate in the decision-making. As previously pointed out, only selected motivated patients have a satisfactory outcome with an insensitive foot—they should be *both able and willing* to comply with foot care to prevent injuries and infections (regular inspection, proper hygiene, moisturizing, appropriate footwear, exercises to enhance proprioception and balance).

Sometimes, FRI patients will have coexisting distal sensory alterations due to comorbidities such as diabetic peripheral neuropathy. Often, only some sensory modalities will be altered, so multiple tests to address each sensory modality (monofilament testing, vibration perception test, thermal sensitivity test, pinprick sensation test, proprioception test, etc.) can be required. In these patients, treatment of their underlying condition is fundamental to prevent further sensory loss and favor limb salvage.

When Is a Satisfactory Functional Outcome After Amputation Considered Likely?

Evidence on this matter is limited and has low methodological quality, with heterogeneous protocols, study populations, and outcome variables [31]. This has been attributed to the abundance of variable interrelated factors that affect outcome after amputation, including residual limb characteristics (amputation level, length of residual bone, soft tissue thickness, etc.), prosthesis characteristics (degree to which it replaces the function of the amputated limb, socket design, suspension mechanism, liner type, etc.), and factors pertaining to the patient-prosthesis interface (such as fit and comfort) [31]. However, there is widespread consensus that for a satisfactory functional outcome after an amputation, the use of a well-fitting prosthesis is key [9, 13–15, 31].

Good Socket Fit (and the residual limb itself) requires lifelong attention, so a high degree of patient commitment is needed for a satisfactory functional outcome after an amputation [13]. Prosthetic fitting is an iterative, never-ending process that is more difficult the higher the level of amputation [14, 15, 32]. Each residual limb is different and irregular in different ways (e.g., shape, soft tissue coverage, bony prominences) that can change in the long- and short-term, worsening fit [14, 15, 31]. This is especially true for stump volume, which, in some patients, has intraday variability, making socket fit and comfort inconsistent throughout the same day [13–15]. These fluctuations result in socket pistoning and excessive shear, leading to sores among other problems, and are especially troublesome in patients with comorbidities such as diabetes mellitus or renal dysfunction [13–15, 31]. Moreover, since the residual limb's skin is tightly occluded for prolonged periods of time and undergoes friction and pressure with prosthesis use, skin issues are frequent, and perspiration, as well as causing skin irritation, can disrupt patient-socket interface, deteriorating the prosthesis' mechanics [31, 33]. Additionally, other problems can arise, such as poor suspension or load transfer, so patients must undergo routine socket revisions every few years [34].

Several strategies have been proposed to improve socket fit and the mechanics of prosthesized limb. For example, myoplasty (suturing agonist to antagonist muscles) or myodesis (anchoring the muscle to the residual bone) are important in amputation to restore the normal length-tension of the muscles, increase the surface area available for prosthetic fitting, help stabilize the residual limb, provide good soft tissue coverage, and increase rehabilitation potential. However, no clinical studies have been found comparing myodesis or myoplasty to techniques without muscle stabilization [35]. Amputation osteomyoplasty, or bone-bridging, was developed in an attempt create a larger and more stable end-bearing construct, as well as preventing fibular instability in transtibial amputations. Multiple research groups have studied the utility of bone bridging procedures in amputees, but the evidence remains conflicting. Functional differences seem to be small, and up to one-third of patients have complications related to the bone-bridge, including delayed union and internal fixation-related complications [36–38]. No randomized trials exist comparing bone-bridging amputations with conventional amputation.

Another option to address the problems described with conventional sockets, including lack of stability, comfort, and increased sweating and irritation, are osseointegrated prostheses. They have been increasingly used in the past two decades, particularly in transfemoral and transhumeral amputees. They can be considered in patients in whom a good socket fit is not possible, but who are very compliant and willing to undertake the lifelong care of a stoma [32, 33]. Osseointegrated prostheses are anchored directly into the remaining bone, a technique that is well-established in dentistry. Although the concept of a bone-anchored implant conflating the outside world to the bone has been met with skepticism, studies report low rates of deep infections and implant removal. Nevertheless, superficial infection has been reported in 1% to 77% of patients over the first 5 postoperative years, and research efforts are directed toward improving the skin-implant interface and antibacterial coating of the implants [32–34]. Experience is limited to case series, several of them related to posttraumatic injury but none specifically to FRI. In addition to superficial infection, which is usually resolved with oral antibiotics, concerns regarding the use of ossteo-integrated prostheses include peri-prosthetic fractures (>60% in the first 5 years after implantation) and mechanical loosening (the second most common cause of implant removal, together with infection). However, physical function and quality of life seem to improve in patients with osseointegrated prostheses compared to patients with traditional socket designs [32, 34, 39, 40]. Survivorship until osseointegrated prosthesis revision is reported to be >90% at 5 years, and until change of abutment 35% at 7 years [33, 41, 42]. It is worth noting that a small number of amputees (around 5%) reported *worsening* with respect to their presurgical status [42]. Only a few case series report on osseointegration in small numbers of patients who were amputated for infectious causes, with promising results at 1 year [40, 43], but more research is needed to appraise the risks of this procedure, both in general and specifically for FRI patients.

Other advancements for amputees include targeted muscle innervation and the use of haptic technologies to restore some form of sensation [34].

Even with a Perfect Fit, Prosthesis Use Is Not Guaranteed Patients will only use the prosthesis if they feel that its usefulness compensates for the multiple troubles related with wearing the prosthesis, including donning and doffing it, a more laborious and time-consuming task the more proximal the level of amputation. As many as one third of patients consider that their prosthesis does not help them with daily activities, highlighting the need for training in how to make the best use of the prosthesis each time the patient receives a new prosthesis. Amputees need to modify their motion patterns and habits to adapt to their prosthesis, and, over time, may acquire anomalous postures or movement sequences with prosthetic use. This mental and physical process of relearning and continuous training is more successful in younger, more active patients. In addition, prostheses are heavy, so weak proximal musculature will hinder the patient's ability to lift the prosthesis in order to use it and to tolerate wearing it for long periods of time [13–15]. As a result of all this, the likelihood that a patient will wear a prosthesis has been found to be closely associated with the patients' age (patients over 70 years are unlikely to wear external prostheses) and pre-amputation mobility [9, 44]. It is important to assess the patient's physical and mental condition and their baseline functionality to gauge their potential for prosthesis wearability.

The Degree to Which the Available External Prostheses Can Replace the Amputated Limb's Function will also influence the functional outcome [13, 15, 45]. A high degree is more likely to be achieved with more distal amputations, and if the functions of the amputated limb are easier to replace. The functions of the lower limb (mostly, related to an upright position and locomotion) are less complex and thus easier to replace prosthetically than those of the upper limb, which encompass not only manipulation of different-sized objects, but also social behaviors such as self-expression. Some types of prostheses can assist more activities (e.g., myoelectric prostheses can generally generate stronger movements in more planes than body-powered prostheses). A further consideration is whether or not the patient has received appropriate training with the device [13–15].

Psychosocial Considerations of Amputation

When proposing amputation, it is important to address the psychosocial issues associated to it [46–49]:

- Most patients see amputation as a mutilation, a perception which affects amputees' body image and the likelihood that they will accept it as a treatment.
- Many patients wonder how the amputation will affect their career and personal relationships.
- Sometimes, amputation is considered a disgrace culturally or religiously. Most amputees report perceived social sigma and increased social isolation after the amputation.

Talking to other amputees (e.g. expert patient programs) can be useful [49].

Patients Best Benefited by Amputation

The decision to opt for limb salvage or amputation is nuanced and depends on multiple factors.

Based on the previously discussed points, the FRI patients best benefited by amputation are R1–3 hosts in whom a satisfactory functional outcome after limb salvage is considered unlikely (because healing of the fracture is considered impossible or because the distal hand or foot does not and is not expected to have at least protective sensation), the patient is committed to residual limb care and would be a good candidate for prosthetic rehabilitation (they are in a good physical and mental condition), the baseline functionality of the affected area is poor, and the available prosthetics are expected to replace the amputated limb's functions well (e.g., transtibial amputations). Additionally, amputation should be contemplated as an option in patients who:

- Are not suitable/fit enough for major reconstructions or multiple procedures. For example, a cohort of 196 patients with lower limb FRI found that chronic kidney disease sufferers were almost 30 times more likely to undergo amputation [4].
- Suffer from sepsis due to FRI.
- Prefer amputation (expectation for cure after failure of other procedures). Most patients who accept amputation do so in an attempt to rid themselves of the need of medical and surgical treatments associated to long-standing FRI [50]. In the abovementioned 196-patient cohort, amputated patients had undergone an average of 6.8 procedures (vs. 2.9 in the no-amputation group) [4].
- Those in whom soft tissue reconstruction is not possible, because the probability of reconstruction failure and/or potential morbidity of the reconstruction are unacceptable (I5), or because a free flap would be required for limb salvage but the patient is not fit enough for it (I4 R4).

Satisfaction of amputated non-rehabilitated patients is very poor, so patients who are unlikely to wear a prosthesis or unwilling to commit to the lifelong care it requires are usually best served by other treatment options [42].

Clinical Cases

Case 8.1

A 47-year-old female without a significant prior history suffered a motorcycle accident with polytrauma (Injury Severity Score 29). She had the following injuries: unstable pelvic fracture with active bleeding, closed comminuted left proximal humerus fracture, Gustilo type II open left intraarticular distal radius fracture, Gustilo type IIIA open right proximal tibia fracture, and Gustilo IIIB open left floating knee injury (tibial plateau + distal femur + patella) with disruption and loss of substance of the extensor mechanism (Fig. 8.1). A damage control strategy was initially applied, with successive debridements and vancomycin-loaded bone cement in the left distal femur and proximal. Serial debridements were performed until the patient was fit for provisional fixation and coverage with an anterolateral thigh flap anastomosed to the posterior tibial artery (Figs. 8.2, 8.3, and 8.4). The patient suffered unsalvageable thrombosis of the vascular anastomosis 24 h later, so a latissimus dorsi flap, anastomosed to a vascular loop to the superficial femoral artery and vein, was used to reconstruct the soft tissue defect (Fig. 8.5).

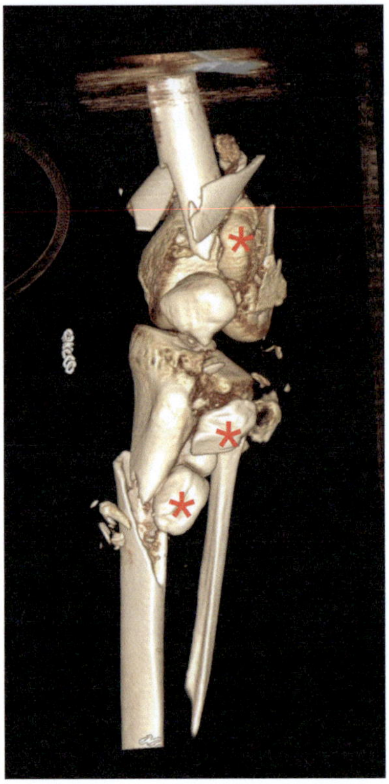

Fig. 8.1 Case 8.1, computed tomography three-dimensional reconstruction image taken after initial damage control surgery with a temporary external fixator. The asterisks signal the location of antibiotic-loaded bone cement beads in the bone defects

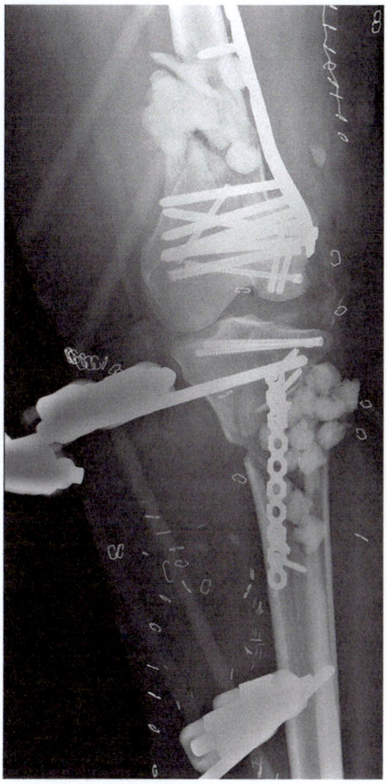

Fig. 8.2 Case 8.1, anteroposterior X-ray after initial internal-external fixation of the fractures. The distal femoral fracture has been stabilized with a VA-LCP condylar plate (DePuy Synthes, Raynham, Massachusetts, United States of America). The attachment of the extensor mechanism to the proximal tibia has been provisionally stabilized with a 3.5 mm EVOS plate (Smith & Nephew, London, United Kingdom) and a temporary external fixator, with the intention of exchanging it for a circular external fixator once the soft tissue defect had been covered. The antibiotic loaded bone cement beads have been exchanged at both fracture sites

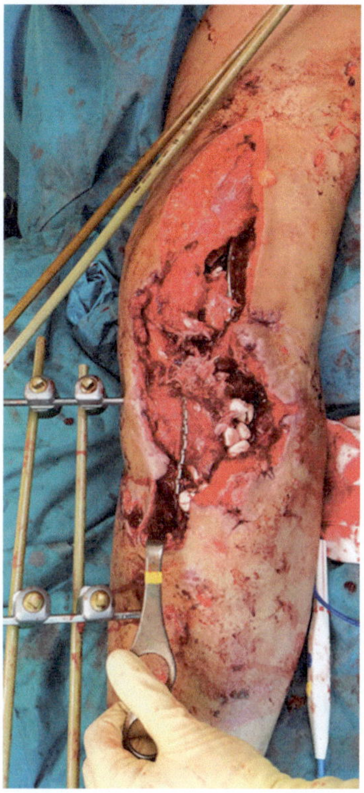

Fig. 8.3 Case 8.1, intraoperative photograph of the soft tissue defect after initial provisional stabilization, before coverage with a free flap

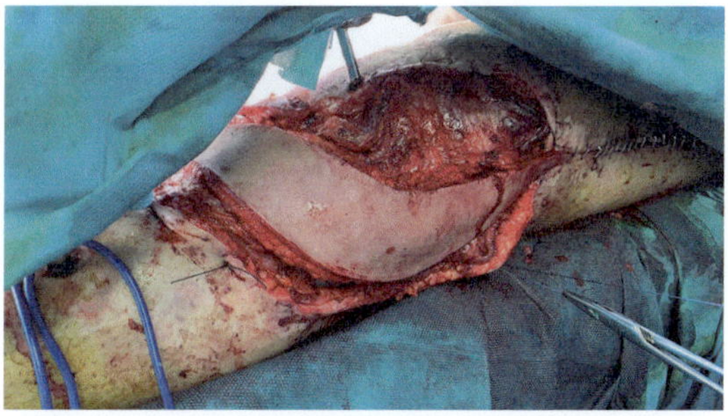

Fig. 8.4 Case 8.1, postoperative photograph of the defect covered with an anterolateral thigh flap

The patient developed a polymicrobial infection of both fractures, with several difficult-to-treat pathogens (including *Enterococcus* spp., VIM carbapenemase-producing *Klebsiella pneumoniae*, VIM carbapenemase-producing *Enterobacter cloacae*, and *Pseudomonas aeruginosa*). Several debridements while retaining the internal fixation were performed, and colistin and vancomycin-loaded bone cement spacers were left in the fracture sites. The infection eventually affected the vascular anastomosis at the superficial femoral artery (F5 R1 I5).

An above-the-knee amputation of the left leg was performed including myodesis of the adductors to the distal femur (Fig. 8.6). The amputation required one further soft tissue debridement, but the level of amputation could be maintained. The patient was able to recover from the rest of her injuries, but suffered phan-

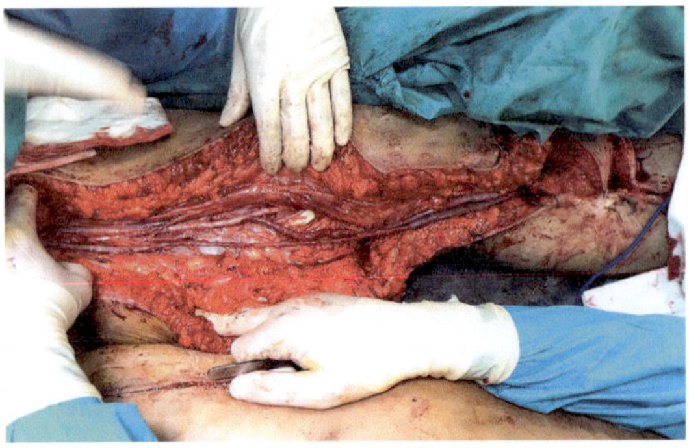

Fig. 8.5 Case 8.1, anastomosis of the latissimus dorsi flap to the superficial femoral vessels with two long vein grafts, after loss of the anterolateral thigh flap

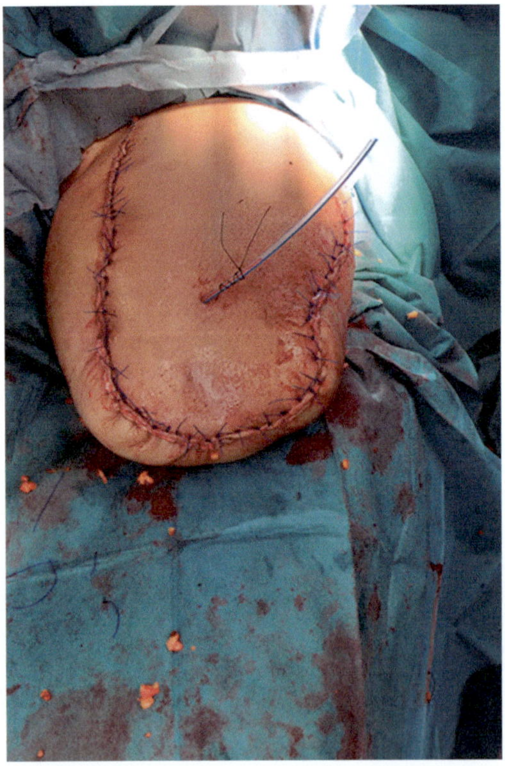

Fig. 8.6 Case 8.1, postoperative photograph after transfemoral amputation

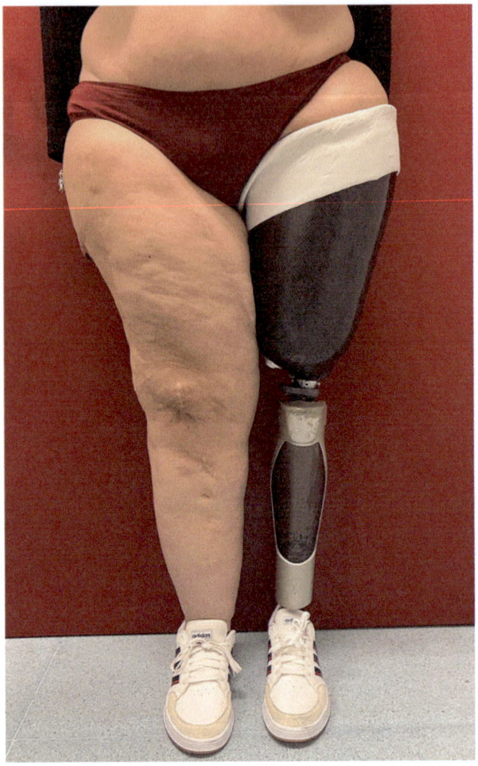

Fig. 8.7 Case 8.1, clinical appearance of the patient 4 years after the initial injury, with an external prosthesis including a mechanical knee joint

tom limb pain which required treatment with gapapentinoids and selective serotonin reuptake inhibitors for approximately one year.

Four years after her accident, she is infection-free, has a painless residual limb, and has a functional prosthesis (Figs. 8.7 and 8.8), which allows her to walk without technical aids, travel abroad, and engage in family activities with her children. She has also returned to her previous job, which involves long periods of standing and walking.

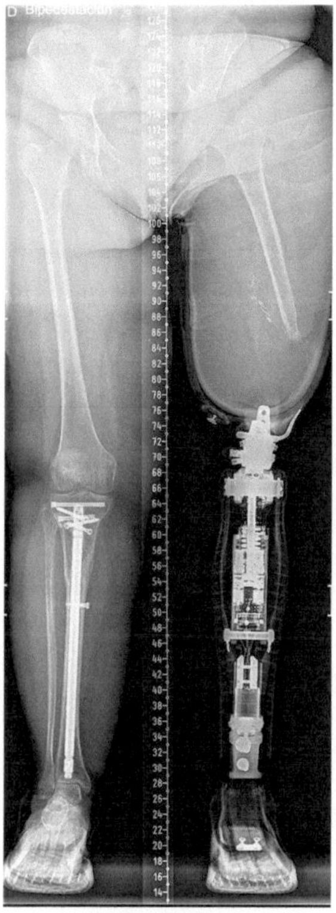

Fig. 8.8 Case 8.1, standing long-leg X-ray of the patient 4 years after injury and wearing her prosthesis. Note the abduction of the residual femur despite having performed an adductor myodesis, due to the force exerted by the hip abductors

Conclusions

Amputation is a therapeutic option, not necessarily a failure, because it can achieve the goal of surgical treatment of FRI, which is an infection-free functional limb. The question is not whether the limb can be saved but whether saving it is in the patient's best interest.

Amputation can provide a *better* functional outcome than a poorly salvaged limb. However, a limb with good sensory feedback is preferable to a prosthesis, because the currently available prosthetic options provide an inferior functional outcome to a well-reconstructed limb. This is because it will provide continuous and dynamic sensory feedback, which is crucial for enhanced mobility, adaptative responses to environmental changes, and adjusting pressure distribution dynamically. It is important to look out for critically important factors that will allow good limb salvage (e.g., early nerve repair).

A satisfactory functional outcome after limb salvage is unlikely when the procedure is not expected to achieve bone union and a minimum of protective sensitivity distally.

A satisfactory functional outcome after amputation is likely when the patient is expected to be able to wear a well-fitting prosthesis, and the prosthesis can replace the amputated limb's functions to a high degree. It is important to assess the patient's physical and mental condition and their baseline functionality to gauge their potential for prosthesis wearability.

The FRI patients best benefited by amputation are R1–3 hosts in whom the functional outcome after limb salvage is expected to be unsatisfactory, the amputation level is below-knee, the patient is a good candidate for prosthetic rehabilitation, and they are committed to lifelong residual limb care. Amputation is also an option in patients who are unsuitable or not fit enough for major reconstructions, in which limb salvage is precluded by the condition of the soft tissues, or who wish for amputation to avoid needing any more treatments for FRI.

References

1. Azoury SC, Stranix JT, Kovach SJ, Levin LS. Principles of Orthoplastic surgery for lower extremity reconstruction: why is this important? J Reconstr Microsurg. 2021;37:42–50. https://doi.org/10.1055/s-0039-1695753.
2. McNally M, Corrigan R, Sliepen J, et al. What factors affect outcome in the treatment of fracture-related infection? Antibiotics (Basel). 2022;11:946. https://doi.org/10.3390/antibiotics11070946.
3. Bezstarosti H, Metsemakers WJ, van Lieshout EMM, et al. Management of critical-sized bone defects in the treatment of fracture-related infection: a systematic review and pooled analysis. Arch Orthop Trauma Surg. 2021;141:1215–30. https://doi.org/10.1007/s00402-020-03525-0.
4. Carter KJ, Yeager MT, Rutz RW, et al. Lower extremity amputation in fracture-related infection. J Orthop Trauma. 2024;38:504–9. https://doi.org/10.1097/BOT.0000000000002853.
5. Iliadis AD, Shivji F, Debuka E, et al. Current concepts in the prevention, diagnosis and treatment of

fracture-related infection (FRI). Eur J Orthop Surg Traumatol. 2021;31:957–66. https://doi.org/10.1007/s00590-021-02956-8.
6. Barla M, Gavanier B, Mangin M, et al. Is amputation a viable treatment option in lower extremity trauma? Orthop Traumatol Surg Res. 2017;103:971–5. https://doi.org/10.1016/j.otsr.2017.05.022.
7. Tsang S-TJ, Ferreira N, Simpson AHRW. The reconstruction of critical bone loss : the holy grail of orthopaedics. Bone Joint Res. 2022;11:409–12. https://doi.org/10.1302/2046-3758.116.BJR-2022-0186.
8. Doukas WC, Hayda RA, Frisch HM, et al. The military extremity trauma amputation/limb salvage (METALS) study: outcomes of amputation versus limb salvage following major lower-extremity trauma. J Bone Joint Surg Am. 2013;95:138–45. https://doi.org/10.2106/JBJS.K.00734.
9. Hungerer S, Kiechle M, von Rüden C, et al. Knee arthrodesis versus above-the-knee amputation after septic failure of revision total knee arthroplasty: comparison of functional outcome and complication rates. BMC Musculoskelet Disord. 2017;18:443. https://doi.org/10.1186/s12891-017-1806-8.
10. Busse JW, Jacobs CL, Swiontkowski MF, et al. Complex limb salvage or early amputation for severe lower-limb injury: a meta-analysis of observational studies. J Orthop Trauma. 2007;21:70–6. https://doi.org/10.1097/BOT.0b013e31802cbc43.
11. Mitchell SL, Hayda R, Chen AT, et al. The military extremity trauma amputation/limb salvage (METALS) study: outcomes of amputation compared with limb salvage following major upper-extremity trauma. J Bone Joint Surg Am. 2019;101:1470–8. https://doi.org/10.2106/JBJS.18.00970.
12. Dickens JF, Kilcoyne KG, Kluk MW, et al. Risk factors for infection and amputation following open, combat-related calcaneal fractures. J Bone Joint Surg Am. 2013;95:e24. https://doi.org/10.2106/JBJS.L.00003.
13. National Academies of Sciences E, Division H and M, Services B on HC, et al. Upper-extremity prostheses. In: The promise of assistive technology to enhance activity and work participation. National Academies Press (US); 2017.
14. Fiedler G, Akins J, Cooper R, et al. Rehabilitation of people with lower-limb amputations. Curr Phys Med Rehabil Rep. 2014;2:263–72. https://doi.org/10.1007/s40141-014-0068-8.
15. Gailey RS, Kirk-Sanchez N, Clemens S, et al. Evidence-based amputee rehabilitation: a systematic approach to the restoration of function in people with lower limb loss. Curr Phys Med Rehabil Rep. 2022;10:17–26. https://doi.org/10.1007/s40141-021-00335-2.
16. Liston JM, Forster GL, Samuel A, et al. Estimating the impact of Postamputation pain. Ann Plast Surg. 2022;88:533–7. https://doi.org/10.1097/SAP.0000000000003009.
17. Bui G, Buckwalter J, Wilken J, et al. Comparison of early versus late below knee amputation after trauma with standardized prosthetic care. Iowa Orthop J. 2022;42:89–96.
18. Krueger CA, Rivera JC, Tennent DJ, et al. Late amputation may not reduce complications or improve mental health in combat-related, lower extremity limb salvage patients. Injury. 2015;46:1527–32. https://doi.org/10.1016/j.injury.2015.05.015.
19. Trouillez T, Faure PA, Martinot P, et al. Above-the-knee amputation versus knee arthrodesis for revision of infected total knee arthroplasty: recurrent infection rates and functional outcomes of 43 patients at a mean follow-up of 6.7 years. Orthop Traumatol Surg Res. 2021;107:102914. https://doi.org/10.1016/j.otsr.2021.102914.
20. Morgenstern M, Clauss M, Sendi P, et al. Treatment of fracture-related infections. In: Textbook of Polytrauma management: a multidisciplinary approach. 3rd ed. Berlin, Germany: Springer; 2022. p. 573–81.
21. Barla JD. Fracture-related infections. In: Slullitel P, Rossi L, Camino-Willhuber G, editors. Orthopaedics and trauma: current concepts and best practices. Cham: Springer; 2024. p. 805–10.
22. Marais LC, Zalavras CG, Moriarty FT, et al. The surgical management of fracture-related infection. Surgical strategy selection and the need for early surgical intervention. J Orthop. 2024;50:36–41. https://doi.org/10.1016/j.jor.2023.11.033.
23. Lu V, Zhang J, Patel R, et al. Fracture related infections and their risk factors for treatment failure-a major trauma Centre perspective. Diagnostics (Basel). 2022;12:1289. https://doi.org/10.3390/diagnostics12051289.
24. Giannoudis PV, Einhorn TA, Marsh D. Fracture healing: the diamond concept. Injury. 2007;38(Suppl 4):S3–6. https://doi.org/10.1016/s0020-1383(08)70003-2.
25. Wildemann B, Ignatius A, Leung F, et al. Non-union bone fractures. Nat Rev Dis Primers. 2021;7:57. https://doi.org/10.1038/s41572-021-00289-8.
26. Emara KM, Ghafar KAA, Al Kersh MA. Methods to shorten the duration of an external fixator in the management of tibial infections. World J Orthop. 2011;2:85–92. https://doi.org/10.5312/wjo.v2.i9.85.
27. Aszmann OC, Vujaklija I, Roche AD, et al. Elective amputation and bionic substitution restore functional hand use after critical soft tissue injuries. Sci Rep. 2016;6:34960. https://doi.org/10.1038/srep34960.
28. Raffin E. The various forms of sensorimotor plasticity following limb amputation and their link with rehabilitation strategies. Rev Neurol (Paris). 2021;177:1112–20. https://doi.org/10.1016/j.neurol.2021.09.003.
29. Momoh AO, Kumaran S, Lyons D, et al. An argument for salvage in severe lower extremity trauma with posterior Tibial nerve injury: the ganga hospital experi-

ence. Plast Reconstr Surg. 2015;136:1337–52. https://doi.org/10.1097/PRS.0000000000001814.
30. Bosse MJ, McCarthy ML, Jones AL, et al. The insensate foot following severe lower extremity trauma: an indication for amputation? J Bone Joint Surg Am. 2005;87:2601–8. https://doi.org/10.2106/JBJS.C.00671.
31. Safari R. Lower limb prosthetic interfaces: clinical and technological advancement and potential future direction. Prosthetics Orthot Int. 2020;44:384–401. https://doi.org/10.1177/0309364620969226.
32. Gerzina C, Potter E, Haleem AM, Dabash S. The future of the amputees with osseointegration: a systematic review of literature. J Clin Orthop Trauma. 2020;11:S142–8. https://doi.org/10.1016/j.jcot.2019.05.025.
33. Kunutsor SK, Gillatt D, Blom AW. Systematic review of the safety and efficacy of osseointegration prosthesis after limb amputation. Br J Surg. 2018;105:1731–41. https://doi.org/10.1002/bjs.11005.
34. Tintle SM, LeBrun C, Ficke JR, Potter BK. What is new in trauma-related amputations. J Orthop Trauma. 2016;30(Suppl 3):S16–20. https://doi.org/10.1097/BOT.0000000000000668.
35. Fabre I, Thompson D, Gwilym B, et al. Surgical techniques of, and outcomes after, distal muscle stabilization in Transfemoral amputation: a systematic review and narrative synthesis. Ann Vasc Surg. 2024;98:182–93. https://doi.org/10.1016/j.avsg.2023.07.105.
36. Tintle SM, Keeling JJ, Forsberg JA, et al. Operative complications of combat-related transtibial amputations: a comparison of the modified burgess and modified Ertl tibiofibular synostosis techniques. J Bone Joint Surg Am. 2011;93:1016–21. https://doi.org/10.2106/JBJS.J.01038.
37. Plucknette BF, Krueger CA, Rivera JC, Wenke JC. Combat-related bridge synostosis versus traditional transtibial amputation: comparison of military-specific outcomes. Strategies Trauma Limb Reconstr. 2016;11:5–11. https://doi.org/10.1007/s11751-015-0240-4.
38. Keeling JJ, Shawen SB, Forsberg JA, et al. Comparison of functional outcomes following bridge synostosis with non-bone-bridging transtibial combat-related amputations. J Bone Joint Surg Am. 2013;95:888–93. https://doi.org/10.2106/JBJS.L.00423.
39. Muderis MA, Aschoff HH, Bosley B, et al. Direct skeletal attachment prosthesis for the amputee athlete: the unknown potential. Sports Eng. 2016;19:141–5. https://doi.org/10.1007/s12283-016-0196-8.
40. Al Muderis M, Lu W, Li JJ. Osseointegrated prosthetic limb for the treatment of lower limb amputations : experience and outcomes. Unfallchirurg. 2017;120:306–11. https://doi.org/10.1007/s00113-016-0296-8.
41. Reif TJ, Khabyeh-Hasbani N, Jaime KM, et al. Early experience with femoral and Tibial bone-anchored Osseointegration prostheses. JB JS Open Access. 2021;6(e21):00072. https://doi.org/10.2106/JBJS.OA.21.00072.
42. Hagberg K, Ghassemi Jahani S-A, Kulbacka-Ortiz K, et al. A 15-year follow-up of transfemoral amputees with bone-anchored transcutaneous prostheses. Bone Joint J. 2020;102-B:55–63. https://doi.org/10.1302/0301-620X.102B1.BJJ-2019-0611.R1.
43. Corona PS, Vargas Meouchi EA, García Hernández JM, et al. Single-stage transcutaneous osseointegrated prosthesis for above-knee amputations including an antibiotic-loaded hydrogel. Preliminary results of a new surgical protocol. Injury. 2024;55:111424. https://doi.org/10.1016/j.injury.2024.111424.
44. Mundell BF, Kremers HM, Visscher S, et al. Predictors of receiving a prosthesis for adults with above-knee amputations in a well-defined population. PM R. 2016;8:730–7. https://doi.org/10.1016/j.pmrj.2015.11.012.
45. Metsemakers W-J, Morgenstern M, Senneville E, et al. General treatment principles for fracture-related infection: recommendations from an international expert group. Arch Orthop Trauma Surg. 2020;140:1013–27. https://doi.org/10.1007/s00402-019-03287-4.
46. National Academies of Sciences E, Division H and M, Services B on HC, Impairments C on the U of SAP and T in E or R the E of, Flaubert JL, Spicer CM, et al. Upper-Extremity Prostheses. The Promise of Assistive Technology to Enhance Activity and Work Participation, National Academies Press (US); 2017
47. Fiedler G, Akins J, Cooper R, Munoz S, Cooper RA. Rehabilitation of People with Lower-Limb Amputations. Curr Phys Med Rehabil Rep 2014;2:263–72. https://doi.org/10.1007/s40141-014-0068-8.
48. Gailey RS, Kirk-Sanchez N, Clemens S, Symsack A, Gaunaurd I. Evidence-Based Amputee Rehabilitation: a Systematic Approach to the Restoration of Function in People with Lower Limb Loss. Curr Phys Med Rehabil Rep 2022;10:17–26. https://doi.org/10.1007/s40141-021-00335-2.
49. Aschoff HH, Örgel M, Sass M, Fischer D-C, Mittlmeier T. Transcutaneous Osseointegrated Prosthesis Systems (TOPS) for Rehabilitation After Lower Limb Loss: Surgical Pearls. JBJS Essent Surg Tech 2024;14:e23.00010. https://doi.org/10.2106/JBJS.ST.23.00010
50. Lerner RK, Esterhai JL, Polomano RC, et al. Quality of life assessment of patients with posttraumatic fracture nonunion, chronic refractory osteomyelitis, and lower-extremity amputation. Clin Orthop Relat Res. 1993;295:28–36.

9 Soft Tissue Management and Obtention of Reliable Wound Coverage in Fracture-Related Infection

Alberto Pérez-García, Pedro Alvedro, Iván Heredia, Nieves Vanaclocha, Alessandro Thione, and Leonard Marais

Introduction

Achieving a healthy soft tissue envelope is one of the cornerstones for successful management of fracture-related infection (FRI) due to its direct effect on outcome, both in terms of bone healing and, especially, infection eradication [1–3]. Well-vascularized soft tissues provide a favorable environment for bone healing and regeneration, while also decreasing reinfection and recurrence risk by [4, 5]:

- Delivering host immune cells, systemic antimicrobials, growth factors, and nutrients to the FRI site.
- Serving as an antimicrobial barrier, which prevents recontamination.
- In cases of tissue transfer, obliterating dead space as well.

The soft tissues surrounding FRI sites are often fibrotic due to trauma and prolonged inflammation. These tissues are unhealthy and unreliable, and tend toward wound instability and breakdown, which increases the risk of further contamination. As a result, up to 40% of FRI patients require tissue transfer [6]. Achieving a well-vascularized tissue envelope as soon as possible is critical for good outcomes, for which an orthoplastic approach is essential [4].

In this chapter, we will discuss the different possibilities for soft tissue management in FRI to obtain a healthy soft tissue envelope that will support bone healing and help eradicate infection. The nature and timing of soft tissue reconstruction with flaps, as well as the role of negative pressure wound therapy (NWPT), will be discussed.

A. Pérez-García (✉)
Department of Surgery, Universitat de València, Valencia, Spain

Orthoplastics Unit and Department of Plastic and Reconstructive Surgery, University and Polytechnic Hospital La Fe, Valencia, Spain

P. Alvedro · I. Heredia
Department of Plastic and Reconstructive Surgery, University and Polytechnic Hospital La Fe, Valencia, Spain

N. Vanaclocha · A. Thione
Orthoplastics Unit and Department of Plastic and Reconstructive Surgery, University and Polytechnic Hospital La Fe, Valencia, Spain

L. Marais
Department of Orthopaedic Surgery, School of Clinical Medicine, College of Health Sciences, University of KwaZulu-Natal, Durban, South Africa

N. Vanaclocha (ed.), *Treatment of Fracture-Related Infection*,
https://doi.org/10.1007/978-3-031-92452-1_9

When Direct Closure Is Possible (I1–2)

Few FRI cases have well-vascularized soft tissues surrounding the fracture that allow realiable tension-free direct closure after debridement (I1). These cases are amenable to simple direct closure, and infection may be eradicated in over 85% of such cases [7]. Very rarely, acute shortening of the bone following bony debridement may assist in obtaining direct closure.

Much more often, direct closure is possible but with some difficulty, or the coverage is not robust because it relies on compromised soft tissues (e.g., by scarring or vascular insufficiency) (I2) [8]. This fibrotic, fragile skin is unpredictable and wound breakdown is common. In these cases, reinforcing the closure with a flap (local or free) is a safer approach to prevent exposure of underlying bone and/or hardware, which would lead to treatment failure, and increase the chance of infection eradication [7, 8]. This "prophylactic flap" approach is especially appropriate in anatomical regions with thin, vulnerable soft tissues, such as the distal tibia, clavicle, or patella, where the risk of complications is inherently higher, as well as in implant retention strategies, due to the higher risk of infection recurrence (higher load of residual pathogens after debridement) [9]. Despite the logistic challenges that this early orthoplastic approach presents, the available evidence suggests that its results are worth the effort for both patients and the teams treating them, as it is associated to less treatment failures and avoids the need for semi-urgent soft tissue coverage due to wound breakdown, which is even more troublesome to organize [7, 10].

It is worth remembering that some techniques developed for other aspects of FRI treatment can aid in wound closure. For example, acute shortening can often downgrade a case that would have originally needed a flap for wound closure to one with a partially exposed muscle requiring only some skin grafting, significantly simplifying closure. As has been mentioned in other chapters, the strategies to manage stability, dead space, and the soft tissues are closely interrelated.

Options for Tissue Transfer in Fracture-Related Infection (I3–I4)

In about 30–40% FRIs, after debridement, direct closure of the wound is not possible and tissue transfer is required [6, 7].

Flap reconstruction involves transfer of tissue(s), such as skin, muscle, and/or bone, *together with their nutrient artery and vein(s)* from one anatomic location to another. In locoregional flaps, the flap pedicle remains uninterrupted and united to its original proximal vessels, so they can only be used for nearby sites (as far as the pedicle will allow the flap to reach). Free flaps are not limited in this way, as their nutrient artery and vein(s) are severed at their origin and microanastomosed to recipient vessels at recipient site. Regardless of whether the flap is locoregional or free, its intrinsic blood supply ensures blood flow to it, and thus, transportation of immune cells, systemic antibiotics, and growth factors to the recipient (FRI) site.

The threshold for the use of flaps in FRI should be low, due to the benefits they offer that directly address the challenges posed by FRI [7, 11]. This is especially true of infection eradication, because flaps effectively replace fibrotic and nonviable tissues with a healthy soft tissue envelope, which serves as an antimicrobial barrier and reduces the risk of infection recurrence by facilitating the delivery of growth factors, immune cells, and systemic antibiotics to the FRI site [12, 13]. This soft tissue-mediated delivery of oxygen, growth factors, and nutrients into the FRI site also promotes fracture consolidation, the other main objective in FRI. Beyond infection control and bone healing, flaps provide stable and durable soft tissue coverage, which is crucial for subsequent orthopedic interventions, such as bone transport or other staged reconstructions. Furthermore, by ensuring robust and adaptable wound coverage, flaps play a pivotal role in restoring both form and function, laying the foundation for optimal long-term outcomes in patients with FRI [12].

No single flap or flap type has been proven superior in FRI management [1, 3]. The choice of flap is guided by many factors, including the characteristics of the defect (which tissues are missing, and should the flap also manage dead space or a bone defect?), the availability of local tissues, specific regional requirements (e.g., shoe-fitting for foot and ankle defects), patient preferences (especially, regarding donor morbidity), and the surgeon's proficiency (given the importance of a healthy soft tissue envelope and the consequences of wound breakdown in FRI, it is important to select a flap that the surgeon can reliably harvest).

Correct patient assessment and optimal surgical planning are critical in the management of FRI. Multidisciplinary preoperative discussion of the surgical plan is advisable, in order for the team responsible for soft tissue reconstruction to be well informed of the skeletal reconstruction and fixation plan. Acute shortening at the fracture site, for example, may change the shape and size of the soft tissue defect, and wire placement needs to be carefully considered if circular external fixation is planned. Moreover, as in any reconstructive procedure, a careful assessment of the vascular status of the affected area is essential to evaluate the viability of locoregional flaps and to determine the suitability of potential recipient vessels for microsurgical reconstruction. Although detailing the methods for vascular examination and selection of recipient vessels lies beyond the scope of this chapter, it is worth highlighting that the vascular integrity of the FRI area is often compromised as a result of prior trauma, previous surgical procedures and/or or chronic infection. Thus, the team must ensure the presence of healthy recipient vessels (often, distant from the zone of injury) and/or that the vascular supply to a potential regional flap is intact. This assessment and multidisciplinary planning are fundamental to the success of reconstruction.

Note that, as for other aspects of FRI management, patient comorbidities such as smoking, peripheral arterial disease, venous insufficiency, or diabetes mellitus significantly increase the risk of flap failure. Thus, preoperative patient optimization is a must.

Locoregional Flaps (I3)

Locoregional flaps are typically chosen when local tissues are abundant and well-preserved, as is often the case in the genicular region. Commonly used flaps in this area include the medial and lateral gastrocnemius, saphenous, and sural flaps (see Case 9.1 in the *Clinical cases* section below). The use of propeller flap is also quite extended, owing to their versatility. However, venous congestion and distal necrosis are not uncommon, potentially leading to flap failure and the need for a second reconstruction. The use of indocyanine green for intraoperative perfusion assessment can improve their reliability [14, 15].

The main advantage of locoregional flaps is that they are significantly easier and faster to perform than free flaps. Moreover, no additional anatomical areas (other than the FRI-affected area) will be surgically affected. The main tradeoff is a higher complication rate than that for free flaps (mostly, distal necrosis) [9]. Given its technical and logistic advantages, if a suitable locoregional flap is available, it is usually preferred over a free flap.

Free Flaps (I4)

When local tissues are compromised or when extensive dead space needs to be addressed, free flaps are preferred. This is often the case when the affected location is the distal tibia, due to the scarcity of local soft tissues in that location. Free flap surgery has been associated with high rates of both fracture union and infection eradication (>90%) [6, 7]. Specifically in tibia FRIs, free flaps have been associated with a 12% increase in the likelihood of bone union and a marked reduction in the infection eradication rate in comparison with patients that did not receive a free flap (20% no free flap vs. 8% free flap group) [7]. Moreover, studies have shown that donor-site morbidity is comparable to that of locoregional flaps, with patients reporting similar quality of life [12, 16].

In FRI, the most often used free flaps are fasciocutaneous flaps, muscle flaps, and osteocutaneous flaps.

Fasciocutaneous flaps are composed mostly of skin and fat tissue. Commonly used ones in FRI include the anterolateral thigh (ALT) flap (see Case 9.2 below), thoracodorsal artery perforator (TDAP) flap, and the superficial circumflex iliac artery perforator (SCIP) flap. They provide a healthy soft tissue envelope, with lower donor-site morbidity than the other two kinds of flaps described, and easier re-elevation for secondary procedures, such as hardware removal or bone grafting.

Muscle flaps are composed of muscle, musculocutaneous flaps including both muscle and the soft tissues above it. Commonly used ones in FRI include the latissimus dorsi, gracilis (see Case 9.3 below), vastus lateralis, and rectus abdominis flaps. These flaps are bulky, so as well as providing reliable wound coverage, they are very useful to manage dead space. Muscle flaps have been traditionally favored over fasciocutaneous flaps for their ability to manage dead space and adapt to three-dimensional defects, particularly over joints where minimal bulk is needed (a muscle flap will atrophy over time). These flaps are typically resurfaced with sheet skin grafts, providing durable coverage and good cosmetic results. Although no randomized controlled trials have definitively compared muscle and fasciocutaneous flaps, which have lower donor site morbidity, large series in lower limb reconstruction suggest both types are equally effective in terms of bony healing and infection eradication when used appropriately [6, 9]. Often, muscle flaps are opted for in cases of complex, three-dimensional defects while fasciocutaneous flaps are preferred for simpler wounds or those requiring future secondary procedures [17, 18]. However, achieving reliable wound coverage *early* appears to be more important than the type of flap used, and both types of flaps can be successful [9].

Osteocutaneous flaps are composed of bone and a skin island. They are used for combined soft tissue and critical bone defects, providing both reliable wound coverage and structural support. They are particularly useful in the upper extremity (e.g., humeral defects). Out of them, the osteocutaneous fibula flap is the most notable, optimizing the chances of successful limb salvage and functional recovery in FRI [19]. The reader is referred to Chaps. 5 and 6 for more information on bone flaps.

In rare cases, other flaps may be appropriate. For instance, free omental flaps may be considered for extremely large defects that cannot be addressed with conventional options such as a latissimus dorsi flap [20]. The omentum offers unique advantages, including its bacteriostatic properties, promotion of angiogenesis and lymphatic drainage, and ability to conform to large, three-dimensional defects. However, disruption of the abdominal cavity can lead to complications like ventral hernia or bowel obstruction, limiting its use.

Free flap revision in the lower limb is not rare, with reported revision rates in excess of 10% [6, 21]. However, revision often achieves flap salvage, with a free flap failure rate in FRI of under 5% in experienced hands [6]. When vascular compromise does happen, it almost always happens early due to a thrombotic event, with late failures being rare. In addition, both free and locoregional flap failure does not appear to be a risk factor for nonunion or for infection recurrence, and secondary flap reconstruction after one failed flap is usually successful [6].

Timing of Flap Reconstruction

Optimal timing of soft tissue reconstruction plays a critical role in the management of FRI. Whenever feasible, a single-stage approach combining debridement and definitive soft tissue reconstruction is preferred [5, 8, 22]. This strategy is associated with lower infection recurrence rates, improved fixation stability, and reduced hospital stay and overall costs. Additionally, it reduces the risks of colonization, biofilm persistence, and antimicrobial resistance, which are more common in multistage reconstructions [12, 23].

Unfortunately, delays are not uncommon. On one hand, this is partly due to the limited availability of plastic surgeons in many FRI treatment teams [24, 25]. Early involvement of plastic surgeons is associated with better outcomes, but publications report the presence in only a minority of teams treating FRI, mostly due to logistic constraints [10, 26]. This is especially true if transfer to another hospital is needed for an orthoplastic approach. A set of criteria on which to base said transfer to a center with orthoplastic capabilities has been proposed to facilitate early transfers in patients who needed them [10], but so far these criteria have not been validated and there is scarce evidence of their use in the literature. On the other hand, in complex infections, some teams prefer to defer definitive reconstruction until negative cultures from intraoperative samples of the FRI site are obtained. This prerequisite of negative microbiological cultures is controversial. The limited available evidence suggests that *adequate surgical debridement* is required to perform soft tissue reconstruction, but negative microbiological cultures are not, as waiting for them to perform soft tissue reconstruction does not improve outcomes [5, 27]. Simultaneously, early wound closure has been associated to lower infection recurrence, fixation failure, and amputation rates, so it is the preferred approach [9].

Soft Tissue Reconstruction in FRI

The selection of the optimal reconstructive approach in FRI cases requires careful consideration of defect characteristics, patient factors, and available resources. The goal is to achieve stable, functional, and durable coverage while minimizing the risk of complications and optimizing long-term outcomes.

1. **Flap selection in FRI**: Choose well-vascularized flaps that replace nonviable tissue, obliterate dead space, and promote infection control.
2. **Timing in reconstruction**: A single-stage approach is preferred. In complex cases, delayed reconstruction may be necessary. The available evidence suggests that negative cultures are not necessary for flap coverage, but adequate surgical debridement is.
3. **Surgical expertise**: Surgeons must have experience in reconstructive and microsurgical techniques to select the best option among regional or free flaps and between muscle, fasciocutaneous, osseous, or combined flaps.
4. **Bone and soft tissue integration**: Osteocutaneous flaps, like the fibula, can address combined bone and soft tissue defects effectively.

Role of Negative Pressure Wound Therapy

When soft tissue coverage must be deferred due to logistic or clinical constraints, wound management can be supported using moist dressings, antibiotic-impregnated PMMA bead pouches or NPWT, in combination with local antibiotic carriers, to control the infection and maintain the wound environment [2, 23, 28].

There is ample evidence that NWPT should be used only as a bridge until definitive coverage and for as few *days* as possible [2, 7]. Use of NWPT for more than 1 week has been associated with significant bacterial colonization, higher risk of antimicrobial resistance, and increased risk of infection by promoting the migration of skin flora into the hardware [23, 29]. In a prospective study on 433 FRIs, NWPT use prior to any method of skin closure was associated with a 3.5-times increase in the treatment failure rate [7].

In summary, NWPT cannot substitute for adequate soft tissue coverage, and definitive wound closure should be performed as promptly as possible.

No Soft Tissue Reconstruction Possible (I5)

Seldom, soft tissue reconstruction will not be possible due to absent vascularity (e.g., consequence of the initial, high-energy trauma), or will be unadvisable due to unacceptably high potential morbidity or risk of reconstruction failure. These patients are usually only candidates for amputation or long-term wound care, with or without antibiotic suppression [8]. For more information on indications for amputation, refer to Chap. 8.

Clinical Cases

Case 9.1

A 58-year-old male consulted for a long-standing FRI of the proximal tibia (Fig. 9.1), after a proximal tibial open fracture on a motorbike accident 40 years prior, which had healed (F1 R2 I3). He had been operated on multiple times, but the FRI kept recurring. Computed tomography imaging showed a lytic lesion with bone sequestra inside and a broken cortex, among other signs suggestive of FRI (Fig. 9.2). He underwent single-stage surgery including debridement and a pedicled medial gastrocnemius flap (Figs 9.3, 9.4, and 9.5). The gastrocnemius flap was chosen because it was an available regional option, there was no bone instability (no need for bone reconstruction), and it simultaneously managed dead space and provided reliable wound coverage (of all the unstable scar tissue was removed). Postoperative cultures were positive for *Pseudomonas aeruginosa*, *Staphylococcus aureus,* and *Staphylococcus warneri,* so he received antimicrobial therapy with ciprofloxacin, rifampicin, and daptomycin (he was beta-lactam allergic). The postoperative recovery was satisfactory. He achieved aidless gait and was able to return to work (Fig. 9.6). At

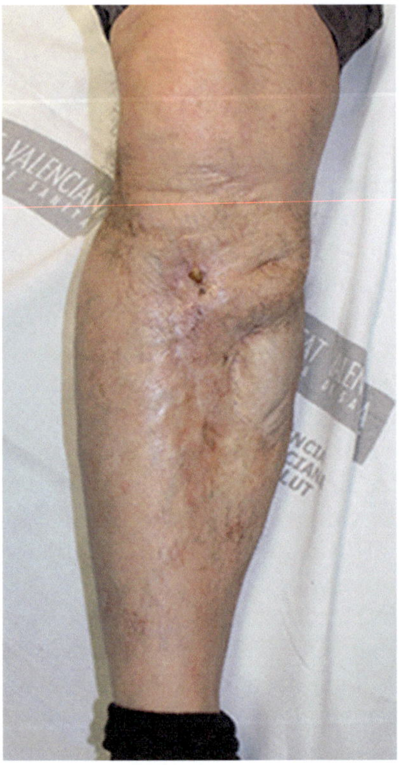

Fig. 9.1 Case 9.1, clinical image showing the post-traumatic scarring and fistula at the anterior proximal tibia

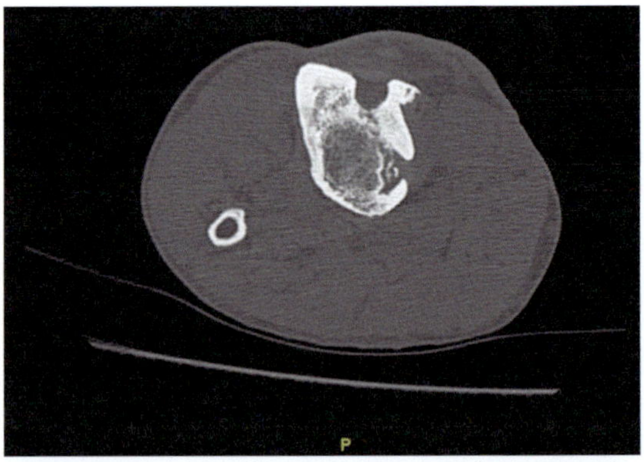

Fig. 9.2 Case 9.1, preoperative computed tomography image of the proximal right tibia, showing osteolysis and bone sequestra

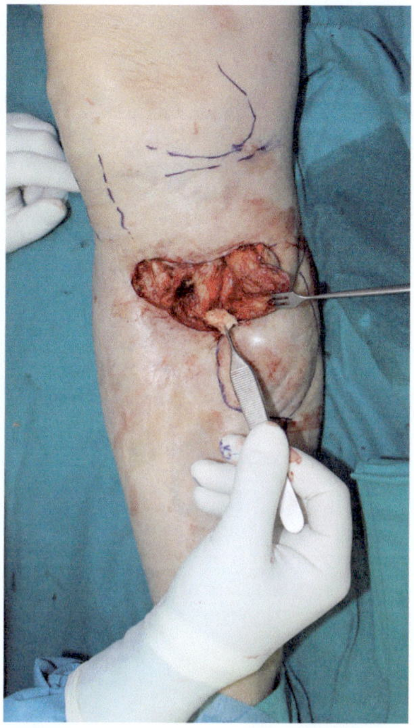

Fig. 9.3 Case 9.1, intraoperative photograph after debridement showing the defect

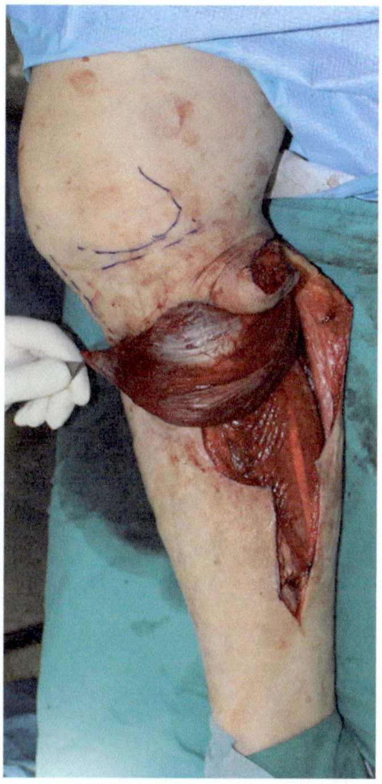

Fig. 9.4 Case 9.1, intraoperative photograph showing the medial gastrocnemius, rotated into the defect

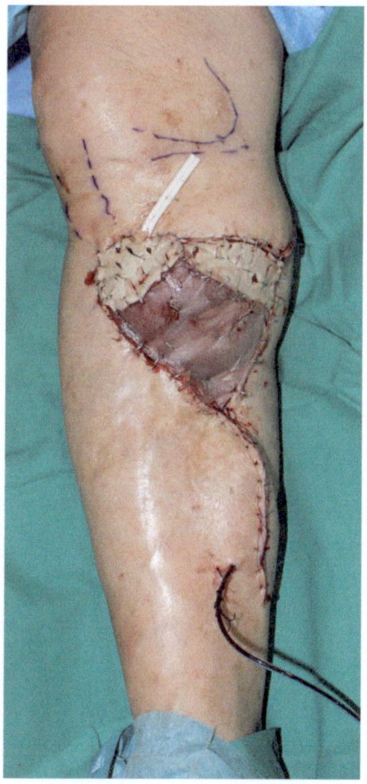

Fig. 9.5 Case 9.1, intraoperative photograph after medial gastrocnemius insetting and skin grafting

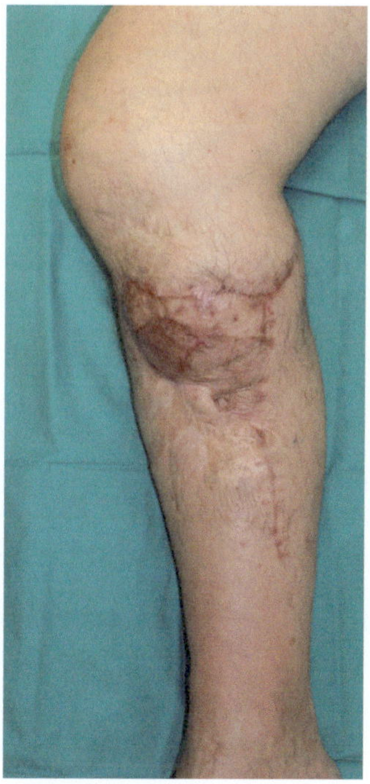

Fig. 9.6 Case 9.1, clinical image at 6 months postoperatively

5 years postoperatively, there have been no signs of infection recurrence, and his gait is normal without pain or need for walking aids.

Case 9.2

A 48-year-old male suffered a motorcycle accident resulting in an open fracture of the left tibia and fibula (Gustilo–Anderson type II, Fig. 9.7), as well as a Lisfranc fracture-dislocation of the left foot (Fig. 9.8). Emergency surgery was performed, which included intramedullary nailing of the tibial fracture, Kirschner wire fixation of the foot, and wound closure. Two weeks later, the patient was referred to our Institution with skin necrosis and infection at both wound sites (F2 R1 I4). We performed debridement, sampling, implant retention, and two free anterolateral thigh flaps harvested from the same thigh to reconstruct the soft tissue defects (Figs. 9.9, 9.10, and 9.11). All wounds healed uneventfully (Fig. 9.12), and the fractures consolidated (Fig. 9.13).

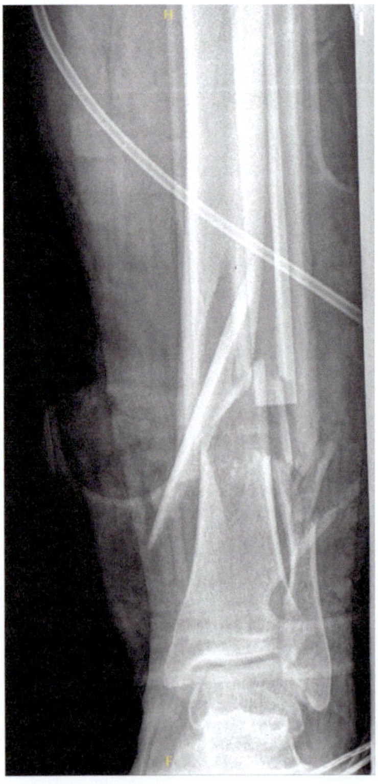

Fig. 9.7 Case 9.2, anterior-posterior X-ray of the leg fracture

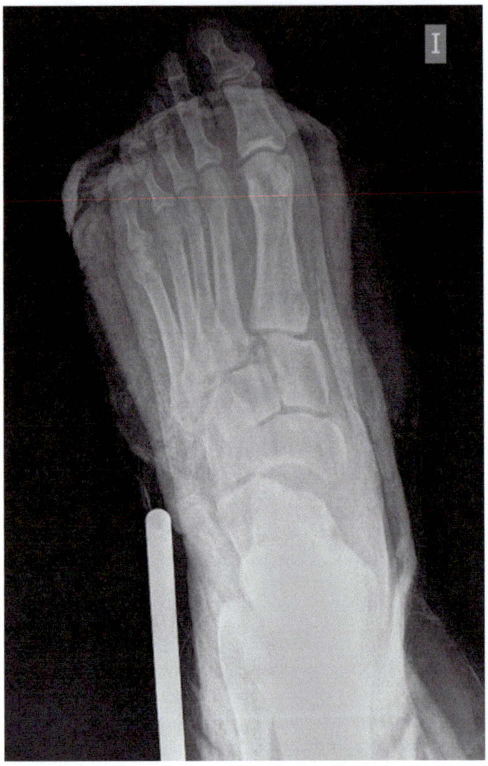

Fig. 9.8 Case 9.2, anterior-posterior X-ray showing a Lisfranc injury of the left foot

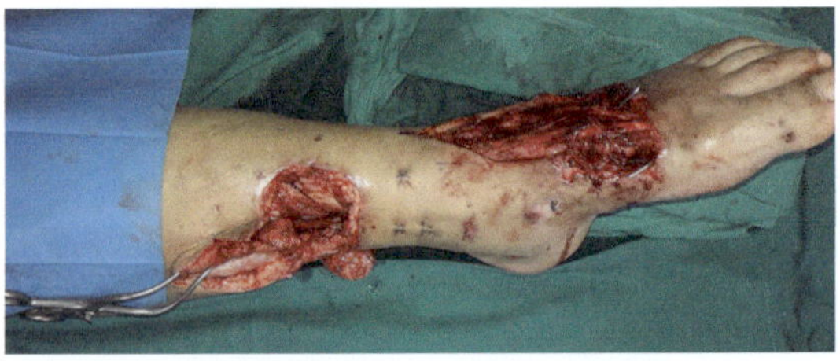

Fig. 9.9 Case 9.2, intraoperative photograph after debridement showing the soft tissue defects

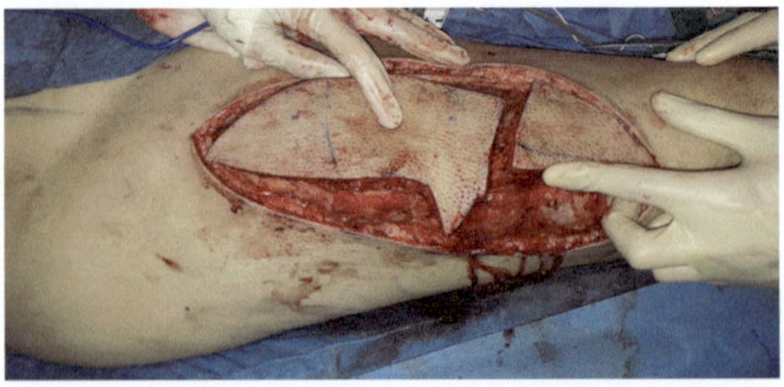

Fig. 9.10 Case 9.2, intraoperative photograph showing the two anterolateral thigh flap islands

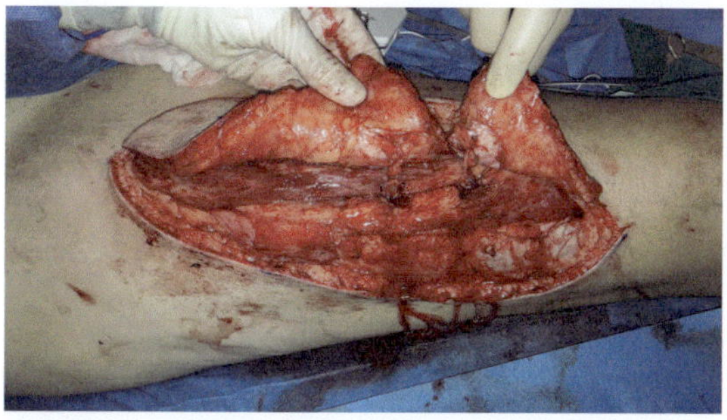

Fig. 9.11 Case 9.2, intraoperative photograph showing the two anterolateral thigh flap perforators, one based proximally and the other one based on the distal segment of the lateral circumflex femoral artery. They were anastomosed separately to the posterior tibial and anterior tibial vessels, respectively

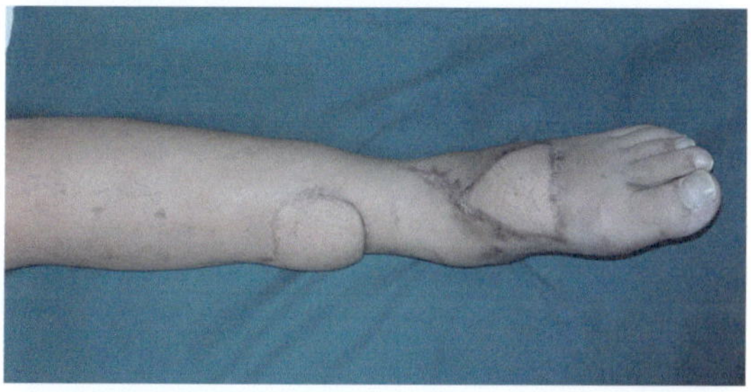

Fig. 9.12 Case 9.2, clinical image at 1 year postoperatively. The wounds have healed; there are some contour irregularities, but the patient was able to wear footwear and did not wish for further surgery to correct them

After 16 months, the patient experienced an episode of cellulitis and fistula affecting the leg flap, caused by a *Staphylococcus epidermidis* infection of the intramedullary nail. This was resolved with nail removal and antibiotic therapy consisting of levofloxacin and rifampin (Fig. 9.14). The patient recovered uneventfully and returned to work. Six years after the initial injury, he remains infection-free, ambulates without crutches, and reports no pain.

Case 9.3

A 45-year-old male presented with FRI after an open calcaneal fracture due to a motorbike accident, 27 years prior. A local flap had been performed at the time of the accident for coverage, but FRI ensued, and a fistula developed

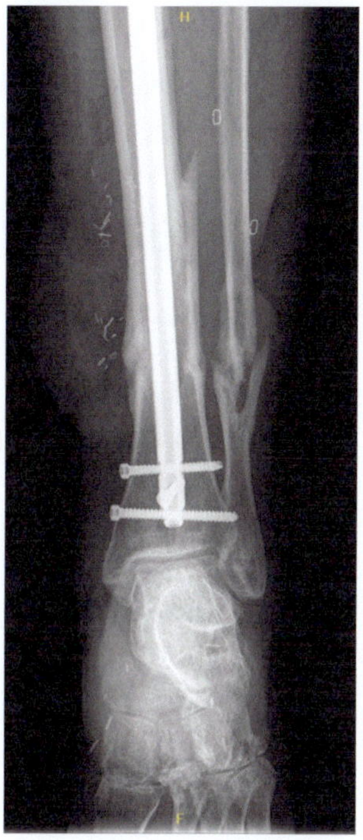

Fig. 9.13 Case 9.2, anterior-posterior X-ray of the left leg showing a healed fracture, 14 months postoperatively

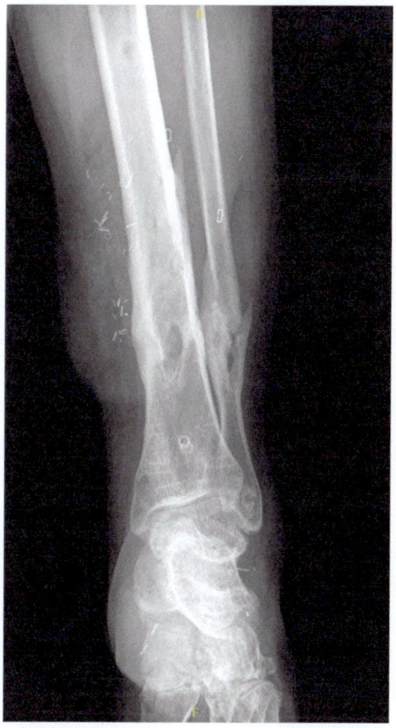

Fig. 9.14 Case 9.2, anterior-posterior X-ray of the left leg, 6 months after tibial nail removal

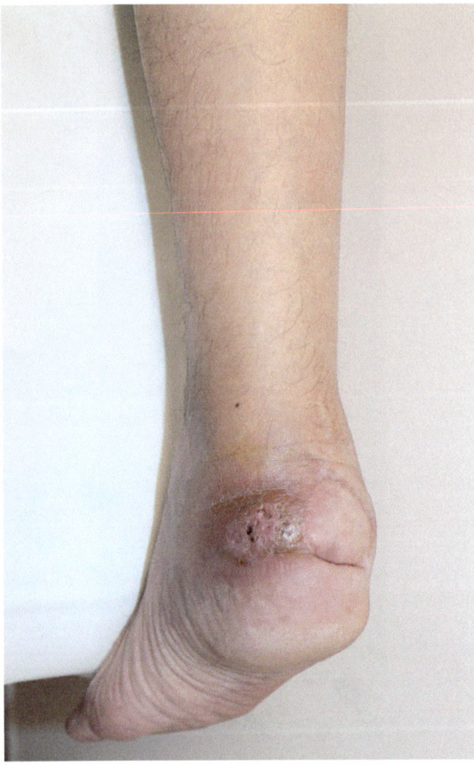

Fig. 9.15 Case 9.3, clinical image showing the posttraumatic scarring and fistula at the medial side of the right calcaneus

(Fig. 9.15). Preoperative X-ray showed osteitis (Fig. 9.16). He was treated with antibiotics, debridement and reconstruction with a free gracilis flap (Fig. 9.17). This flap was chosen because it managed simultaneously dead space and reliable wound coverage, the defect was located over a joint (need for a non-bulky reconstruction), and the short pedicle could comfortably be anastomosed to the posterior tibial vessels. The postoperative outcome was satisfactory (Fig. 9.18). One year postoperatively, he experienced an isolated episode of cellulitis, which resolved with oral antibiotics. At the 6-year postoperative visit, he remained free from infectious recurrences, had a painless, independent gait, and lead an active lifestyle.

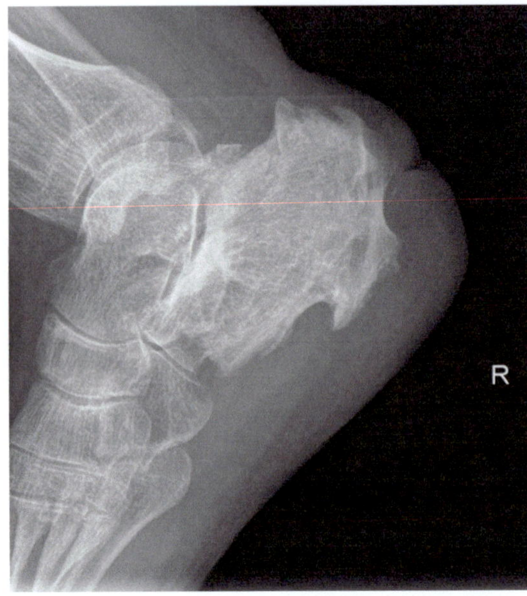

Fig. 9.16 Case 9.3, lateral X-ray of the right foot, showing sequelae after the calcaneal fracture (27 years prior to this X-ray), including subtalar osteoarthritis

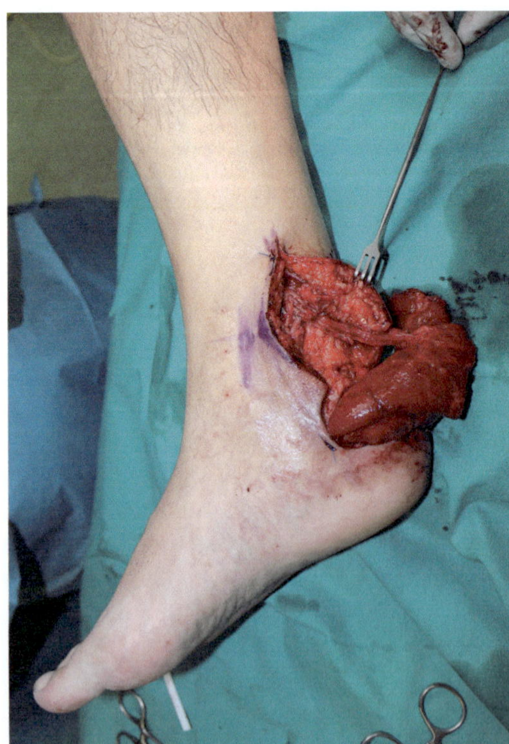

Fig. 9.17 Case 9.3, intraoperative photograph showing the free gracilis flap, after microanastomosis to the posterior tibial vessels

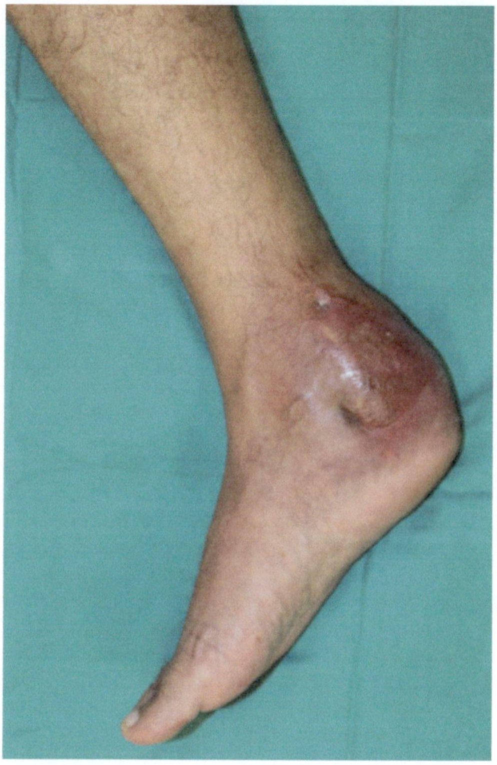

Fig. 9.18 Case 9.3, clinical image at 6 months postoperatively

Conclusions

Achievement of a healthy soft tissue envelope early is critical for a good outcome in FRI, both in terms of infection eradication and bone healing. Accordingly, early orthoplastic approaches provide better outcomes.

Often in FRI, direct closure is only possible with some difficulty, or the tissues used for coverage are compromised due to extensive scarring. In such cases, consider reinforcing the closure with a flap, especially in anatomical regions with thin, vulnerable soft tissues, such as the distal tibia.

Up to 40% of FRI cases will require tissue transfer to obtain reliable wound coverage. The threshold for flaps in FRI should be low, due to the importance of a healthy soft tissue envelope for a good outcome (infection eradication and fracture consolidation). They replace nonviable tissue, obliterate dead space, and facilitate infection control. No single flap or flap type has been proven superior in FRI management, both fasciocutaneous and muscle flaps are equally effective when used appropriately. A single-stage approach is preferred as it is associated with lower rates of infection recurrence, biofilm persistence, and antimicrobial resistance, as well as improved fixation stability and reduced hospital stay and costs. When logistic or clinical constraints prevent prompt reliable wound coverage, every effort should be made to obtain robust soft tissue coverage as soon as possible.

NWPT use has been associated with a higher risk of treatment failure. It cannot substitute for adequate soft tissue coverage. Definitive wound closure should be performed as promptly as possible, NWPT being used only as a bridge until definitive soft tissue reconstruction for as few days as possible, if at all.

References

1. Depypere M, Morgenstern M, Kuehl R, Senneville E, Moriarty TF, Obremskey WT, Zimmerli W, Trampuz A, Lagrou K, Metsemakers W-J. Pathogenesis and management of fracture-related infection. Clin Microbiol Infect. 2020;26:572–8.
2. Metsemakers W-J, Morgenstern M, Senneville E, et al. General treatment principles for fracture-related infection: recommendations from an international expert group. Arch Orthop Trauma Surg. 2020;140:1013–27.
3. Chan JKK, Ferguson JY, Scarborough M, McNally MA, Ramsden AJ. Management of post-traumatic osteomyelitis in the lower limb: current state of the art. Indian J Plast Surg. 2019;52:62–72.
4. Morgenstern M, Clauss M, Sendi P, Cadosch D, Osinga R, Metsemakers W-J. Treatment of fracture-related infections. In: Textbook of polytrauma management: a multidisciplinary approach. 3rd ed. Berlin: Springer Nature; 2022. p. 573–81.
5. Marais LC, Zalavras CG, Moriarty FT, Kühl R, Metsemakers W-J, Morgenstern M. The surgical management of fracture-related infection. Surgical strategy selection and the need for early surgical intervention. J Orthop. 2024;50:36–41.
6. Müller SLC, Morgenstern M, Kuehl R, Muri T, Kalbermatten DF, Clauss M, Schaefer DJ, Sendi P, Osinga R. Soft-tissue reconstruction in lower-leg fracture-related infections: an orthoplastic outcome and risk factor analysis. Injury. 2021;52:3489–97.
7. McNally M, Corrigan R, Sliepen J, Dudareva M, Rentenaar R, Ijpma F, Atkins BL, Wouthuyzen-

Bakker M, Govaert G. What factors affect outcome in the treatment of fracture-related infection? Antibiotics (Basel). 2022;11:946.

8. Alt V, McNally M, Wouthuyzen-Bakker M, Metsemakers W-J, Marais L, Zalavras C, Morgenstern M. The FRI classification – a new classification of fracture-related infections. Injury. 2024;55:111831.
9. Marais LC, Hungerer S, Eckardt H, Zalavras C, Obremskey WT, Ramsden A, McNally MA, Morgenstern M, Metsemakers W-J, FRI Consensus Group. Key aspects of soft tissue management in fracture-related infection: recommendations from an international expert group. Arch Orthop Trauma Surg. 2024;144:259–68.
10. Azoury SC, Stranix JT, Kovach SJ, Levin LS. Principles of orthoplastic surgery for lower extremity reconstruction: why is this important? J Reconstr Microsurg. 2021;37:42–50.
11. Lu V, Zhang J, Patel R, Zhou AK, Thahir A, Krkovic M. Fracture related infections and their risk factors for treatment failure-a major trauma centre perspective. Diagnostics (Basel). 2022;12:1289.
12. Chan JK-K, Harry L, Williams G, Nanchahal J. Soft-tissue reconstruction of open fractures of the lower limb: muscle versus fasciocutaneous flaps. Plast Reconstr Surg. 2012;130:284e–95e.
13. Nasser A, Azimi T, Ostadmohammadi S, Ostadmohammadi S. A comprehensive review of bacterial osteomyelitis with emphasis on Staphylococcus aureus. Microb Pathog. 2020;148:104431.
14. Gir P, Cheng A, Oni G, Mojallal A, Saint-Cyr M. Pedicled-perforator (propeller) flaps in lower extremity defects: a systematic review. J Reconstr Microsurg. 2012;28:595–601.
15. Iida T, Yoshimatsu H, Koshima I. Reconstruction of anterolateral thigh defects using perforator-based propeller flaps. Ann Plast Surg. 2017;79:385–9.
16. Hotchen AJ, Dudareva M, Corrigan RA, Ferguson JY, McNally MA. Can we predict outcome after treatment of long bone osteomyelitis? Bone Joint J. 2020;102-B:1587–96.
17. Yazar S, Lin C-H, Lin Y-T, Ulusal AE, Wei F-C. Outcome comparison between free muscle and free fasciocutaneous flaps for reconstruction of distal third and ankle traumatic open tibial fractures. Plast Reconstr Surg. 2006;117:2468–75. discussion 2476–2477
18. Cho EH, Shammas RL, Carney MJ, Weissler JM, Bauder AR, Glener AD, Kovach SJ, Hollenbeck ST, Levin LS. Muscle versus fasciocutaneous free flaps in lower extremity traumatic reconstruction: a multicenter outcomes analysis. Plast Reconstr Surg. 2018;141:191–9.
19. Viaud-Ambrosino S, Bargemon JBV, Kachouh N, Gay A, Mayoly A, Legre R, Jaloux C, Curvale C. Free fibula flap in traumatic femoral bone reconstruction: a 10-year review. Strategies Trauma Limb Reconstr. 2023;18:44–50.
20. Trapero A, Pérez-García A, Thione A, Carpio MA, Oliete JB. Omental free flap for surgical treatment of chronic osteomyelitis of lower limb: a technical note. Injury. 2021;52:1065–8.
21. Serra PL, Boriani F, Khan U, Atzeni M, Figus A. Rate of free flap failure and return to the operating room in lower limb reconstruction: a systematic review. J Clin Med. 2024;13:4295.
22. McNally MA, Ferguson JY, Scarborough M, Ramsden A, Stubbs DA, Atkins BL. Mid- to long-term results of single-stage surgery for patients with chronic osteomyelitis using a bioabsorbable gentamicin-loaded ceramic carrier. Bone Joint J. 2022;104-B:1095–100.
23. Iliadis AD, Shivji F, Debuka E, Trompeter A, Narayan B, Heidari N. Current concepts in the prevention, diagnosis and treatment of fracture-related infection (FRI). Eur J Orthop Surg Traumatol. 2021;31:957–66.
24. Bezstarosti H, Metsemakers WJ, van Lieshout EMM, Voskamp LW, Kortram K, McNally MA, Marais LC, Verhofstad MHJ. Management of critical-sized bone defects in the treatment of fracture-related infection: a systematic review and pooled analysis. Arch Orthop Trauma Surg. 2021;141:1215–30.
25. Olesen UK, Juul R, Bonde CT, Moser C, McNally M, Jensen LT, Elberg JJ, Eckardt H. A review of forty five open tibial fractures covered with free flaps. Analysis of complications, microbiology and prognostic factors. Int Orthop. 2015;39:1159–66.
26. Bezstarosti H, Van Lieshout EMM, Voskamp LW, Kortram K, Obremskey W, McNally MA, Metsemakers WJ, Verhofstad MHJ. Insights into treatment and outcome of fracture-related infection: a systematic literature review. Arch Orthop Trauma Surg. 2019;139:61–72.
27. Alt V, Rupp M, Kerschbaum M, Prantl L, Geis S. Treatment strategies for fracture-related infections with concurrent soft tissue damage. Unfallchirurgie (Heidelb). 2024;127:103–9.
28. Patterson JT, Becerra JA, Brown M, Roohani I, Zalavras C, Carey JN. Antibiotic bead pouch versus negative pressure wound therapy at initial management of AO/OTA 42 type IIIB open tibia fracture may reduce fracture related infection: a retrospective analysis of 113 patients. Injury. 2023;54:744–50.
29. Olesen UK, Pedersen NJ, Eckardt H, Lykke-Meyer L, Bonde CT, Singh UM, McNally M. The cost of infection in severe open tibial fractures treated with a free flap. Int Orthop. 2017;41:1049–55.

10 Antimicrobial Therapy in Fracture-Related Infections

Eva Calabuig, María Tasias, Nieves Vanaclocha, and Miguel Salavert

Introduction

Fracture-related infections (FRIs) are a major complication in orthopedic surgery, often resulting in delayed healing, high morbidity, and extended hospital stays. Their occurrence ranges from 1% to 2% after closed fractures to over 30% after Gustilo–Anderson type III open tibia fractures [1, 2].

Depending on the time of onset of symptoms after fracture fixation, FRIs can be classified as early (<2–3 weeks), delayed (3–10 weeks), or late (>10 weeks), representing time-dependent pathophysiological changes such as biofilm maturation [3]. Late infections are caused by either bloodstream seeding or by recurrence of an inadequately treated early FRI [4]. In any case, the combination of surgery and antimicrobial therapy remains the mainstay of treatment [5].

Effective antimicrobial therapy is crucial in managing FRIs. Its goals are to eliminate pathogens, reduce inflammation, disrupt biofilm, and facilitate bone healing. The choice of antimicrobial agents is influenced by several factors including timing of the infection, the patient's immune status, the presence of biomedical devices, and the presence of biofilm. This chapter provides an overview of the complexities surrounding antimicrobial therapy in FRIs, emphasizing the need for tailored approaches based on individual patient circumstances and microbiologic surgical findings. Preventative strategies are also discussed.

E. Calabuig (✉)
Infectious Diseases Unit, University and Polytechnic Hospital La Fe. IIS-La Fe. Medicine Department, University of Valencia, Valencia, Spain
e-mail: calabuig_eva@gva.es

M. Tasias
Medicine Department, University of Valencia, Valencia, Spain

N. Vanaclocha
Orthoplastics Unit and Department of Plastic and Reconstructive Surgery, University and Polytechnic Hospital La Fe, Valencia, Spain

M. Salavert
Infectious Diseases, Medicine Department, Catholic University of Valencia San Vicente Martir, Valencia, Spain

Microbiological Considerations

Many pathogens are implicated in the development of FRIs (refer to Chap. 1 for more detailed information on pathogenesis). Some studies suggest that early FRIs tend to be caused by highly virulent microorganisms, whereas in delayed and late FRIs the proportion of low-virulency bacteria, such as coagulase-negative *Staphylococci* (CNS), increases [6, 7]. Other research groups have been unable to corroborate these findings [8].

Overall, the most common causative pathogens are Gram-positive cocci, which are usually part of the skin microbiome. Specifically, *Staphylococcus*

N. Vanaclocha (ed.), *Treatment of Fracture-Related Infection*,
https://doi.org/10.1007/978-3-031-92452-1_10

aureus is the most common causative pathogen. It is the culprit for over half of FRI cases regardless of symptom duration, BACH score, anatomical location, age, or body mass index [6, 9].

Less-frequent causative microbes include Gram-negative bacilli, polymicrobial, anaerobic and fungal infections. *Mycobacteria* spp. cause a minority of FRIs, but they must be ruled out in patients with a history of previous active or latent tuberculosis. Atypical mycobacteria have occasionally been found to be associated with previously contaminated antiseptic fluids or surgical soaps, sometimes causing clusters of cases or small outbreaks.

Regardless of the causative pathogen, accurate identification and susceptibility testing are crucial for targeted therapy. For information on appropriate sampling, the reader is referred to Chap. 2.

Biofilm Formation

Infections that occur following internal fixation of a fracture are typically caused by biofilm-forming bacteria, which adhere to the fixation implants and devascularized tissues [10, 11]. Biofilm plays a pivotal role in FRI pathogenesis and persistence, because its development on any natural (e.g., fractured bone) or synthetic surface (foreign bodies, such as orthopedic hardware) is the main barrier to infection eradication. Thus, understanding biofilm dynamics is essential for effective therapeutic strategies.

Biofilm is an organized multicellular community of bacteria with a complex structure, formed by bacterial cells of multiple phenotypes and their self-produced extracellular matrix. Its creation and maintenance are enabled by the ability of biofilm-forming bacteria to exist in 3 distinct phenotypic states depending on the degree of their attachment to surfaces at the FRI site: planktonic state (unattached cells floating freely), quasi-sessile state (semi-attached), and sessile state (attached) (Fig. 10.1). These phenotypic states also correspond to different metabolic states: planktonic bacteria are very active and have fast replication rates, whereas sessile bacteria are less metabolically active and exhibit stationary growth. Bacteria in a quasi-sessile state detach and reattach easily, and are credited with

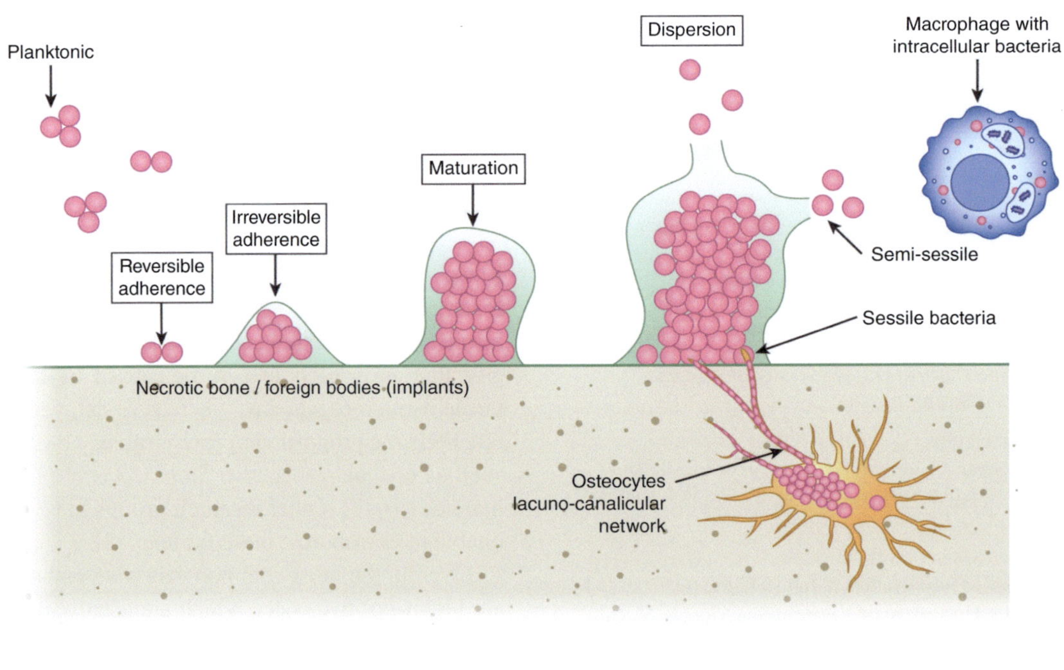

Fig. 10.1 Development of biofilm and other immune-privileged bacterial reservoirs in fracture-related infections

reactivation of previously latent FRIs, cross-contamination and other forms of dissemination. Bacteria can change between these phenotypic states depending on environmental cues, amongst other factors.

The development of mature biofilm is a quick process, which can be completed in 12 to 18 h [11, 12]. After approximately 1 week, biofilm is established, and the bacteria within it are more protected from host defenses and antibiotics than bacteria in the planktonic state [13]. In fact, animal studies suggest that biofilms are up to 1000-fold more tolerant to antibiotics than their planktonic counterpart [14]. Additionally, susceptibility to antibiotics decreases as biofilm age increases [15]. This is because bacteria within the biofilm undergo physiological changes that enhance their resistance (they turn into less metabolically active phenotypes) and due to the maturation of the biofilm structure and the accumulation of extracellular polymeric substances, which, over time, create a physical barrier that restricts antibiotic penetration. The consequence of these simultaneous changes is that the longer the duration of the FRI, the higher the causative pathogens' abilities for persistence and immune evasion.

Principles of Antimicrobial Therapy

Therapeutic success is primarily determined by the antimicrobials' activity against the infecting pathogen. Note that this is not only influenced by the pathogen's susceptibility to the administered antimicrobials, but also by the ability of the antimicrobials to reach the site of infection, which is indispensable for the antimicrobials to be effective. Thus, debridement of all necrotic tissue and ensuring a healthy, well-vascularized soft tissue envelope surrounding the infected bone are critical for good outcomes. The role of retained osteosynthesis material in persistent infections should be considered; it is estimated that just under a third of patients with retained implants suffer prolonged FRI [15, 16].

Other aspects such as the route of antimicrobial administration, dosing regimen, and potential drug interactions should be carefully evaluated in order to optimize treatment outcomes, prevent the development of antimicrobial resistance, and minimize the risk of adverse effects [5, 17]. The results of preclinical studies on antibiotics' pharmacokinetics and pharmacodynamics suggest that for FRI treatment, initial high-loading doses and prolonged infusions of antibiotics with time-dependent bactericidal activity, such as beta-lactams, are best, and that therapeutic drug monitoring should be carried out when available. The patient's clinical condition, site of FRI, and relevant comorbidities also influence posology choices (Table 10.1).

Table 10.1 Patient features that influence antibiotic treatment

Age and weight
Underlying diseases (diabetes, liver disease, kidney disease)
Previous infection
Recent surgery
Recent hospitalization
Previous travel
Immunodeficiency
Type of implant used for bone fixation
Site of infection

Note that *no antimicrobial* or combination thereof *can compensate for inadequate surgery*. The principles outlined in Chap. 3, including a thorough debridement, are critical to achieve a good outcome.

Empirical Treatment

Empiric antibiotic treatment, without knowledge of individual microbiology, should be administrated promptly in patients with a suspected FRI to achieve rapid reduction of bacterial load at the FRI site [11]. To maximize culture yields, antibiotic therapy should be delayed until deep tissue samples have been obtained, especially during the 2 weeks prior to the surgery [3, 10]. An exception is patients with sepsis, in whom immediate antibiotic therapy should be initiated after obtaining blood samples for microbiological culture [18]. In cases with a low suspicion of FRI, it is safe to administer empiric antibiotic therapy until

Table 10.2 Antimicrobial therapy against different bacterial osteoarticular infections (initial empiric regimen and ensuing pathogen-specific treatments)

Microorganism	Initial IV regimen	Oral treatment
Staphylococcus spp.	Methicillin-susceptible: (Cloxacillin or cefazolin) ± Daptomycin Methicillin-resistant: Vancomycin (alone) or Daptomycin + (Cloxacillin or Fosfomycin)	Levofloxacin + rifampicin Alternatively: Linezolid/Tedizolid, co-trimoxazole, clindamycin or doxycycline
Streptococcus spp.	Ceftriaxone or penicillin	Amoxicillin or levofloxacin ± rifampicin
Enterococcus faecalis	Ampicillin ± ceftriaxone	Amoxicillin ± rifampicin
Enterococcus faecium	Vancomycin or Daptomycin	Linezolid/Tedizolid
Enterobacteriaceae	Ceftriaxone	Ciprofloxacin
Pseudomonas aeruginosa	Ceftazidime or Cefepime + ciprofloxacin	Ciprofloxacin

Table 10.3 Risk factors associated with methicillin-resistant *Staphylococcus aureus* (MRSA) infections, including community acquired-MRSA

Risk factor	Description of high-risk subgroup for MRSA infection
Ethnicity	African American and Hispanic populations (compared to Caucasian).
Recent travel	Travel to regions with high MRSA prevalence (e.g., Africa, Latin America, Southeast Asia).
Socioeconomic factors	Lower socioeconomic status, poor hygiene, overcrowded living conditions, and incarceration.
Previous antibiotic therapy	Antibiotic use within the past 3 months.
History of MRSA	Previous MRSA colonization or infection.
Exposure factors	Hospitalization within the previous 12 months, intensive care unit admission, residence in long-term care facilities, and high-risk household contacts.
Surgical history	Previous minor or major surgery, particularly when involving devices or invasive procedures.
Instrumental and procedural exposure	Use of central vascular catheters, implantable devices, or invasive radiological studies.
Contact activities	High-risk activities include daycare for young children, contact sports, military service, contact with farm animals, and insect bite injuries.
Comorbidities	Presence of underlying conditions such as diabetes, peripheral vascular disease, cardiovascular disease, chronic wounds (often open), chronic renal disease, dialysis dependence, or IV drug use.
Pre-existing skin lesions	Any disturbance of the skin barrier, such as that resulting from burns, eczema or dermatitis, can serve as an entry point for infection.
Purulent cellulitis	A history of purulent cellulitis.
Immunocompromised state	Genetic immunodeficiencies, iatrogenic neutrophil disorders, and immunosuppressive therapy (e.g., chemotherapy).

culture results and histopathology are available. Therapy should be stopped as soon as infection is ruled out [18].

Broad-spectrum antibiotics that cover both Gram-positive and Gram-negative bacteria are recommended [15, 18]. Most often, this includes a beta-lactam antibiotic, such as ceftazidime, cefepime, piperacillin-tazobactam, or meropenem, together with cloxacillin, vancomycin, or daptomycin, conditioned by the presence of a previous FRI or bacterial resistance (Table 10.2) [19]. No beta-lactam has proven superior to the rest, the only requirement is that concentrations above the pathogen's minimal inhibitory concentration (MIC) are kept. When there is a high suspicion of infection by methicillin-resistant *Staphylococcus aureus* (MRSA) (Table 10.3), empirical therapy should provide coverage against MRSA strains.

Intravenous (IV) administration is recommended until full antimicrobial susceptibility test results are available, because it avoids malabsorption related to gastric intolerance, increases bioavailability of certain drugs, and allows the administration of higher doses [3]. In some cases, continuous or extended IV infusion allows efficacy optimization of time-dependent antibiotics, such as beta-lactams, vancomycin, or clindamycin. Their prolonged IV administration generates therapeutic plasma concentrations that exceed the pathogen's MIC during much more time daily and are associated with a lower risk of resistance development than if these antibiotics are administered orally. However, there is increasing evidence for the non-inferiority of oral antibiotics with good bioavailability once stable plasma concentrations have been achieved, with some randomized controlled trials showing no differences in outcomes between patients treated with up to 7 days of IV antibiotics followed by oral therapy and those treated with prolonged IV therapy [20], so teams are increasingly switching early to oral therapies.

Targeted Treatment

Once the microorganism causing the infection is identified, selection of the most appropriate antimicrobial agent to target the specific pathogen is compulsory. This step is crucial to improve outcomes and minimize the development of antimicrobial resistance. It includes adhering to local guidelines and recommendations, as well as monitoring treatment response and adjusting therapy as needed (Table 10.2) [5, 21].

As in Empirical Treatment, Beta-lactam Antibiotics play a major role in targeted therapy. In the case of Gram-negative bacilli, the choice of beta-lactam agent depends on the species and mechanisms of resistance. Carbapenems, the new beta-lactam antibiotics (ceftazidime-avibactam, ceftolozane-tazobactam, ceftobiprole, cefiderocol, etc.), tigecycline, or the novel long-acting intravenous antibiotics (see *Novel Antimicrobial Agents* below) are suggested against multidrug-resistant microbes. Alternative antibiotics in patients allergic to beta-lactams are:

- Vancomycin, daptomycin, linezolid, or tedizolid in Gram-positive cocci infections.
- Aztreonam, fosfomycin, or colistin for Gram-negative bacilli.
- Tigecycline, along with other newer tetracycline derivatives, for selected cases of polymicrobial FRIs caused by both Gram-positive and Gram-negative bacteria.

Due to the Importance of Biofilm in the Pathogenesis of FRI, Anti-biofilm Agents Are a Must Among these, fluoroquinolones and rifampicin stand out.

Fluoroquinolones are the best studied antibiotic group for bone infections, both for Gram-negative and Gram-positive bacteria, with reported infection curation rates of 60–80% [22]. They have patient-friendly posology, often only requiring administration once or twice a day, and high oral bioavailability. Rifampicin, though somewhat less-studied, can target intracellular bacterial reservoirs (as well as biofilm) and has been observed to improve outcomes when used against chronic *Staphylococcus aureus* bone infections in combination with either fluoroquinolones or other active agents (daptomycin, linezolid, cefazolin, cloxacillin, vancomycin, gentamicin) [22]. Drawbacks to rifampicin use include its numerous drug interactions, which must be reviewed before its administration to a particular patient, and the rapid development of resistance to it, which forbids monotherapy with rifampicin, especially when the bacterial load is high. Rifampicin should always be administered with another anti-staphylococcal drug and started a few days after surgery, once the bacterial burden has been reduced [5, 15]. In addition, rifampicin therapy can produce severe adverse effects, such as allergic reactions or acute renal failure, which cause treatment discontinuation in almost 20% of patients [23], as well as the more common gastrointestinal symptoms. The occurrence of these adverse events is known to increase with increasing dose of rifampicin, without an apparent improvement in outcomes, but there is controversy as to the optimal posology of rifampicin.

Other compounds that have some activity against biofilm-forming bacteria include daptomycin, linezolid, ceftaroline (a new parenteral fifth-generation cephalosporin with activity against methicillin-resistant *Staphylococcus*), and colistin (a peptide with anti-biofilm action when used in combination with fosfomycin). The combination of colistin and fosfomycin has proven useful in long-standing infections of multidrug-resistant Gram-negative bacteria [24], but since it mostly targets sessile bacteria, concomitant use of agents that are effective against planktonic bacteria is mandatory. As with rifampicin, colistin toxicity is frequent and, though reversible, can lead to discontinuation in over 20% of patients undergoing treatment with it, mostly in relation to high blood levels [25].

Fungal FRIs are generally considered very difficult to eradicate and removal of all implants is the recommended strategy [5]. The use of amphotericin and echinocandins is associated with better outcomes than azoles in the presence of biofilm, particularly in cases of yeast infections [26]. This is especially true of those caused by *Candida* spp.

Principles of Antimicrobial Therapy in FRI

Empirical treatment should be administered promptly (after deep tissue samples have been obtained, whenever possible) and preferably intravenously. It should provide broad coverage for both Gram-positive and Gram-negative bacteria. Initial high-loading doses and prolonged infusions of antibiotics with time-dependent bactericidal activity are best. Therapeutic drug monitoring should be performed if available.

Once the causative pathogen is identified and sensitivity test results are available, the antimicrobial treatment must be adapted accordingly to best target that specific microorganism.

The use of beta-lactams is widespread. No beta-lactam has proven superior to the rest, the only requirement is that concentrations above the pathogen's minimal inhibitory concentration are kept.

Due to biofilm's crucial role in bacterial persistence and antimicrobial evasion, anti-biofilm agents, such as rifampicin or fluoroquinolones, are a must. Rifampicin has many drug interactions and resistance to it develops rapidly, so it must always be used in combination with another agent and started a few days after surgery.

Duration of Therapy

The optimal duration of antimicrobial therapy for FRI remains uncertain [27, 28]. The decision depends on multiple factors, including microorganism sensitivities, host response, levels of inflammatory biomarkers, and, especially, the surgical strategy regarding hardware (retention, exchange, removal). This strategy should be decided with advice from a multidisciplinary team, as it improves outcomes.

In general, a minimum of 6 weeks is often recommended, but individual patient factors and the presence of biofilm may extend this duration up to 12 weeks (Fig. 10.2) [10, 29]. Consider also that clinical, biochemical, and radiological monitoring is important to decide the best moment to stop antimicrobial treatment [30].

When the Strategy Is Based on Implant Retention (DAIR, debridement, antimicrobial therapy, and implant retention), FRI treatment requires prolonged antibiotic suppressive therapy. Some experts recommend a minimum duration of 12 weeks of antimicrobial therapy in DAIR cases, given the presence of residual biofilm in the retained implant, but there is controversy as to the optimal duration [10]. In any case, suppressive antimicrobial therapy must be tailored to the microorganism's susceptibility and, if possible, should be orally available, able to control the infection with minimal side effects and toxicity, and have low propensity to induce

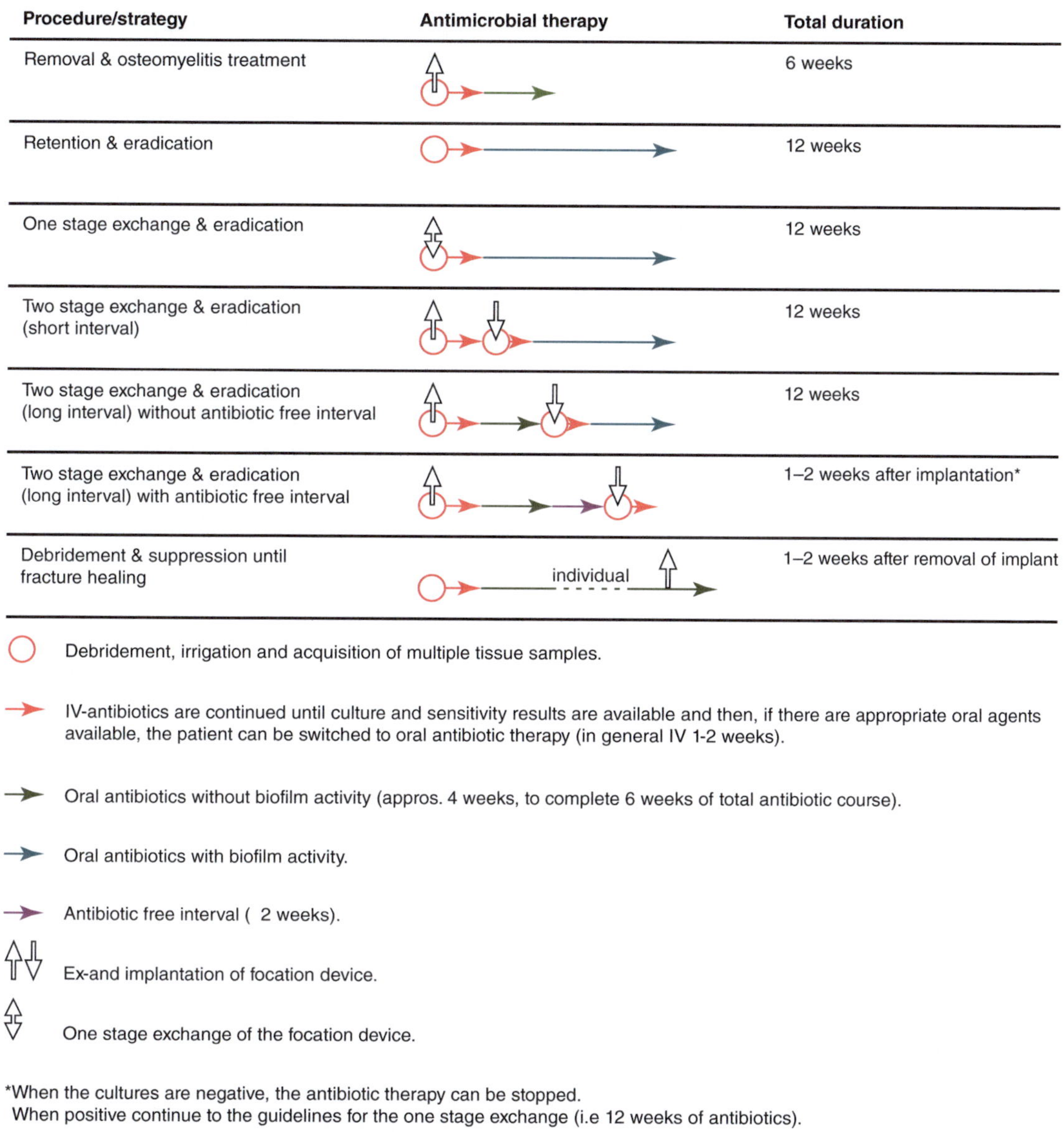

Fig. 10.2 Duration of antimicrobial therapy in different treatment strategies. (from Depypere M, Kuehl R, Metsemakers WJ, et al. (2020) Recommendations for Systemic Antimicrobial Therapy in Fracture-Related Infection: A Consensus from an International Expert Group. J Orthop Trauma. 34(1):30–41)

resistance. In patients with a Gram-positive FRI for which there is no option of oral antibiotics, new therapeutic agents like long-acting intravenous antibiotics are a good alternative (see section *Novel Antimicrobial Agents* below) [31].

In patients in whom DAIR has been performed, anti-biofilm agents are especially important, because eradication is generally only possible in these patients if anti-biofilm agents are used [10, 22]. Rifampicin and other rifamycins can be effective adjuvant agents in suppressing Gram-positive organisms, while ciprofloxacin (fluoroquinolones) is preferred to suppress Gram-negative bacilli [15]. In patients in whom no biofilm-active antibiotics are available due to potential drug interactions, intolerance, or antimicrobial resistance, the FRI is considered "difficult-to-treat," and antibiotic administration continues until the fracture heals and the implants can be removed. In this situation, the FRI can usually be suppressed but not eradicated as long as the implants are retained, so the goal is to achieve sufficient bacterial load reduction (through debridement and long-term antibiotic therapy) to allow fracture consolidation, after which the implant can be removed without functional loss. This strategy is only appropriate for patients with good bone healing potential (F2), and conversion to external fixation should be considered (refer to Chap. 4 for more information on which patients best benefit from DAIR) [11, 32].

When Implants Are Exchanged the duration of antimicrobial therapy is strongly influenced by whether the surgical strategy is a single-stage (12 weeks) or two-stage (two 6-week regimes) approach [33]. The absence of internal fixation (e.g., osteogenic distraction with a circular frame) also favors short antimicrobial regimes.

When Implants Are Removed 6 weeks of antimicrobial therapy are considered sufficient [10, 33]. This is especially true of united fractures (F1), as the removal of fixation hardware greatly decreases the available surface for biofilm formation and thus eases eradication [34].

Long-Term Suppressive Antimicrobial Treatment

Long-term suppression is considered mainly in two scenarios: a DAIR approach (as a bridge until the implant can be removed), or patients who can only be treated conservatively.

In DAIR, the objective of antimicrobial suppression is to prevent or delay infection recurrence until the fracture has consolidated and the implants can be safely removed (as previously pointed out, after implant removal the potential for biofilm formation decreases and eradication is easier). This strategy fails in about a fourth of well-selected patients, it being challenging to predict beforehand in which patients it will fail, but the remainder will be healed [35, 36].

Long-term suppressive antimicrobial treatment can also be indicated in severely compromised patients (R4–5) despite optimization, or those who decline surgical treatment [37]. Surgical treatments of FRI are aggressive, so patients in a poor condition to face surgery, with a high risk of both medical and surgical complications, may benefit best from conservative treatments. This is especially true if they have a limited lifespan, as they are less likely to suffer complications of antimicrobial suppression, including side effects and toxicity derived from their prolonged use. The available evidence suggests that the benefit of antimicrobial suppression plateaus at about 1–2 years, after which the suppressive effect wanes and the side effects increase.

Note that overall, side effects are common (especially gastrointestinal), and discontinuation of treatment due to toxicity is not rare. Furthermore, in addition to toxicity, drug interactions and/or patient comorbidities may limit the application of continuous suppressive treatment. Consequently, some patients can only be treated with antimicrobials when they suffer an exacerbation of the FRI.

Use of Local Antimicrobials

In FRI, the delivery and tissue penetration of systemic antimicrobials are impaired due to the presence of immune-privileged bacterial reservoirs and the poor perfusion of FRI sites [11, 28]. This impairment limits the doses that can be reached at the FRI site, and the potential for successfully tackling immune-privileged bacterial reservoirs, including biofilm, the osteocyte-cannalicular network, and intracellular reservoirs, among others. To address these problems, local administration routes have been developed.

Local delivery of antimicrobials through carriers such as antibiotic-impregnated polymethyl methacrylate (PMMA) or biodegradable ceramics allows the administration of very high doses of several antimicrobials directly to the FRI site, with low systemic exposure [38, 39]. These doses are high enough to affect the sessile bacteria biofilm populations, which have a low metabolic rate, while simultaneously minimizing systemic toxic effects [39]. The direct delivery to the FRI site also allows antimicrobials to reach immune-privileged bacterial reservoirs. Delivery is usually maximally high within the first days after implantation of the carrier, and decreases thereafter throughout the following weeks.

The use of local antibiotic therapy has been associated with a 9% decrease in infection recurrence rate, which corresponds to the risk of recurrence almost halving [35]. It is recommended by expert panels and overall, commonly done [18, 27]. Local antibiotics should cover the germs that are commonly involved in that geographical location, such as gentamycin and vancomycin, a synergistic combination with improved elution and coverage of almost all usual pathogens, including MRSA [39]. Other antimicrobials applied locally include tobramycin, protein synthesis inhibitors (clindamycin, erythromycin, linezolid), bactericides for Gram-positive (cefazolin, daptomycin) or Gram-negative bacteria (polymyxin), and antifungals (amphotericin, voriconazole).

However, there is currently no evidence to support the use of any specific antibiotic, optimal dosing, application technique, or carrier [18, 28]. For example, though it is clear that higher doses achieve higher rates of infection eradication, there is concern over the cytotoxic effects of these very high antimicrobial doses on nearby bone cells, especially in the case of fluoroquinolones. This is based on preclinical studies that have found decreased osteoblast proliferation rates with increasing dose of local antibiotics, which could then compromise fracture consolidation [39]. Further research is needed to assess the effects of local antimicrobials on bone healing. In addition, the elution profiles for different local antimicrobial carriers are still under investigation, and some carriers impose limitations on the antimicrobials that they can successfully carry. For instance, PMMA has a highly exothermic polymerization process, so it can only carry thermally stable antibiotics such as aminoglycosides, glycopeptides, tetracyclines, and quinolones [15, 39]. Beta-lactams are *not* heat-stable, they degrade quickly as temperature increases. For more information on local antibiotic carriers, the reader is referred to Chap. 3.

The risk of systemic toxicity with locally administered antibiotics, though considerably lower than with enteral or parenteral administration, still exists. This risk should be weighed in the context of patient characteristics (e.g., age, comorbidities) to adapt the antibiotic dosing accordingly.

The direct application of antibiotic powder (without a carrier) is so far experimental, and more evidence is needed to make recommendations [39].

Note that the use of local antibiotics is part of a complex treatment plan but does not replace the need for systemic parenteral antibiotics, or proper debridement [10].

Future Directions

Novel Antimicrobial Agents

Research into new antimicrobial agents and combinations, as well as alternative therapies such as bacteriophage therapy, shows promise in overcoming difficult-to-treat FRIs.

The Use of New Antibiotics (Table 10.4) is particularly appealing when prolonged therapy, early discharge, or avoidance of long-term intravascular catheter access are desired, in patients with poor or nonadherence to oral therapy, or when multidrug-resistant bacteria are suspected.

For example, long-acting lipoglycopeptide intravenous antibiotics, such as dalbavancin and oritavancin, have emerged recently against a broad spectrum of Gram-positive pathogens, including methicillin-resistant *Staphylococcus* and vancomycin-resistant *Enterococcus*. They have extended half-lives and excellent tissue penetration, which allows prolonged high therapeutic concentrations at the site of infection, even in challenging sites such as bone. Moreover, these antibiotics have demonstrated in vitro efficacy against biofilm. They are well-tolerated and do not require therapeutic drug monitoring [31]. They must be administered IV and the lit-

Table 10.4 New antimicrobial agents for the treatment of fracture-related infections. MRSA: methicillin-resistant *Staphylococcus aureus*

Class/family	Antibiotic	Antimicrobial spectrum
Oxazolidinones	Tedizolid	Gram-positive (MRSA included)
Long-acting lipoglycopeptides	Dalbavancin, oritavancin	Gram-positive (MRSA included)
Anti-MRSA cephalosporins (fifth generation)	Ceftaroline, Ceftobiprole	Gram-positive and gram-negative bacteria
Fluoroquinolones (fourth generation)	Delafloxacin	Gram-positive (MRSA included) and gram-negative bacteria
Cephalosporins and beta-lactamase inhibitor	Ceftazidime/avibactam, ceftolozane/tazobactam	Multidrug-resistant gram-negative bacteria
Cephalosporin (siderophore)	Cefiderocol	Multidrug-resistant gram-negative bacteria
Carbapenem	Meropenem/vaborbactam	Multidrug-resistant gram-negative bacteria

erature on their use for osteoarticular infections is yet limited, but their broad spectrum, anti-biofilm activity, synergism with rifampicin, and safety profile make them appealing for the treatment of FRIs.

Another new antimicrobial of interest for FRI treatment is a new, fourth-generation fluoroquinolone, delafloxacin. Delafloxacin is the only anionic fluoroquinolone, so it is highly active in acidic mediums (e.g., abscesses or skin necrosis), and has shown excellent penetration into tissues including bone and biofilms. It has demonstrated high potency against Gram-positive bacilli, in addition to efficacy against multidrug-resistant Gram-negative bacterial strains, including isolates resistant to levofloxacin and moxifloxacin. In Gram-positive bacteria, delafloxacin, as well as targeting DNA topoisomerase that other fluoroquinolones target, also targets DNA gyrase, providing this drug with potent antibacterial activity and decreased risk of resistance selection [40]. Given these characteristics, delafloxacin holds potential for use in the treatment of FRIs.

Bacteriophage Therapy (viruses targeting the infecting bacteria) is developing as a promising treatment to eradicate difficult-to-treat microbes or patients with severe comorbidities (R4–5 hosts) [41, 42]. In these cases, phage therapy is typically applied locally through a drain to obtain the highest concentration of phages at the site of infection, although intravenous applications have been described. The drain allows therapeutic phage monitoring and facilitates treatment optimization. After the final phage administration, the drain is removed, thereby minimizing the risk of superinfection [41]. A few case series have reported good outcomes after the administration of selected bacteriophages combined with surgical debridement in patients with recurrent *Staphylococcus aureus* and *Pseudomonas aeruginosa* prosthetic joint infections (PJI), with only some case reports of bacteriophage application in FRI [41]. Based on this limited available literature, the main benefits of phage therapy are a higher probability of success of suppressive antimicrobial therapy and potential to delay the development of resistance to suppressive antimicrobials, which can then delay aggressive surgical treatments such as amputation or resection arthroplasty in cases of multidrug-resistant pathogens. However, prolonged suppressive antibiotic therapy must be maintained, and bacteria can (and do, over time) become resistant to bacteriophages. Furthermore, knowledge gaps remain regarding the optimal treatment protocol, and given that this therapy is only being applied to selected patients, it is likely that these knowledge gaps will remain in the near future.

Additional Strategies Have Been Tested Preclinically aiming to destroy biofilm in situ. Citric acid used as a cytotoxic agent, bioactive enzymes (as dispersin B), electrical stimulation, pulsed electromagnetic fields, and electrolytic cleaning of the retained implant have been experimented with promising results [43, 44].

Thanks to advances in basic and translational pharmacological research, as well as the development of novel mechanisms for the targeted delivery and controlled release of active molecules at precise concentrations, we are poised to significantly improve the management of FRI. A key factor in this progress is the advent of nanotechnology, alongside innovations in fields such as encapsulation microparticles, biodegradable polymers, and microfluidics. These emerging technologies offer promising solutions for optimizing therapeutic efficacy and minimizing systemic side effects.

Stewardship Programs

The rise of antimicrobial resistance has prompted the development of antimicrobial stewardship programs. Appropriate use of antimicrobials not only allows effective treatment of infections, thus improving patient outcomes, but also reduces hospital admissions and the length of hospital stays (both of which tend to be long in FRI patients). Accordingly, it is one of the emerging research trends.

In this matter, local antimicrobials have been a popular strategy, as they have been reported to enable a reduction in the duration of systemic therapy and the amount of systemic drugs needed (with a concomitant reduction in side effects), reduced risk of antimicrobial resistance, and improved patient compliance [15, 45].

Antibiotic Strategies for Prevention

Preventative measures, including prophylactic antibiotics and improved surgical techniques, are critical in reducing the incidence of FRIs.

Antibiotics should be administered as soon as possible after any open fracture. They should be administered for no more than 24 h for Gustilo–Anderson type I and II fractures, and for no more than 72 h for type III fractures [33]. They should mainly target Gram-positive organisms because they are the microorganisms that most frequently cause FRI. Additional coverage for Gram-negative organisms should be considered for patients with high-energy open fractures. Cephalosporins with a broad range of antibacterial activities against Gram-positive and Gram-negative bacteria are often used as first-line prophylaxis [15].

Patients who are methicillin-resistant *Staphylococcus aureus* carriers or are allergic to penicillin should receive glycopeptides, like vancomycin. However, glycopeptides only cover Gram-positive bacteria, so they are often combined with a first-generation cephalosporin or with an aminoglycoside (gentamicin), with higher risk of acute kidney damage in patients with baseline altered renal function. Decisions on using single versus dual-agent prophylaxis should depend on local epidemiology and resistant rates, adapted to the lesion and the patient [15, 33]. A randomized controlled trial comparing vancomycin and cefazolin versus only cefazolin in patients with open fractures found no significant differences in the infection rates between both groups (19% vs. 15%, respectively) [46].

In open fractures with potential clostridial contamination (e.g., fecal contamination), anaerobic coverage (penicillin, clindamycin or metronidazole) is compulsory. Anaerobic coverage is also recommended in cases of farm and vascular injuries.

Recently, osteosynthesis material with resorbable antibiotic-impregnated coatings are being developed in an attempt to reduce the risk of FRI. To date, the only commercialized product is a tibia nail with gentamycin-impregnated poly(D,L-lactide) (PDLLA), which releases the gentamycin over the first 2 weeks [39]. The published results are promising but so far, the studies evaluating this material are very few, further evaluation is warranted [28].

Clinical Cases

Case 10.1

A 56-year-old woman suffered a trimaleolar luxation-fracture of her left ankle after a fall from her own height (Figs. 10.3 and 10.4). She had no medical history. The fracture was treated with open reduction and internal fixation with a plate and screws (Fig. 10.5) through bilateral surgical incisions in the distal third of the ankle. A middle

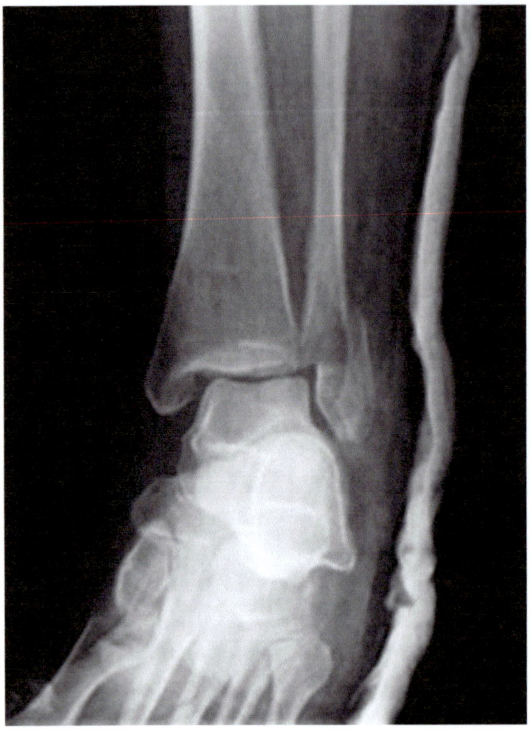

Fig. 10.3 Case 10.1, conventional X-ray image at presentation in the emergency room, showing a trimaleolar luxation-fracture in her left ankle

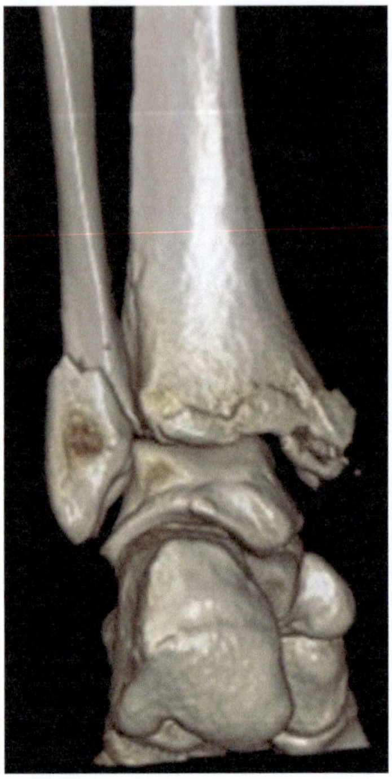

Fig. 10.4 Case 10.1, computed tomography images of the left ankle at presentation

ankle arthroscopy was performed as well to ensure anatomic reduction.

One week after the surgery, a blister appeared on the anteromedial skin of the ankle, near the arthroscopy portal. It was treated conservatively with wound care. However, increasing pain and swelling over the following days led the patient to consult in the emergency room. She denied any systemic symptoms such as fever or shivering, but the ankle was swollen and had an erythematous area 2 cm in diameter around the arthroscopic wound. Upon opening the wound, purulent drainage suffused and was sent for bacterial cultures. The patient's laboratory evaluation revealed a normal white blood cell count, C-reactive protein (2.1 mg/L), and erythrocyte sedimentation rate (ESR, 45 mm/h, with the normal range being 0–20 mm/h in our laboratory).

Methicillin-susceptible *Staphylococcus aureus* grew on cultures of intraoperative samples, so an arthroscopic debridement and irrigation were performed within 2 weeks of the initial

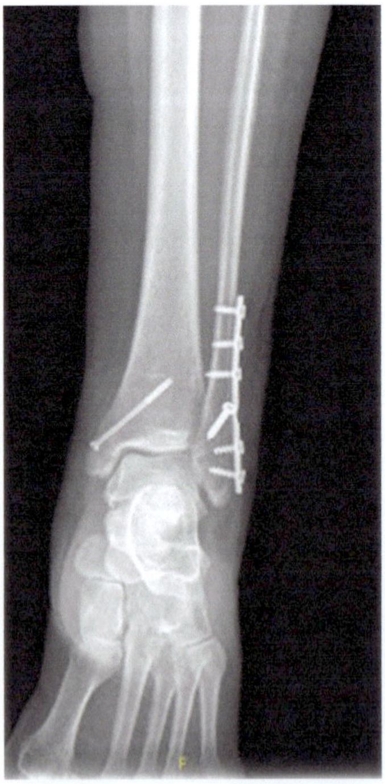

Fig. 10.5 Case 10.1, ankle X-ray on the first postoperative day after ankle fracture fixation

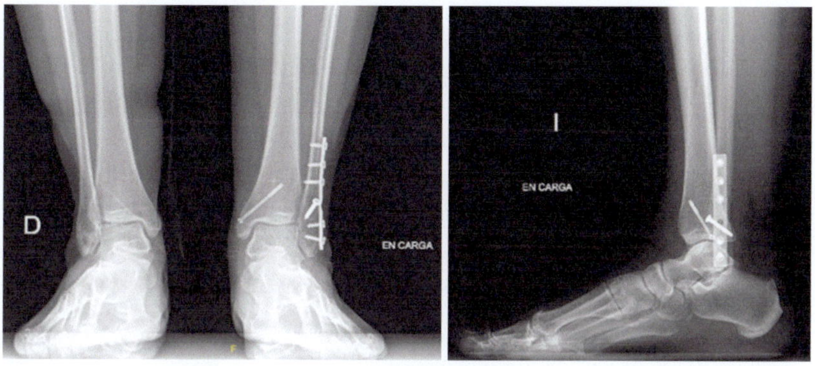

Fig. 10.6 Case 10.1, anteroposterior (left) and lateral (right) standing ankle X-ray images at 6 months postoperatively

surgery. The bone healing potential was deemed good (F2 R1 I2), so the implant was retained. After a 10-day IV course of cefazoline and daptomycin, the patient was discharged on oral levofloxacin and rifampicin.

Progressive healing was noted at routine follow-up appointments. She completed 12 weeks of antibiotics. Bone union was noted at 6 months postoperatively, so she underwent early removal of the implants. At 2 years postoperatively, she has painless gait (Fig. 10.6).

Conclusions

Antimicrobial therapy (systemic and/or local) cannot compensate for inadequate surgery.

In FRI, empirical treatment should be administered promptly *after* deep tissue samples have been obtained (except for patients with sepsis, in whom immediate antibiotic therapy should be initiated after obtaining blood samples for microbiological culture). High-loading intravenous doses and prolonged infusions of antibiotics with time-dependent bactericidal activity that have a broad-spectrum including coverage of both Gram-positive and Gram-negative bacteria are recommended. Therapeutic drug monitoring should be performed if available.

Once the causative pathogen is identified and antimicrobial sensitivity results are available, targeted treatment should be initiated. Anti-biofilm agents are essential.

The optimal duration of antimicrobial therapy for FRI remains uncertain. It is often between 6 and 12 weeks, with factors like implant retention favoring extended regimes.

Long-term suppressive antimicrobial treatment can be appropriate as a bridge in a DAIR approach until bone union and removal of the implant, or in patients who can only be treated conservatively (R5). The benefits seem to plateau after about 1–2 years.

Local antimicrobials decrease the risk of infection recurrence as the administered doses can be high enough to affect biofilm, with low systemic exposure.

New antimicrobial agents such as long-acting lipoglycopeptides or delafloxacin have potential for FRIs, with improved penetration, anti-biofilm action, and favorable safety profiles. Bacteriophage therapy also holds promise, but further research is needed to clarify the optimal treatment protocol and what role it will play in FRI treatment. Other research focuses include antimicrobial stewardship programs and preventative strategies.

Multidisciplinary teams involved in all stages of FRIs care are an effective way to improve results, as well as to save resources and time for the benefit of patients and the health system.

References

1. Trampuz A, Zimmerli W. Diagnosis and treatment of infections associated with fracture-fixation devices. Injury. 2006;37(Suppl 2):S59–66.
2. Metsemakers W-J, Moriarty TF, Morgenstern M, et al. The global burden of fracture-related infection: can we do better? Lancet Infect Dis. 2024;24:e386–93.

3. Depypere M, Morgenstern M, Kuehl R, Senneville E, Moriarty TF, Obremskey WT, Zimmerli W, Trampuz A, Lagrou K, Metsemakers W-J. Pathogenesis and management of fracture-related infection. Clin Microbiol Infect. 2020;26:572–8.
4. Ochsner P, Sirkin M, Trampuz A. Acute infections. In: AO principles of fracture management (Volume I). Stuttgart and New York: Thieme; 2016. p. 520–40.
5. Depypere M, Kuehl R, Metsemakers W-J, Senneville E, MA MN, Obremskey WT, Zimmerli W, Atkins BL, Trampuz A, Fracture-Related Infection (FRI) Consensus Group. Recommendations for systemic antimicrobial therapy in fracture-related infection: a consensus from an international expert group. J Orthop Trauma. 2020;34:30–41.
6. Depypere M, Sliepen J, Onsea J, Debaveye Y, Govaert GAM, FFA IJ, Zimmerli W, Metsemakers W-J. The microbiological etiology of fracture-related infection. Front Cell Infect Microbiol. 2022;12:934485.
7. Kuehl R, Tschudin-Sutter S, Morgenstern M, Dangel M, Egli A, Nowakowski A, Suhm N, Theilacker C, Widmer AF. Time-dependent differences in management and microbiology of orthopaedic internal fixation-associated infections: an observational prospective study with 229 patients. Clin Microbiol Infect. 2019;25:76–81.
8. Corrigan RA, Sliepen J, Dudareva M, FFA IJ, Govaert G, Atkins BL, Rentenaar R, Wouthuyzen-Bakker M, McNally M. Causative pathogens do not differ between early. Delayed or Late Fracture-Related Infections Antibiotics (Basel). 2022;11:943.
9. Masters EA, Ricciardi BF, de Bentley KLM, Moriarty TF, Schwarz EM, Muthukrishnan G. Skeletal infections: microbial pathogenesis, immunity and clinical management. Nat Rev Microbiol. 2022;20:385–400.
10. Morgenstern M, Clauss M, Sendi P, Cadosch D, Osinga R, Metsemakers W-J. Treatment of fracture-related infections. In: Textbook of Polytrauma management: a multidisciplinary approach. 3rd ed. Berlin, Germany: Springer; 2022. p. 573–81.
11. Moriarty TF, Metsemakers W-J, Morgenstern M, Hofstee MI, Vallejo Diaz A, Cassat JE, Wildemann B, Depypere M, Schwarz EM, Richards RG. Fracture-related infection. Nat Rev Dis Primers. 2022;8:67.
12. Busscher HJ, van der Mei HC. How do bacteria know they are on a surface and regulate their response to an adhering state? PLoS Pathog. 2012;8:e1002440.
13. Stojicic S, Shen Y, Haapasalo M. Effect of the source of biofilm bacteria, level of biofilm maturation, and type of disinfecting agent on the susceptibility of biofilm bacteria to antibacterial agents. J Endodont. 2013;39:473–7.
14. Pettygrove BA, Kratofil RM, Alhede M, et al. Delayed neutrophil recruitment allows nascent Staphylococcus aureus biofilm formation and immune evasion. Biomaterials. 2021;275:120775.
15. Foster AL, Moriarty TF, Trampuz A, Jaiprakash A, Burch MA, Crawford R, Paterson DL, Metsemakers W-J, Schuetz M, Richards RG. Fracture-related infection: current methods for prevention and treatment. Expert Rev Anti-Infect Ther. 2020;18:307–21.
16. Morgenstern M, Kuehl R, Zalavras CG, McNally M, Zimmerli W, Burch MA, Vandendriessche T, Obremskey WT, Verhofstad MHJ, Metsemakers WJ. The influence of duration of infection on outcome of debridement and implant retention in fracture-related infection. Bone Joint J. 2021;103-B:213–21.
17. Vicenti G, Buono C, Albano F, Ladogana T, Pesare E, Colasuonno G, Passarelli AC, Solarino G. Early Management for Fracture-Related Infection: a literature review. Healthcare (Basel). 2024;12:1306.
18. Metsemakers W-J, Morgenstern M, Senneville E, et al. General treatment principles for fracture-related infection: recommendations from an international expert group. Arch Orthop Trauma Surg. 2020;140:1013–27.
19. Baertl S, Walter N, Engelstaedter U, Ehrenschwender M, Hitzenbichler F, Alt V, Rupp M. What is the Most effective empirical antibiotic treatment for early, delayed, and late fracture-related infections? Antibiotics (Basel). 2022;11:287.
20. Li H-K, Rombach I, Zambellas R, et al. Oral versus intravenous antibiotics for bone and joint infection. N Engl J Med. 2019;380:425–36.
21. He S-Y, Yu B, Jiang N. Current concepts of fracture-related infection. Int J Clin Pract. 2023;2023:4839701.
22. Spellberg B, Lipsky BA. Systemic antibiotic therapy for chronic osteomyelitis in adults. Clin Infect Dis. 2012;54:393–407.
23. Nguyen S, Robineau O, Titecat M, Blondiaux N, Valette M, Loiez C, Beltrand E, Migaud H, Senneville E. Influence of daily dosage and frequency of administration of rifampicin-levofloxacin therapy on tolerance and effectiveness in 154 patients treated for prosthetic joint infections. Eur J Clin Microbiol Infect Dis. 2015;34:1675–82.
24. Corvec S, Furustrand Tafin U, Betrisey B, Borens O, Trampuz A. Activities of fosfomycin, tigecycline, colistin, and gentamicin against extended-spectrum-β-lactamase-producing Escherichia coli in a foreign-body infection model. Antimicrob Agents Chemother. 2013;57:1421–7.
25. Mancheño-Losa M, Murillo O, Benavent E, et al. Efficacy and safety of colistin plus beta-lactams for bone and joint infection caused by fluoroquinolone-resistant gram-negative bacilli: a prospective multicenter study. Infection. 2025;53:359–72.
26. Pappas PG, Kauffman CA, Andes DR, et al. Clinical practice guideline for the Management of Candidiasis: 2016 update by the Infectious Diseases Society of America. Clin Infect Dis. 2016;62:e1–50.
27. Prada C, Bengoa F, Bhandari M. The management of fracture related infections: what practices can be supported by high-level evidence? J Orthop Surg (Hong Kong). 2022;30:10225536221119580.
28. Iliadis AD, Shivji F, Debuka E, Trompeter A, Narayan B, Heidari N. Current concepts in the prevention,

diagnosis and treatment of fracture-related infection (FRI). Eur J Orthop Surg Traumatol. 2021;31:957–66.
29. Mauffrey C, Herbert B, Young H, Wilson ML, Hake M, Stahel PF. The role of biofilm on orthopaedic implants: the "holy grail" of post-traumatic infection management? Eur J Trauma Emerg Surg. 2016;42:411–6.
30. Kanakaris NK, Tosounidis TH, Giannoudis PV. Surgical management of infected non-unions: an update. Injury. 2015;46(Suppl 5):S25–32.
31. Cooper CC, Stein GE, Mitra S, Abubaker A, Havlichek DH. Long-acting Lipoglycopeptides for the treatment of bone and joint infections. Surg Infect. 2021;22:771–9.
32. Foster AL, Moriarty TF, Zalavras C, et al. The influence of biomechanical stability on bone healing and fracture-related infection: the legacy of Stephan Perren. Injury. 2021;52:43–52.
33. Rupp M, Walter N, Bärtl S, Heyd R, Hitzenbichler F, Alt V. Fracture-related infection-epidemiology, etiology, diagnosis, prevention, and treatment. Dtsch Arztebl Int. 2024;121:17–24.
34. Kanakaris NK, Giannoudis PV. Biofilm and its implications postfracture fixation: all I need to know. OTA Int. 2021;4:e107(1–7).
35. McNally M, Corrigan R, Sliepen J, Dudareva M, Rentenaar R, IJpma F, Atkins BL, Wouthuyzen-Bakker M, Govaert G. What factors affect outcome in the treatment of fracture-related infection? Antibiotics (Basel). 2022;11:946.
36. Lu V, Zhang J, Patel R, Zhou AK, Thahir A, Krkovic M. Fracture related infections and their risk factors for treatment failure-a major trauma Centre perspective. Diagnostics (Basel). 2022;12:1289.
37. Alt V, McNally M, Wouthuyzen-Bakker M, Metsemakers W-J, Marais L, Zalavras C, Morgenstern M. The FRI classification – a new classification of fracture-related infections. Injury. 2024;55:111831.
38. Hussain SA, Walters S, Ahluwalia AK, Trompeter A. Fracture-related infections. Br J Hosp Med (Lond). 2023;84:1–10.
39. Metsemakers W-J, Fragomen AT, Moriarty TF, Morgenstern M, Egol KA, Zalavras C, Obremskey WT, Raschke M, McNally MA. Evidence-based recommendations for local antimicrobial strategies and dead space Management in Fracture-Related Infection. J Orthop Trauma. 2020;34:18–29.
40. Tulkens PM, Van Bambeke F, Zinner SH. Profile of a novel anionic fluoroquinolone-Delafloxacin. Clin Infect Dis. 2019;68:S213–22.
41. Ferry T, Onsea J, Roussel-Gaillard T, Batailler C, Moriarty TF, Metsemakers W-J. Bacteriophage therapy in musculoskeletal infections: from basic science to clinical application. EFORT Open Rev. 2024;9:339–48.
42. Walter N, Bärtl S, Alt V, Rupp M. Recent advancements and future directions in fracture related infections: a scoping review. Injury. 2024;55:111902.
43. Muniyasamy R, Manjubala I. Synergistic combination of baicalein and rifampicin against Staphylococcus aureus biofilms. Front Microbiol. 2024;15:1458267.
44. Kizhner V, Krespi YP, Hall-Stoodley L, Stoodley P. Laser-generated shockwave for clearing medical device biofilms. Photomed Laser Surg. 2011;29:277–82.
45. Unsworth A, Young B, Ferguson J, Scarborough M, McNally M. Local antimicrobial therapy with combined aminoglycoside and vancomycin compared to aminoglycoside monotherapy in the surgical Management of Osteomyelitis and Fracture-Related Infection. Antibiotics (Basel). 2024;13:703.
46. Saveli CC, Morgan SJ, Belknap RW, Ross E, Stahel PF, Chaus GW, Hak DJ, Biffl WL, Knepper B, Price CS. Prophylactic antibiotics in open fractures: a pilot randomized clinical safety study. J Orthop Trauma. 2013;27:552–7.

Fine-Tuning Postoperative Care of Fracture-Related Infection

11

Elena Armas and Nieves Vanaclocha

Introduction

Exquisite postoperative care is essential to achieve the best functional result in fracture-related infection (FRI) patients. Postoperative care can be the deciding factor between success and failure after an otherwise perfect procedure, and can promote or prevent the occurrence of postoperative complications depending on what postoperative care is provided and how. Therefore, it is wise to pay proper attention to it and be intentional in the chosen postoperative regimen for each patient in their individual context.

In this chapter, we will address:

- Postoperative wound care, depending on the soft tissue reconstruction modality.
- Postoperative rehabilitation, including weight-bearing and limb dangling.

E. Armas (✉)
Department of Plastic and Reconstructive Surgery, University General Hospital Gregorio Marañón, Madrid, Spain
e-mail: elena.armas@salud.madrid.org

N. Vanaclocha
Orthoplastics Unit and Department of Plastic and Reconstructive Surgery, University and Polytechnic Hospital La Fe, Valencia, Spain

Antimicrobial therapy is discussed at length in Chap. 10, to which the reader is referred for information on this subject.

Postoperative Wound Care

As pointed out in Chap. 9, stable wound coverage is essential to preventing reinfection of the FRI site. Thus, wound care is one of the core elements of postoperative care in FRI.

Direct Closure and Pin Care

When direct closure has been possible, standard postoperative wound care is appropriate. Common practices include dressing changes every 48 hours, applying topical antiseptics such as chlorhexidine, and to allow showering between 3 and 10 days after surgery depending on the quality of the closure and whether the patient has drains. However, the evidence on many of these practices is very scarce, and their application is based more on general consensus after long-term experience with them and/or team habits than on the limited available evidence. The evidence to support the use of specific surgical dressings (e.g., hydrocolloids, silver-containing dressings) to reduce the risk of complications such as surgical site infection is weak [1].

N. Vanaclocha (ed.), *Treatment of Fracture-Related Infection*,
https://doi.org/10.1007/978-3-031-92452-1_11

If an external fixator has been implanted, to avoid pin tract infections (the most common complication of distraction osteogenesis techniques), it is essential to convey the importance of good pin care, show the patient how it is properly done, and have the patient explain how they do it on outpatient visits to check that the patient is taking good care of the pins at home.

Skin Grafts

In FRI patients that have been skin-grafted, standard skin graft care is appropriate.

After skin grafting, immobilization of the grafted area during the first postoperative week is recommended to avoid skin graft displacement, which interferes with graft take [2]. In the limbs, compressive bandages and explaining to the patient on which area they should avoid shearing forces usually suffice. In areas where semi-compressive bandaging would be challenging, such as the clavicle, a bolster with compressive gauze or sterile sponges can be applied for the first postoperative 5–7 days [2]. After the first 5–7 days, checking the status of the grafted tissue is mandatory to address the current necessities of the wound (e.g., removal of excess fluid or fibrin).

There are several techniques to treat skin graft donor areas, which tend to be highly exudative, including meshed gauzes impregnated with petroleum-based products, hydrocolloids, and foams [3]. No specific dressing has demonstrated superiority over others, but for gauze-based dressings, which are reported to be the least favorable [4].

Locoregional Flaps

Pedicled flaps are often unavailable in FRI patients because nearby tissues are often damaged either by the initial trauma or the subsequent surgeries, but when they are performed, the key postoperative point is avoiding compression of pedicle. This implies avoiding highly compressive bandages on the skin paddle and the trajectory of the pedicle. If there are any signs of ischemia or congestion, pedicle kinking or compression by a hematoma should be suspected [3]. Often, it is possible to resolve the problem in the hospital ward. Otherwise, urgent surgical revision to salvage the flap is warranted.

Free Flaps

Free flaps are the most laborious bone and/or soft tissue reconstruction method, and as such require the most complex postoperative care out of all the reconstructive modalities. Microanastomotic thrombosis of free flaps performed by experienced teams is infrequent (see section *Flap failure* below) [5], but flaps performed on the limbs (especially, the lower limb) are more prone to needing revision that flaps on other areas such as the trunk, and, given that the salvage rate drops as the delay between identification of flap compromise and surgical revision lengthens, close postoperative monitoring of all free flaps is recommended [5, 6].

Clinical monitoring of free flaps (color, capillary refill, and temperature) is subjective, but widely available [6, 7]. Many teams rely on residents for clinical monitoring of free flaps, but there is evidence supporting that trained nurses are able to correctly monitor free flaps as well [8]. Though in many institutions free flap patients will routinely spend the first night in the intensive care unit to facilitate clinical monitoring, there are no differences in free flap salvage rate between patients that stay in an intensive care unit and patients that stay in a ward [9].

Doppler auscultation is used in conjunction with clinical monitoring in most institutions [5, 6, 10]. The principle is that if the pedicle flow is heard, the flap is not compromised. The required device is generally inexpensive and widely available. However, in certain anatomical locations it may be challenging to distinguish the flow through the pedicle from flow in nearby vessels, and venous flow (the most often affected when a flap is compromised) is much harder to evaluate than arterial flow. Sometimes, due to the small caliber of the veins and the slow flow, it is not possible to evaluate venous flow with Doppler auscultation at all. Additionally, it is subjective and operator-dependent.

In most FRI patients in whom a free flap is performed, the flap will be required for soft tissue reconstruction (whether bone reconstruction is needed as well or not), so a skin paddle will be available for monitorization. In this situation, clinical monitoring by a trained team is effective [6]. However, at some institutions a trained team is not always available for 24/7 monitorization, and in some patients the soft tissue envelope is adequate and no skin paddle is needed. These issues, together with the subjectivity inherent in clinical monitoring and the limitations of Doppler auscultation, have sparked the development of free flap monitoring devices that seek to detect flap compromise earlier, more precisely, and in a nonoperator dependent way, potentially leading to higher flap salvage rates. The ideal device would be noninvasive and user-friendly, provide real-time data on flap perfusion, and have good sensitivity and specificity for detecting microvascular thrombosis [6]. So far, the ideal device has not been found.

Color duplex ultrasound adds visual ultrasound information to the auditive information provided by Doppler auscultation, thus increasing precision in targeting blood flow through the pedicle specifically [6]. It is a reliable method to evaluate free flap vascularity, with some publications reporting a false-positive rate of 0% when used by trained professionals [11–14]. However, it is subjective and user-dependent (like Doppler auscultation), it requires specific training, and the equipment needed is considerably more expensive than for Doppler auscultation [6].

Near-infrared spectroscopy (NIRS) allows monitorization of changes in tissue perfusion and oxygenation status based on absorption of infrared light by tissue chromophores contained in hemoglobin [6]. It allows real-time measurement of oxygenated (StO_2) and deoxygenated hemoglobin [6, 7]. The most common thresholds to consider that flap vascularization is compromised are $StO_2 \leq 30\%$ or a drop in $StO_2 > 20\%$ lasting for 30 min [7]. Systematic reviews have found that flap compromise is detected earlier with NIRS than when free flaps are monitored clinically, and flap salvage ratio is higher (89%), with a lower flap loss rate [6, 7]. This monitorization modality can be especially useful for free muscle flaps without a skin paddle [15], since a correct clinical assessment of this type of flaps is more difficult than when a skin paddle is present [16].

The implantable Doppler, or Cook-Swartz Doppler, is a piezoelectric crystal embedded in a silicon sheath connected to an acoustic Doppler device [6, 17]. It is wrapped around either the pedicle vein or its artery and converts the flow detected through the vessel into a sound signal in real time [6]. Free flap failure risk is lower (risk ratio 0.4) and successful salvage rate is higher (risk ratio 1.73) when the implantable Doppler is used for monitorization than with clinical assessment and Doppler auscultation [4, 10, 18]. However, a wide range (0.75–37%) of false positives (signal loss without free flap malfunction) has been reported [17], the higher end corresponding to studies with buried flaps, in which a clinical assessment to compliment implantable Doppler information is not possible. False positives can happen due to probe dislodgement, fibrin coating, or device malfunction, and result in unnecessary surgical revisions. There appear to be fewer false positives when the implantable Doppler is wrapped around arteries instead of veins [19], but as previously pointed out, venous compromise is more frequent than arterial thrombosis so measuring venous flow is of more interest. Thus, many teams will combine the implantable Doppler information with clinical assessment and/or color duplex ultrasound to reduce the false-positive rate [12]. Additionally, vascular compromise needing surgical revision after pulling on the device's wire to cut it (the piezoelectric crystal and part of the wire stays inside the patient) has been described [20]. These limitations result in that currently, the main use of the implantable Doppler is to monitor buried flaps, in which most other forms of monitoring are not available (this circumstance is rare in the setting of FRI) [21].

Flow Coupler devices combine a traditional Coupler with an incorporated ultrasonic micro-Doppler probe that then measures blood flow through the anastomosis [6]. The intention behind their development was to improve upon the implantable Doppler's false positive rate. So far, flap survival rates and rates of surgical revisions have been observed to be no different than those for flaps monitored with an implantable Doppler [22]. However, one study reported a higher rate of venous thrombosis than when non-flow Coupler devices are used [23]. More evidence is needed to understand the effects of flow Coupler devices on the risk of thrombosis.

Laser Doppler flowmetry is based on detecting the reflections of emitted laser light by blood cells circulating through static free flap tissues (the patterns differ depending on blood cell velocity) [6]. Laser Doppler flowmetry has been found to allow detection of vascular events earlier than when clinical monitoring is used, with a consequent higher free flap salvage ratio (70% clinical monitoring vs. 83% laser Doppler flowmetry) [24, 25]. Some investigators have suggested that laser Doppler flowmetry can differentiate arterial from venous compromise depending on how the pattern changes [25]. However, laser Doppler flowmetry does not provide exact numbers but a pattern based on erythrocyte movement, and measurements can be affected due to vibration or motion of either the probe or the free flap, the location of the probe over a macroscopic blood vessel, or partial detachment of the probe [6, 24, 25]. These limitations have so far prevented its widespread use, in favor of other modalities such as NIRS.

Thermal imaging is based on measuring heat radiation, which is proportional to the body temperature, creating visible images and heat maps [6]. Images provide information about surface temperature but cannot display blood flow [26], so flap assessment is based on comparing the flap's temperature to that of surrounding tissues [27]. Flaps with vascular compromise appear to be colder [26–28]. A difference of ≥ 2 °C between surrounding tissue and flap has been proposed to determine flap vascularity compromise, with a sensitivity of around 90% and a specificity of 85–99% [27, 28]. Its main advantages are its accessibility (a smartphone camera can be used), its low cost, and the fact that no contact with the flap is needed. Further studies to determine the optimal temperature difference to detect microvascular failure are needed, but its wide availability and little to no extra cost make it a promising tool.

Free Flap Monitoring Methods

Clinical monitoring coupled with Doppler auscultation by a trained team is the most frequently used method of flap monitoring. However, the limitations associated with this combined modality (mostly, subjectivity and user-dependency) have sparked the development of other monitoring methods to detect flap compromise earlier and more precisely:

- Color duplex ultrasound combines visual and auditive information, but it is subjective and user-dependent.
- NIRS monitors tissue perfusion by measuring oxygenated and deoxygenated hemoglobin. So far, results with it are promising.
- The implantable Doppler converts the flow through the vessel that it is wrapped around to an acoustic signal. The rate of false positives when used alone are high, so it is often reserved for buried flaps.
- Flow Coupler devices provide an acoustic signal corresponding to blood flow detection through the anastomosis for which the Coupler device was used. More evidence is needed to understand their effects on risk of microthrombosis.
- Laser Doppler flowmetry detects erythrocyte movement through the cells' laser light reflection. The patterns differ depending on blood cell velocity, but no numbers are provided and interpretation can be challenging, limiting widespread adoption.
- Thermal imaging is accessible and cheap, but further studies are needed to determine which threshold for temperature difference between the flap and the surrounding tissues best identifies those flaps requiring revision.

Flap Failure

Global survival of free flaps is reported to be from 90% to 97% [5]. However, in the lower limb, it is estimated 4–13% of free flaps must return to the operating room (OR) because of suspected vascular compromise [29, 30]. For those that are revised surgically, a wide range of flap salvage rates (22–100%) is reported [5, 30]. Free flap salvage rates in recipients located in the extremities (the most common scenario in FRI patients) are similar to those for flaps on the head and neck region, and lower than salvage rates of free flaps in the trunk region [5]. In the limbs, venous compromise is more likely to be successfully managed when compared to arterial compromise [5].

In the event of *partial* flap failure, it may not be possible to identify the cause of the failure precisely, but often simple techniques such as skin grafts or locoregional flaps, or even secondary healing depending on the case, suffice to achieve wound coverage [31].

In the event of *total* flap failure where flap salvage has not been possible, the underlying problem that caused the flap failure must be addressed before further reconstructive measures are undertaken. For example, if the cause of the failure was an arterial thrombosis, an angiography is appropriate to check for potential abnormalities of the recipient artery [31, 32]. If the recipient's flow is normal, the same recipient vessel can be used again, whereas when poor flow is seen, a different recipient should be chosen (or a bypass to a more proximal section with normal flow, if no better nearby recipients are available) [31]. If venous thrombosis occurs, another vein from a different system (e.g., a superficial vein, if previously a deep vein had been used) should be selected for the new anastomosis [31]. If the recipient pedicle presented an anatomic anomaly or vasospasm, or was compressed extrinsically, the deleterious condition should be addressed when performing a second flap.

When a second free flap is performed, the ratio of survival is lower than with the first one (82% success rate) [32]. The indication for limb reconstruction with a second flap versus an amputation must be revised. Identified risk factors for amputation after failed lower limb salvage with a free flap include residual infection, a high number of preoperative debridements, and comorbidities such as diabetes mellitus or arterial pathology (especially, three-vessel injury) [33]. For more information on indications for amputation, refer to Chap. 8.

Note that when a second free flap is performed after a primary flap failure, infection eradication, and union rates do not change [30].

Postoperative Rehabilitation

Physical therapy and rehabilitation are fundamental to obtain good functional outcomes, preventing joint stiffness and the need for secondary procedures [34].

Treatments are protracted, often with periods of immobility after surgery, especially when joints are involved since their immobilization improves infection control [35]. Thus, without exquisite attention to keeping joints supple, range of motion of nearby joints will decrease [36]. Even with adequate physical therapy, it may be challenging to maintain full range of motion, especially with some treatments that tend to interfere with the range of motion of adjacent joints, such as bone transport [37]. When a joint does become stiff, joint contracture release may be necessary [35]. The optimal time to perform it is after infection eradication and before adjunctive procedures such as nerve, muscle, or tendon transfers [38].

Axial Load and Weight-Bearing

The evidence to aid decision-making on when to allow the patient to load on the affected bone is scarce.

In the lower limb, weight-bearing will depend strongly on the kind of treatment that was applied. For example, cancellous bone autografts provide little mechanical stability, so stability will depend mostly on hardware. Generally, autografted patients are able to start partial weight-bearing at 14 weeks [39]. With techniques based on distraction osteogenesis (acute shortening and re-lengthening, bone transport), partial weight-bearing can be started immediately, gradually increasing the load until full weight-bearing within the first postoperative week or two [40]. If bone flaps are used, weight-bearing must be delayed until bone union (three out of four cortices) is observed. In most patients, this will take about 4 months [41]. After this time, protected weight-bearing with a CAM walker-type boot until adequate hypertrophy of the bone flap is obtained is important to prevent stress fractures. The patient should avoid jumps and plyometric-style exercises, as well as activities in which their lower limb must resist weight additional to their body weight, for a full year minimum [42].

After harvesting a fibula flap, it was traditionally considered necessary to splint the ankle of the donor leg with a cast or an orthopedic boot and forbid weight-bearing on that leg for 2 weeks, after which partial weight-bearing could be initiated [41]. More recent evidence suggests that early weight-bearing on the first postoperative day is associated with a reduction in donor-site complications and shorter length of stay [43, 44].

In the upper limb, where maintaining mobility is key for a good functional result, range of motion exercises should generally be started in the immediate postoperative period (for free flaps and skin grafts, a delay of a few days is wise) [45]. Allowing axial load will depend mostly on the strength of the osteosynthetic construct. If sturdy internal fixation was possible, it is reasonable to allow axial load once the wounds are stable (usually 2–3 weeks) [45].

Limb Dangling

Free flaps on the lower limb are affected by positional hemodynamic changes, which can lead to edema, decreased perfusion, and potential compromise of the reconstruction [46]. Many microsurgeons adopt dangle protocols to avoid this potential outcome, these protocols being highly heterogenic [46–48]. There is no evidence to support any one specific dangling protocol over another.

It has been theorized that early dangling protocols could lead to a faster patient discharge, but there is currently insufficient evidence to support this claim. There is evidence that patients with diabetes, hypertension or smokers can safely tolerate early dangling protocols [48]. Some surgeons have combined early dangling at postoperative day 3 with wrapping of the flap to prevent edema, without increases of flap failure rate [49–51]. If performed, elastic wrapping should be placed with 30 mmHg pressure [52].

Conclusions

Adequate postoperative care of every type of wound is necessary to achieve a good outcome. In general, standard care of postoperative wounds, skin grafts, and flaps is applicable. As we move up on the reconstructive ladder, more resources are necessary to ensure good postoperative care and a successful reconstruction.

Clinical examination by trained professionals can provide adequate information regarding the vascular status of free flaps, but device-based monitoring, such as NIRS or the implantable Doppler, is becoming increasingly popular as early evidence suggests more precise, prompt, and user-independent detection of vascular compromise using these devices.

When free flap failure occurs, performing a second free flap might not always be the best strategy. Reconsider which technique will benefit the patient best in the new scenario. It is important to identify the cause(s) of failure and any factors negatively affecting flap viability.

Physical therapy is essential to achieve a good functional outcome in every trauma patient. When to allow mobilization, axial load, and weight-bearing will depend on where the fracture is located and the treatment applied. For example, in FRIs in the lower limb, many treatment strategies allow early weight-bearing. Constructs with bone flaps are often not stable enough for early weight-bearing, so protected weight-bearing using orthopedic boots is common. In FRIs in the upper limb, which sustain lesser forces and in which maintaining mobility of nearby joints is especially important, controlled range of movement and axial loading are often started as soon as the wounds are stable.

References

1. Dumville JC, Gray TA, Walter CJ, Sharp CA, Page T, Macefield R, et al. Dressings for the prevention of surgical site infection. Cochrane Database Syst Rev. 2016;12(12):Cd003091. https://doi.org/10.1002/14651858.CD003091.pub4.
2. Braza ME, Fahrenkopf FM. Split-thickness skin grafts. StatPearls. 2023. https://www.ncbi.nlm.nih.gov/books/NBK551561/. Accessed July 2024.
3. Nelligan PC. Plastic surgery. 5th ed. Amsterdam: Elsevier; 2023.
4. CADTH Rapid Response Reports. Dressings and care of skin graft sites: a review of clinical evidence and guidelines. Ottawa: Canadian Agency for Drugs and Technologies in Health; 2013.
5. Odorico SK, Reuter Muñoz K, Nicksic PJ, Gunderson KA, Wood K, Nkana ZH, et al. Surgical and demographic predictors of free flap salvage after takeback: a systematic review. Microsurgery. 2023;43(1):78–88. https://doi.org/10.1002/micr.30921.
6. Knoedler S, Hoch CC, Huelsboemer L, Knoedler L, Stögner VA, Pomahac B, et al. Postoperative free flap monitoring in reconstructive surgery-man or machine? Front Surg. 2023;10:1130566. https://doi.org/10.3389/fsurg.2023.1130566.
7. Newton E, Butskiy O, Shadgan B, Prisman E, Anderson DW. Outcomes of free flap reconstructions with near-infrared spectroscopy (NIRS) monitoring: a systematic review. Microsurgery. 2020;40(2):268–75. https://doi.org/10.1002/micr.30526.
8. Patel UA, Hernandez D, Shnayder Y, Wax MK, Hanasono MM, Hornig J, et al. Free flap reconstruction monitoring techniques and frequency in the era of restricted resident work hours. JAMA Otolaryngol Head Neck Surg. 2017;143(8):803–9. https://doi.org/10.1001/jamaoto.2017.0304.
9. Deldar R, Abu El Hawa AA, Gupta N, Truong BN, Bovill JD, Fan KL, et al. Intensive care unit versus floor admission following lower extremity free flap surgery: is there a difference in outcomes? Microsurgery. 2022;42(7):696–702. https://doi.org/10.1002/micr.30935.
10. Han ZF, Guo LL, Liu LB, Li Q, Zhou J, Wei AZ, et al. A comparison of the Cook-Swartz Doppler with conventional clinical methods for free flap monitoring: a systematic review and a meta-analysis. Int J Surg. 2016;32:109–15. https://doi.org/10.1016/j.ijsu.2016.06.034.
11. Vakharia KT, Henstrom D, Lindsay R, Cunnane MB, Cheney M, Hadlock T. Color Doppler ultrasound: effective monitoring of the buried free flap in facial reanimation. Otolaryngol Head Neck Surg. 2012;146(3):372–6. https://doi.org/10.1177/0194599811427377.
12. Rosenberg JJ, Fornage BD, Chevray PM. Monitoring buried free flaps: limitations of the implantable Doppler and use of color duplex sonography as a confirmatory test. Plast Reconstr Surg. 2006;118(1):109–13.; discussion 14-5. https://doi.org/10.1097/01.prs.0000221113.78244.8c.
13. Maeda T, Ishikawa K, Oda Y, Kano S, Tsushima N, Sakashita T, et al. Utility of color Doppler ultrasonography in monitoring of a free jejunal flap. Laryngoscope. 2023;133(12):3361–9. https://doi.org/10.1002/lary.30793.
14. Cowan R, Mann G, Salibian AA. Ultrasound in microsurgery: current applications and new frontiers. J Clin Med. 2024;13(12) https://doi.org/10.3390/jcm13123412.
15. Romeo PB, Graham A, Zwart J, Sørensen K. Near infrared spectroscopy; A novel application of INVOS™ for monitoring muscle only free flaps. J Plast Reconstr Aesthet Surg. 2021;74(3):644–710. https://doi.org/10.1016/j.bjps.2020.08.071.
16. Dat AD, Loh IW, Bruscino-Raiola F. Free-flap salvage: muscle only versus skin paddle – an Australian experience. ANZ J Surg. 2017;87(12):1040–3. https://doi.org/10.1111/ans.13522.
17. Chang TY, Lee YC, Lin YC, Wong ST, Hsueh YY, Kuo YL, et al. Implantable Doppler probes for postoperatively monitoring free flaps: efficacy. A systematic review and meta-analysis. Plast Reconstr Surg Glob Open. 2016;4(11):e1099. https://doi.org/10.1097/gox.0000000000001099.
18. Rozen WM, Enajat M, Whitaker IS, Lindkvist U, Audolfsson T, Acosta R. Postoperative monitoring of lower limb free flaps with the Cook-Swartz implantable Doppler probe: a clinical trial. Microsurgery. 2010;30(5):354–60. https://doi.org/10.1002/micr.20720.
19. Klifto KM, Milek D, Gurno CF, Seal SM, Hultman CS, Rosson GD, et al. Comparison of arterial and venous implantable Doppler postoperative monitoring of free flaps: systematic review and meta-analysis of diagnostic test accuracy. Microsurgery. 2020;40(4):501–11. https://doi.org/10.1002/micr.30564.
20. Ong AA, Ducic Y, Pipkorn P, Wax MK. Implantable Doppler removal after free flap monitoring among head and neck microvascular surgeons. Laryngoscope. 2022;132(3):554–9. https://doi.org/10.1002/lary.29810.
21. Dunklebarger MF, McCrary H, King B, Carpenter P, Buchmann L, Hunt J, et al. Success of implantable Doppler probes for monitoring buried free flaps. Otolaryngol Head Neck Surg. 2022;167(3):452–6. https://doi.org/10.1177/01945998221082533.
22. Um GT, Chang J, Louie O, Colohan SM, Said HK, Neligan PC, et al. Implantable cook-Swartz Doppler probe versus synovis flow coupler for the postoperative monitoring of free flap breast reconstruction. J Plast Reconstr Aesthet Surg. 2014;67(7):960–6. https://doi.org/10.1016/j.bjps.2014.03.034.

23. Kempton SJ, Poore SO, Chen JT, Afifi AM. Free flap monitoring using an implantable anastomotic venous flow coupler: analysis of 119 consecutive abdominal-based free flaps for breast reconstruction. Microsurgery. 2015;35(5):337–44. https://doi.org/10.1002/micr.22341.
24. Yuen JC, Feng Z. Monitoring free flaps using the laser Doppler flowmeter: five-year experience. Plast Reconstr Surg. 2000;105(1):55–61. https://doi.org/10.1097/00006534-200001000-00009.
25. Heller L, Levin LS, Klitzman B. Laser Doppler flowmeter monitoring of free-tissue transfers: blood flow in normal and complicated cases. Plast Reconstr Surg. 2001;107(7):1739–45. https://doi.org/10.1097/00006534-200106000-00015.
26. Phillips CJ, Barron MR, Kuckelman J, Derickson M, Sohn VY, Paige KT, et al. Mobile smartphone thermal imaging characterization and identification of microvascular flow insufficiencies in deep inferior epigastric artery perforator free flaps. J Surg Res. 2021;261:394–9. https://doi.org/10.1016/j.jss.2020.12.044.
27. Singla P, Dixit PK, Kala PC, Katrolia D, Karmakar S, Humnekar A, et al. Free flap monitoring using infrared thermography: an objective adjunct to clinical monitoring. Indian J Plast Surg. 2024;57(3):179–83. https://doi.org/10.1055/s-0044-1786742.
28. Cruz-Segura A, Cruz-Domínguez MP, Jara LJ, Miliar-García Á, Hernández-Soler A, Grajeda-López P, et al. Early detection of vascular obstruction in microvascular flaps using a thermographic camera. J Reconstr Microsurg. 2019;35(7):541–8. https://doi.org/10.1055/s-0039-1688749.
29. Serra PL, Boriani F, Khan U, Atzeni M, Figus A. Rate of free flap failure and return to the operating room in lower limb reconstruction: a systematic review. J Clin Med. 2024;13(15) https://doi.org/10.3390/jcm13154295.
30. Müller SLC, Morgenstern M, Kuehl R, Muri T, Kalbermatten DF, Clauss M, et al. Soft-tissue reconstruction in lower-leg fracture-related infections: an orthoplastic outcome and risk factor analysis. Injury. 2021;52(11):3489–97. https://doi.org/10.1016/j.injury.2021.07.022.
31. Perrot P, Bouffaut AL, Perret C, Connault J, Duteille F. Risk factors and therapeutic strategy after failure of free flap coverage for lower-limb defects. J Reconstr Microsurg. 2011;27(3):157–62. https://doi.org/10.1055/s-0030-1268855.
32. Koster ITS, Borgdorff MP, Jamaludin FS, de Jong T, Botman M, Driessen C. Strategies following free flap failure in lower extremity trauma: a systematic review. JPRAS Open. 2023;36:94–104. https://doi.org/10.1016/j.jpra.2023.03.002.
33. Piwnica-Worms W, Stranix JT, Othman S, Kozak GM, Moyer I, Spencer A, et al. Risk factors for lower extremity amputation following attempted free flap limb salvage. J Reconstr Microsurg. 2020;36(7):528–33. https://doi.org/10.1055/s-0040-1710358.
34. Bond TJ, Lundy J. Physical therapy following peripheral nerve surgeries. Clin Podiatr Med Surg. 2006;23(3):651–66. https://doi.org/10.1016/j.cpm.2006.04.006.
35. Fang C, Wong TM, To KK, Wong SS, Lau TW, Leung F. Infection after fracture osteosynthesis – part II. J Orthop Surg (Hong Kong). 2017;25(1):2309499017692714. https://doi.org/10.1177/2309499017692714.
36. Dehghan N, McKee MD, Jenkinson RJ, Schemitsch EH, Stas V, Nauth A, et al. Early weightbearing and range of motion versus non-weightbearing and immobilization after open reduction and internal fixation of unstable ankle fractures: a randomized controlled trial. J Orthop Trauma. 2016;30(7):345–52. https://doi.org/10.1097/bot.0000000000000572.
37. Giannikas KA, Maganaris CN, Karski MT, Twigg P, Wilkes RA, Buckley JG. Functional outcome following bone transport reconstruction of distal tibial defects. J Bone Joint Surg Am. 2005;87(1):145–52. https://doi.org/10.2106/jbjs.C.01550.
38. Giuffre JL, Bishop AT, Spinner RJ, Shin AY. The best of tendon and nerve transfers in the upper extremity. Plast Reconstr Surg. 2015;135(3):617e–30e. https://doi.org/10.1097/prs.0000000000001071.
39. Gupta G, Ahmad S, Mohd Z, Khan AH, Sherwani MK, Khan AQ. Management of traumatic tibial diaphyseal bone defect by "induced-membrane technique". Indian J Orthop. 2016;50(3):290–6. https://doi.org/10.4103/0019-5413.181780.
40. Ilyas MS, Sattar A, Zehra U, Aziz A. Management of femoral shaft infected nonunion through customised Ilizarov external fixator assembly in a morbidly obese patient. BMJ Case Rep. 2022;15(1) https://doi.org/10.1136/bcr-2021-245824.
41. Wei FC, Mardini S. Flaps and reconstructive surgery. Elsevier; 2017.
42. Campanacci DA, Totti F, Puccini S, Beltrami G, Scoccianti G, Delcroix L, et al. Intercalary reconstruction of femur after tumour resection: is a vascularized fibular autograft plus allograft a long-lasting solution? Bone Joint J. 2018;100-b(3):378–86. https://doi.org/10.1302/0301-620x.100b3.Bjj-2017-0283.R2.
43. Kim M, Wu MP, Miller LE, Meyer CD, Feng AL, Varvares MA, et al. Early weight-bearing after fibula free flap surgery. JAMA Otolaryngol Head Neck Surg. 2024;150(2):127–32. https://doi.org/10.1001/jamaoto.2023.4024.
44. McCrary HC, Dunklebarger MF, Fechter BJ, Drejet SM, Monroe MM, Buchmann LO, et al. Early ambulation after fibular free flap surgery is associated with reduced length of stay, increased mobility independence, and discharge to home. Head Neck. 2024;46(5):1160–7. https://doi.org/10.1002/hed.27737.
45. Dehghan N, Mitchell SM, Schemitsch EH. Rehabilitation after plate fixation of upper and lower extremity fractures. Injury. 2018;49(Suppl 1):S72–s7. https://doi.org/10.1016/s0020-1383(18)30308-5.

46. Lindelauf A, van Rooij JAF, Hartveld L, van der Hulst R, Weerwind PW, Schols RM. Tissue oximetry changes during postoperative dangling in lower extremity free flap reconstruction: a pilot study. Life (Basel). 2023;13(5) https://doi.org/10.3390/life13051158.
47. Soteropulos CE, Chen JT, Poore SO, Garland CB. Postoperative management of lower extremity free tissue transfer: a systematic review. J Reconstr Microsurg. 2019;35(1):1–7. https://doi.org/10.1055/s-0038-1667049.
48. Lee ZH, Ramly EP, Alfonso AR, Daar DA, Kaoutzanis C, Kantar RS, et al. Dangle protocols in lower extremity reconstruction. J Surg Res. 2021;266:77–87. https://doi.org/10.1016/j.jss.2021.03.028.
49. McGhee JT, Cooper L, Orkar K, Harry L, Cubison T. Systematic review: early versus late dangling after free flap reconstruction of the lower limb. J Plast Reconstr Aesthet Surg. 2017;70(8):1017–27. https://doi.org/10.1016/j.bjps.2017.04.001.
50. Jokuszies A, Neubert N, Herold C, Vogt PM. Early start of the dangling procedure in lower extremity free flap reconstruction does not affect the clinical outcome. J Reconstr Microsurg. 2013;29(1):27–32. https://doi.org/10.1055/s-0032-1326736.
51. Neubert N, Vogt PM, May M, Boyce M, Koenneker S, Budde E, et al. Does an early and aggressive combined wrapping and dangling procedure affect the clinical outcome of lower extremity free flaps?-A randomized controlled prospective study using microdialysis monitoring. J Reconstr Microsurg. 2016;32(4):262–70. https://doi.org/10.1055/s-0035-1568882.
52. Kolbenschlag J, Ruikis A, Faulhaber L, Daigeler A, Held M, Rothenberger J, et al. Elastic wrapping of lower extremity free flaps during dangling improves microcirculation and reduces pain as well as edema. J Reconstr Microsurg. 2019;35(7):522–8. https://doi.org/10.1055/s-0039-1688451.

MIX
Papier aus verantwortungsvollen Quellen
Paper from responsible sources
FSC® C105338
FSC
www.fsc.org

If you have any concerns about our products,
you can contact us on
ProductSafety@springernature.com

In case Publisher is established outside the EU,
the EU authorized representative is:
Springer Nature Customer Service Center GmbH
Europaplatz 3, 69115 Heidelberg, Germany

Printed by Libri Plureos GmbH
in Hamburg, Germany